/C NO:
CCESSION NO:
SELFMARK: 616.890 25/KHO

Dedicated to my wife Lynn and my children Andrea, Andrew, and Adam, without whose help, support, inspiration, and sacrifice this work would not have been possible.
—Hani R. Khouzam

I dedicate this book to my husband Robert Shuttleworth and my children Siyarin, Richard, and Marc Tan-Shuttleworth.
—Doris T. Tan

I dedicate this book to God and Family.
—Tirath S. Gill

VC NO:
CESSION NO. KHO1436
ELLMARK:

A gentle answer turns away wrath, but harsh words stir up anger.

—Proverbs 15:1

616.89025/KHO

;ENERAL
ITAL
RE LIBRARY
184216

return c or before he last da

Handbook of
Emergency
Psychiatry

HSE South Kerry General Hospital
Library

KH01426

Acquisitions Editor: Susan F. Pioli
Editorial Assistant: Joan Ryan
Senior Project Manager: Robin E. Hayward
Publishing Services Manager: Frank Polizzano
Design Direction: Steven Stave

Handbook of
Emergency
Psychiatry

Hani Raoul Khouzam, MD, MPH, FAPA

Interim Chief and Medical Director
Chemical Dependency Treatment Program
Veterans Affairs Central California
Health Care System
Fresno, California

Doris Tiu Tan, DO

Chief
Inpatient Psychiatry and Consultation Liaison Service
Veterans Affairs Central California
Health Care System
Fresno, California

Tirath Singh Gill, MD

Chief
Emergency Psychiatry Service
Veterans Affairs Central California
Health Care System
Fresno, California

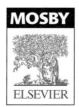

MOSBY

ELSEVIER

MOSBY
ELSEVIER

1600 John F. Kennedy Boulevard
Suite 1800
Philadelphia, PA 19103-2899

HANDBOOK OF EMERGENCY PSYCHIATRY   ISBN: 978-0-323-04088-4

Copyright © 2007 by Mosby, Inc., an affiliate of Elsevier Inc.

All rights reserved. No part of this publication may be reproduced or transmitted in any form or by any means, electronic or mechanical, including photocopying, recording, or any information storage and retrieval system, without permission in writing from the publisher.

Permissions may be sought directly from Elsevier's Health Sciences Rights Department in Philadelphia, PA, USA: phone: (+1) 215 239 3804, fax: (+1) 215 239 3805, e-mail: healthpermissions@elsevier.com. You may also complete your request online via the Elsevier homepage (http://www.elsevier.com), by selecting "Customer Support" and then "Obtaining Permissions."

Notice

Knowledge and best practice in this field are constantly changing. As new research and experience broaden our knowledge, changes in practice, treatment, and drug therapy may become necessary or appropriate. Readers are advised to check the most current information provided (i) on procedures featured or (ii) by the manufacturer of each product to be administered, to verify the recommended dose or formula, the method and duration of administration, and contraindications. It is the responsibility of the practitioner, relying on their own experience and knowledge of the patient, to make diagnoses, to determine dosages and the best treatment for each individual patient, and to take all appropriate safety precautions. To the fullest extent of the law, neither the Publisher nor the Authors assume any liability for any injury and/or damage to persons or property arising out of or related to any use of the material contained in this book.

The Publisher

Library of Congress Cataloging-in-Publication Data
Khouzam, Hani Raoul.
  Handbook of emergency psychiatry/Hani Raoul Khouzam, Tirath S. Gill, Doris T. Tan —1st ed.
    p.; cm.
  Includes bibliographical references and index.
  ISBN 978-0-323-04088-4
  1. Psychiatric emergencies—Handbooks, manuals, etc. 2. Crisis intervention (Mental health services)—Handbooks, manuals, etc.
I. Gill, Tirath S. II. Tan, Doris T. III. Title.
  [DNLM: 1. Mental Disorders—diagnosis—Handbooks. 2. Mental Disorders—therapy—Handbooks. 3. Emergency Services, Psychiatric—methods—Handbooks. WM 34 K45h 2007]
RC480.6.H364 2007
616.89'025—dc22   2006025413

Printed in China

Working together to grow
libraries in developing countries
www.elsevier.com | www.bookaid.org | www.sabre.org

ELSEVIER   BOOK AID International   Sabre Foundation

Last digit is the print number: 9 8 7 6 5 4 3 2 1

PREFACE

Emergency psychiatry is about providing timed, immediate, and planned interventions and treatment for patients in need of urgent care. It involves making quick and accurate psychiatric assessment in order to decide the appropriate level of care that is needed in each emergency.

Although the book title implies that this is a handbook, that may be misleading since the book may not be carried in the clinician's pocket. *Handbook of Emergency Psychiatry* provides comprehensive evaluation, assessment, treatment, and management of psychiatric emergencies, covering an array of topics that are relevant to the ever-growing field of psychiatry with specific emphasis on emergency aspects.

Early chapters deal with specific psychiatric conditions that are assessed in the acute setting of the emergency department. Several chapters describe how to conduct a comprehensive psychiatric evaluation, gather relevant medical and psychiatric historical information, and conduct an accurate but timely diagnostic investigation that explores the underlying medical and psychiatric disorders that precipitated the psychiatric emergency. Each chapter recommends various pharmacological, psychosocial, and, at times, spiritual interventions that are specifically geared toward the management and treatment of urgent and emergent psychiatric signs and symptoms.

Each chapter begins with Key Points that are carefully selected and worded to inform the prospective reader of the salient and important aspects of the chapter. Definitions and epidemiological data are also emphasized to clarify the meaning of various psychiatric terms and to provide information to the emergency department clinicians in regard to the relevance, incidence, and prevalence of the specific psychiatric emergency. Tables, figures, acronyms, mnemonics, and screening and rating scales are also included to help the reader differentiate between the various psychiatric and medical conditions that could present with similar symptoms. Postscript quotations are added at the end of certain chapters with the intention of inspiring and encouraging clinicians who are constantly assessing and managing medical and psychiatric emergencies.

Mental status examination and safety considerations are incorporated throughout the chapters, and updated references and resource lists at the end of each chapter provide guidance for further reading. The approved and off-label indications of psychopharmacological agents that have been commonly used in emergency departments, outpatient settings, or inpatient psychiatric units are described throughout the book. Details of psychopharmacological treatment, dosages, adverse effects, and drug-to-drug interactions are also described.

Early chapters discuss crisis intervention, general psychiatric assessment, medications for general psychiatric emergencies, and the emergency psychiatric manifestation of medical conditions. The emergencies associated with delirium, suicide, depression, bipolar disorder, psychosis, violence, anxiety, personality disorders, and somatizing patients are then addressed in the subsequent chapters. The psychiatric emergencies related to the comorbidities of psychiatric and substance abuse disorders are addressed in two separate chapters that deal with alcohol and drug dependence in the acute setting. They describe how to gather information and give practical and clinical advice for the emergency care of dually diagnosed patients. Another chapter is solely devoted to child and adolescent psychiatric emergencies.

This handbook was originally designed to have 17 chapters. The tragic events that occurred with the 9/11 terrorist attacks and the major disasters that have occurred worldwide, as in the case of the December 2004 Indian Ocean earthquake and resulting tsunami and in the aftermath of hurricanes Katrina and Rita, prompted the inclusion of two more chapters, with special emphasis on posttraumatic stress disorder and the emergency psychiatric care for victims and survivors of terrorism and natural disasters. The new diagnostic category of religious and spiritual problems in the *Diagnostic and Statistical Manual of Mental Disorders* (DSM-IV and DSM-IV-TR) led to the addition of a chapter on the religious and spiritual dimensions of psychiatric emergencies. Because of the ongoing expected increase in the elderly population—and many of them do or would suffer from medical and psychiatric conditions—a rather lengthy but comprehensive chapter related to the psychiatric emergencies of geriatric patients was added. The recent emphasis on the importance of biological treatment of most psychiatric disorders led to the addition of a chapter on emergency psychiatric aspects of drugs and psychotropic medications. Although psychiatry is the medical specialty that is most experienced in the biological treatment of psychiatric disorders, it is uniquely oriented toward a comprehensive medical as well as psychosocial treatment approach. The acuteness and urgency of the emergency department setting require an integration of all available biological, psychological, social, and, in certain situations, spiritual interventions. This aspect of emergency psychiatry led to the addition of a chapter related to the emergency care of patients who are victims of domestic violence or rape. The political and economic influences on the practice of medicine and the increased demand and decreased resources in an era of managed care and dwindling health insurance coverage for mental illness have forced most hospitals' emergency departments to become the de facto providers of medical and psychiatric care of the uninsured and the destitute of our society. These factors led to the addition of a chapter on the medical and legal aspects of psychiatric emergencies.

The idea of this handbook was conceived by Tirath S. Gill, who had a vision of writing a comprehensive and practical text in psychiatric emergencies. Dr. Gill was thinking of a book that could be easily read and would offer emergency department clinicians evidence-based updated and relevant information to guide their steps in managing psychiatric emergencies. Subsequently, Doris T. Tan carried the baton to pursue a publisher for the book. After several attempts Dr. Tan found the listening ear and encouraging support of Susan F. Pioli of Elsevier. Ms. Pioli asked for samples of materials that had been previously published by any of the prospective authors of the proposed handbook. When I was a junior faculty member at the Department of Psychiatry and Behavioral Sciences of the University of Oklahoma College of Medicine, I was encouraged and supported by several of my mentors and senior faculty members to write and publish in the psychiatric literature. So I sent Ms. Pioli a chapter from the *Manual of Emergency Psychiatric Intervention*, which I had written for the Oklahoma County Crisis Intervention Center. Ms. Pioli was graciously positive toward the chapter contents, which addressed the emergency management of suicidal patients. So she offered us the opportunity to write this handbook.

I am sincerely thankful to Ms. Pioli and to my colleagues Dr. Gill and Dr. Tan for allowing me to write several of this book's chapters. I would also like to thank Dr. Gill, who conceived the illustrations to make the book more informative and user friendly. I am also grateful to Elsevier for all of the help and support that was generously provided to get this book published.

In the process of studying, preparing, and writing this handbook, several currently available books on the topic of emergency psychiatry were read, including the following: *The Handbook of Emergency Psychiatry* by Jorge R. Petit; *Emergency Psychiatry* by Randy Hillard and Brook Zitek; *Emergency Psychiatry* (Review of Psychiatry, vol 21) by Michael H. Allen; and *Manual of Psychiatric Emergencies* by Steven E. Hyman and George E. Tesar (editors). These books are well written, organized, informative, comprehensive, and state of the art in the field. They are valuable assets for mental health clinicians who evaluate and treat psychiatric emergencies. This *Handbook of Emergency Psychiatry* is written to complement rather than duplicate these extremely valuable texts.

This handbook provides more information and in-depth discussion than a concise guide, and certain chapters are similar in their contents to psychiatry textbooks. The chapters emphasize the aspects of the emergency presentation of a psychiatric disorder, treatment modality, or a population that is assessed in the emergency department setting. It can be read as a manual of clinical emergency psychiatry or can be read in a random fashion based on the particular encountered emergencies.

Although the title may imply that this book is only intended for psychiatrists treating emergencies, the topics of concern are also relevant for psychiatry residents and medical students who are in training and called upon to learn and be supervised in assessing, managing, and treating psychiatric emergencies. Emergency department clinicians from various disciplines and specialties, mental health professionals, and primary care providers would find the discussed principles to be a practical and helpful reference for the assessment, diagnosis, and treatment of psychiatric disorders in and outside the emergency department setting.

—Hani Raoul Khouzam

ACKNOWLEDGMENTS

To those who have encouraged and supported my writing while growing up in Heliopolis, Egypt; my parents Raoul and Jeannette, my sisters Hoda and Héla, and my brother Hadi; my teachers of the Jesuit school in Cairo, Egypt; my professors at Cairo University Faculty of Medicine, Drs. Mohammed Shaalan and Tarek A. Hassan; my advisors Dr. Bernett L. Cline and Ms. Penny Jessop at the Tulane School of Public Health and Tropical Medicine in New Orleans; Chairmen, Drs. Gordon H. Deckert and Joseph Westermeyer and Residency Training Directors Drs. Jean E. Carlin and Blaine Shaffer of the Department of Psychiatry and Behavioral Sciences at the University of Oklahoma College of Medicine; the Chief of Mental Health Dr. Charles Smith and supervisors Drs. Gloria B. Green and Joseph B. Ruffin at the Veterans Affairs Medical Center in Oklahoma City; the former State of Oklahoma Commissioner of Mental Health, Dr. J. Frank James; the Chief of Mental Health, colleague and mentor Dr. Paul E. Emery; Drs. Edward Gillie, Donald R. Bernard, and Michael F. Mayo-Smith at the Veterans Affairs Medical Center in Manchester and Harvard Medical School in Boston; the Chairman of the Department of Psychiatry, Dr. Peter M. Silberfarb and the Director of Residency Training in Psychiatry, Dr. Ron L. Green at Dartmouth Medical School in Lebanon, New Hampshire; my colleagues here in Fresno, California, Drs. Robert W. Hierholzer, Avak A. Howsepian, Nestor Manzano, Matthew Battista, and Mr. Leonard Williams, PA, at the Veterans Affairs Central California Health Care System, and Hospital Director Mr. Al Perry, FACHE, and Chief of Staff Dr. William Cahill; Drs. Craig C. Campbell and Scott R. Ahles at the University of California, San Francisco, School of Medicine, Fresno Central San Joaquin Valley Medical Education Program.

To all of these and many others I am in great debt and gratitude. I would like also to extend my thanks to my coauthors Dr. Tirath S. Gill, for his idea in writing this book and for his commitment to the expected deadlines, and to Dr. Doris T. Tan, for her attention to detail that kept things moving toward the goal of completing the text.

—HRK

No other way does one communicate validation more than by words of encouragement. I thank the first professor who took an interest in my ability, and that is Professor Darryl D. Coon. Guidance through college at the University of Pittsburgh by Professor Richard Yang and Professor Charles Walsh was invaluable. Mr. Wesley Knollenberg, MS, who taught me the value of consistent work while I was at Iowa State University, along with my major professor, Dr. Kenneth Shaw. Many thanks to Professor Lynwood Clemens of Michigan State University and his wife, Linda Coniglio, DO, PhD, along with Antonio Nunez, PhD, who took me in under their wings. I thank Dr. Coniglio for the inspiration to enter the field of Osteopathic Medicine at Ohio University. There, again, I was inspired by Peter Dane, DO, Jack Brose, DO, John Howell, PhD, and Marjorie Nelson, MD. Supervisors Paul Weiss, DO, and Ned Underwood, DO, of the previous Youngstown Osteopathic Hospital, and previous Chairman of Family Medicine Residency Program at St Joseph's Hospital, Frank Veres, DO. I thank professors and supervisors, now my colleagues, Drs. Hoyle Leigh, Glenn Ikawa, Scott Ahles, Nestor Manzano, Frederick Reinfurt, Robert Hierholzer, Avak Howsepian, Karen Kraus, Mathew Battista, John Donnelley, Burke Bonilla, Petros Ghermay, and Dr. Craig Campbell, Director of Psychiatry Residency Training Program at the University of California, San Francisco, School of Medicine, Fresno Central San Joaquin Valley Medical Education Program. They continue to provide support and encouragement. I also thank Mr. Leonard Williams, PA, Ruben Hunter, LSW, and Ms. Schere Lau, LSW, for their continued support. I would like to extend my gratitude to my coauthors, Tirath S. Gill, and especially to Hani R. Khouzam, who continues to function as our wise mentor.

However, prior to meeting these wonderful people, it is my mother, Tiu Po, who defied cultural norm and sent me packing from the Philippines to the University of Pittsburgh. My sisters Victoria, Florence, Lucy, and Ana, and my brother Johnny, who all knew before I did that I would make it, I thank you from the bottom of my heart.

—DTT

I would like to thankfully acknowledge the assistance of our librarians Daphne Perry and Patricia Kangas. Many colleagues have been helpful with their words of encouragement and discussion. These include Robert Hierholzer, MD, Avak

Howsepian, MD, PhD, Nestor Manzano, MD, and Scott Ahles, MD. I want to acknowledge my residency director, Beverly Sutton, MD, for allowing a rich interaction between the general and child psychiatry programs. Paramjeet Singh, MD, of Jaipur and Harjinder Kaur, MD, provided support and words of wisdom. Alan S. Perry, FACHE, and William Cahill, MD, have also provided encouragement every step of the way. I would also like to thank our coauthor and guiding light, Dr. Khouzam, who guided us through the project with optimism and calm.

I would be remiss if I did not acknowledge the many fine nurses, nurse practitioners, social workers, pharmacists, and fellow physicians with whom I have worked. Some names stand out, such as Stella, Jeff, Scheree, Emma, Viral, Sincerae, Dr. Feldman, and Dr. Lindsey. They represent the very best of human caring and compassion. I would also like to acknowledge and thank Ms. Robin Hayward for her excellent work with us during the final edit and Ms. Susan Pioli and all her staff for their support.

Last but not least are my special people: Baljeet (Fran), Shaleen, Vikram, Savraj (Savy), and Dad. Their love is like a light on rocky shores.

—TSG

Note from the Authors

The authors have worked to ensure that all information in this book, especially that concerning medication dosages, schedules, and routes of administration, is accurate as of the time of publication and consistent with the standards set by the U.S. Food and Drug Administration and the general medical community. As medical research and practice advance, however, therapeutic standards may change. For this reason and because human and mechanical errors sometimes occur, we recommend that nonclinicians and general public readers follow the advice of the physician who is directly involved in their care or the care of their family members.

CONTENTS

CHAPTER 1

Crisis Intervention

Hani R. Khouzam, MD, MPH, FAPA

KEY POINTS

- **When a crisis is perceived as a "danger," it can lead to a decreased level of functioning; however, if the person experiencing the crisis perceives it as an "opportunity," it can lead to a higher level of functioning.**
- Documentation for crisis intervention has special characteristics that differentiate it from the regular emergency psychiatric assessment.
- Persons experiencing a crisis may present with physical, psychological, and interpersonal symptoms.
- The ABC model of crisis intervention provides a problem-focused method of intervening in a brief time period.
- Making referrals for crisis stabilization is an integral component of the overall management of crisis intervention.

Overview

Crisis intervention is an approach and an attitude. Emergency department (ED) clinicians intervening in crisis stabilization have a significant impact on patients in crisis. Taking the crisis out of crisis could have a lasting effect on these patients' lives and livelihood. By applying the ABC principles of crisis intervention, a specific, concrete plan can be developed to reverse the disorganization, immobilization, and demoralization that occur during the time of crisis.

In general, effective crisis intervention should lead to:
- Stabilizing symptoms of distress
- Mitigation of symptoms
- Restoring adaptive level functioning
- Facilitating access to further support.

1

Definitions

 Crisis. An unexpected event or series of events that precipitate a distressful acute response or reaction. During a crisis the person's usual coping mechanisms are disrupted, and subsequently a failure in counteracting the unexpected event occurs, leading to significant distress or social, interpersonal, and vocational impairment. When a crisis is perceived as a "danger," it can lead to a decreased level of functioning; however, if the person experiencing the crisis perceives it as an "opportunity," it can lead to a higher level of functioning.

Critical incident. The stressor event that precedes the crisis response is commonly referred to as the *critical incident*.

Crisis intervention. The provision of acute effective intervention aiming at reversing the crisis status and resumption of the pre-crisis level of functioning.

Documentation for Crisis Intervention

- Documentation should be detailed in terms of present history and the current living situation, but more general in terms of past history.
- In case of suicide, homicide, or violence risk, documentation of the history and mental status relevant to these risks should be detailed and comprehensive.
- All contacts with family members, significant others, and law enforcement agencies should be recorded, as well as previous treatments, including telephone and electronic media contacts.
- Information related to the disposition decision should be specifically recorded; however, information unrelated to disposition decision can be nonspecifically recorded.

Clinical Presentation

Because crisis is a time-limited event, crisis intervention needs to begin immediately to prevent the development of chronic psychological complications. To intervene appropriately, ED clinicians need to be aware of the different types of crisis.

Types of Crises

Developmental Crises

These occur as the individuals proceed through the adjustments they need to make in the various stages of the life cycle. Emergency psychiatric interventions in these crises are covered in different chapters of this handbook.

Situational Crises

These result from unexpected events such as the sudden death of a loved one, divorce, illness, assaults, and disasters. The emergency psychiatric interventions in these crises are covered in different chapters of this handbook.

During the critical incident period, persons experiencing a crisis may present with physical, psychological, or interpersonal symptoms of distress, some of these are summarized in Box 1-1.

Principles of Crisis Intervention

 The ABC model of crisis intervention provides a problem-focused method of intervening in a brief time period. It begins

---

Box 1–1. Symptoms of Distress during Crisis

Physical Symptoms
Sleep disturbances; back, jaw, shoulder, or neck pain
Tension headaches, cramps, heartburn, constipation, diarrhea, eating disturbances
Hair loss, muscle tension, fatigue, sweaty palms or hands, cold hands or feet
Shortness of breath, chest pain, skin problems
Increased vulnerability to colds, flu, and infections

Psychological Symptoms
Anxiety, fear, irritability, hopelessness, helplessness, impatience
Feelings of doom and gloom, nervousness

Interpersonal Symptoms
Increased arguments, isolation from social activities
Job instability, conflict with co-workers or employers
Road rage, domestic or workplace violence, overreactions

with identifying the person's perception of the event that triggered the crisis, a process best started within 4 to 6 weeks of the
crisis event. It is a three-stage process which was developed by
several clinicians. The ABC model is a process in which several
stages of change—that is, A = **A**chieving rapport; B = **B**eginning
of problem identification; and C = **C**oping—are introduced in
order to restore individuals to their pre-crisis level of functioning.

A—Achieving Rapport

The ED clinician, rather than offering interpretations and advice,
creates a safe environment in which talking about the perception
and the meaning of the crisis is encouraged. Listening, eye
contact, and appropriate questioning facilitates the development
of rapport. The use of open-ended questions that begin with
"what" and "how" can help persons in crisis freely express their
personal views and feelings. Closed-ended questions (with
yes/no answers) are not effective in crisis interviewing. Para-
phrasing, reflection of feelings, and summarization can convey
the basic themes of the person's viewpoints and feelings. This
also provides an opportunity for the ED clinician to understand
the perception by persons in crisis of their critical incident experiences, thus allowing for correction of any misperceptions.

B—Beginning of Problem Identification

Problem identification focuses on the person's views in regard to:
- *Precipitating event*: a thorough exploration of the event
  that triggered the crisis from the person's viewpoint.
  Timing and patience by the ED clinician is critical because
  if a full exploration is not allowed, resistance to the
  intervention may result.
- *Perceptions*: meaning of the event as perceived by the
  person in crisis; the perception of stressful situations that
  led to the crisis state and to the loss of the ability to cope
  effectively.
- *Subjective distress*: the emotions that resulted from
  the crisis.
- *Level of functioning*: the degree of impairment in
  occupational, social, academic, interpersonal, and family
  areas as a result of the crisis.

At this stage of intervention, the ED clinician needs to assess
the level of functioning before and after the crisis in order to

motivate the achievement of the pre-crisis level of functioning. Also, at this time, the clinician should note a history of any suicidal or homicidal ideations and intentions, agitation, psychosis, depression, anxiety, and substance and alcohol abuse, as well as current medical conditions. ED clinician interventions for these conditions are described in other sections of this handbook.

C—Coping

This step in the process focuses on the past, present, and future coping behaviors. The ED clinician may use certain techniques to encourage and motivate the improvement of coping abilities. These include:

- Supportive statements to validate the person's feelings and convey understanding and empathy.
- Educational statements offering facts, statistics, and theories to help change misperceptions and normalize daily experiences.
- Empowering statements to regain control.
- Reframing statements about the problems, to envision a solution and dissipate the sense of hopelessness.
- Exploring past coping behaviors to demonstrate "what has and has not worked in the past," and guiding the development of a coping plan for the current crisis.
- Providing referrals to support groups, long-term psychotherapy, counseling, and/or shelters or other agencies; medical and legal resources need to be incorporated as essential components of the development of the coping plan.
- Obtaining a firm commitment for following and pursuing problem solving will add more support to the coping process.

Crisis Intervention in Specific Situations

This section summarizes interventions related to death and dying and to crises related to divorce and separation. Crises related to domestic abuse, disasters, terrorism, substance abuse, and posttraumatic disorder are described in other chapters of this handbook.

For the management of suicide, see Chapter 6; for management of violence, assaultive behavior, agitation, and aggression see Chapters 9 and 17; for management of victims of domestic abuse and rape, see Chapter 19.

Death and Dying

Certain individuals may present to the ED due to crises related to death of a loved one or to anticipation of one's own death.

In her book *On Death and Dying*, Elisabeth Kubler-Ross described five stages related to death and dying:

Stage I: Denial and isolation
Stage II: Anger
Stage III: Bargaining
Stage IV: Depression
Stage V: Acceptance.

Stage I, *denial and isolation*, is a reaction that offers a defense against the initial shock of the loss. The second stage, *anger*, is a reaction to the realization of the depth and magnitude of the loss. In Stage III, *bargaining* is an attempt to seek contact with a higher being to negotiate a change in the situation. Stage IV acknowledges that the loss is final or irreversible. This stage may be associated with sadness, pessimism, and feelings of guilt, worthlessness, and tiredness. *Acceptance*, the final stage, occurs as the depression subsides. This stage can entail either a disengagement from life if one is grieving the impending loss of one's own life or it can be associated with feelings of serenity and peace as one is satisfied with his or her life's journey and accomplishments.

In crisis intervention, a review of these stages by the ED clinician can facilitate the mourning that accompanies the bereavement process. The ED clinician needs to explain to persons in crisis that these stages are generalized suggestions for understanding the grief process and that not everyone experiences each stage in such a predictable, sequential order.

The grief process applies to other forms of loss also. It is important to remember that loss can trigger suicidal thinking in a grieving person.

Divorce and Separation

Relationship breakups (divorce, separation) are personal devastating experiences. Often a person's life/self concept is based on being a couple. How well the person copes with a breakup depends on personal, material, and social resources. The goal of the crisis intervention is to facilitate the initiation of the grieving process. Divorce can be more stressful when children are affected. Crisis intervention is also needed upon remarriage and when new families are blended in order to adjust to the complexity of acquiring new roles.

Transition to the Post-Crisis Stage

 The transition to the post-crisis stage includes facilitation of the tasks of mourning, summarized in Box 1-2 (see also Chapters 19, 20, and 21).

Referrals

- Making referrals for crisis stabilization requires comprehensive knowledge of specialized community resources that meet the unique needs of each person experiencing a crisis.
- Effective networking by multidisciplinary intervention teams is essential, particularly by social work staff, to create linkages with the city's administrative, clinical, and community outreach services.
- Follow-up care and appointments need to be timed and allocated to accurate addresses rather then just provided in the form of telephone numbers.
- Education about the goal and expectations of each individual facing a crisis must be addressed prior to the referral for ongoing psychotherapy.
- If pharmacological interventions are initiated during the crisis intervention process, then a clearly defined follow-up treatment plan must be incorporated in the disposition of the case.
- Hospitalization is necessary if post-crisis stage transition is not achieved.

Box 1–2. The Four Tasks of Mourning	
Task I	Accepting the reality of the loss
Task II	Experiencing the pain of grief
Task III	Adjusting to a new environment
Task IV	Redirecting emotional energy to other relationships

Further Reading

Flannery RB Jr, Everly GS Jr: Crisis intervention: A review. Int J Emerg Mental Health 2000;2:117-123.

Kristi K: A Guide To Crisis Intervention, 2nd ed. Atlanta, Wadsworth/Brooks/Cole, 2003.

Kubler-Ross E: On Death and Dying. New York, Macmillan, 1969.

Puryear DA: Helping People in Crisis. San Francisco, Jossey-Bass, 1979.

Puryear DA: Proposed standards in emergency psychiatry. Hosp Community Psychiatry 1992;43:14-15.

Schatzberg AF, Cole JO, DeBattista C: Manual of Clinical Psychopharmacology, 5th ed. Arlington, VA, American Psychiatric Publishing, 2005.

POSTSCRIPT

I hope that posterity will judge me kindly, not only as to the things which I have explained, but also to those which I have intentionally omitted so as to leave to others the pleasure of discovery.

René Descartes—1596-1650

CHAPTER 2

Assessment of Psychiatric Emergencies

Doris T. Tan, DO

KEY POINTS

- Not every clinician sets out to work in an emergency room; outlined are some personal qualities that may be useful.
- Proper environment and a well-equipped psychiatric evaluation unit (with security officers and an appropriate number of properly trained personnel) are important for the safety of patients and staff.
- Situations that may confuse even the most astute clinicians will arise, and the treatment outcome will not always be the desired one. This, however, should not be an obstacle in striving for success.
- Evaluation of lethality should always be a priority, thus evaluation of suicidal and homicidal ideation, intents, and attempts is always necessary. However, as with many medical conditions, we will not be able to save everyone, even with the most heroic of efforts.
- One must always be mindful of the patient's legal rights so as not to override them. As with medical conditions, psychiatrically impaired patients have the right to make their own decisions unless they are so gravely disabled due to the severity of their mental illness that they do not have this capacity.
- The standard of care in an emergency and the factors that trigger hospitalization are outlined in this chapter.
- Although this is to be avoided as much as possible, the use of physical or chemical restraints may be necessary when the patient's or staff's safety is deemed to be compromised. Prevention of violence is a must.

Overview

Persons that require emergency psychiatric evaluation are not always the most cooperative of patients. They may be brought in by their friends, relatives, or even the police. Different states and even counties may have different laws regarding civil commitment. Emergency department (ED) clinicians must know these laws inside and out in order to apply them with care. They also must know the consequences of civil commitment and how commitment may affect a particular patient. In the state of California, the police-written 72-hour-hold (termed 5150 for the form that is used to write the civil commitment) may limit the ability of the patient to purchase guns or seek employment that requires carrying weapons in the future. This may also extend to acceptability into military service (see Chapter 23 for more details).

Desired Fortitude of Emergency Psychiatry Clinicians

The qualities discussed in this section are vital to efficient performance by emergency psychiatry clinicians.

KNOW THE USE OF ONE'S INSTINCTS FOR DANGER. To know oneself and to be able to use one's own feelings as a gauge, especially in sensing a dangerous situation in the ED. Use one's own sense and feeling of comfort (or discomfort) with a patient. Use one's own instinct and be attuned to it to gauge safety concerns, both for the ED clinician and the patient.

TOLERANCE. To continue to be calm when one needs to deal with difficult physicians, difficult patients, and nursing staff. Be able to tolerate potentially hurtful words given by patients during an exacerbation of their illness. Be able to tolerate potentially frustrating multitasks, inability to obtain collateral information, poorly responsive primary care givers and admitting staff, returning phone calls to family, and converging interests for your attention at the most inopportune of times.

EMPATHY. To be able to put oneself in the patient's shoes—not to be confused with sympathy, which is to feel sorry for the patient. It is a challenge to balance empathy with self-assertion.

Since high achieving physicians may have a higher rate of narcissism, which may hinder their effectiveness in this, all ED clinicians should continue to strive for this balance.

SELF-ASSERTION. To be tough enough to assert oneself and set firm limits, while the situation or the patient is creating havoc in the ED. While your decision is being questioned by either the patients or their representatives, you as the professional, having empathy and tolerance, must still make the best professional decision and disposition for the patient.

HONESTY. To be truthful, but to use gentle care and finesse to avoid causing more ego structure breakdown for the patient. One must continue to like one's patients, even just a little, and be involved in their plight.

RESOURCEFULNESS. To be able to draw on available resources of the community that particularly suit an individual patient—every story is different. The astute emergency clinician is able to accumulate a network of other professionals that may be useful, including other agencies. A social service worker is usually very helpful in this area, but one still needs to have personal knowledge of available resources in order to utilize them as part of the crisis intervention or disposition planning.

CREATIVITY. To be creative about how to use the available resources. As an art, the emergency psychiatric clinician has to accommodate the different types, and presentation of various patients. Relentlessly search for more information in order to synthesize the multitude of information to come up with a working diagnosis and make treatment and disposition plans.

ENDURANCE. The ability to sustain a prolonged stressful effort or activity. The emergency clinician has to last a little longer than the patient in the battle for sanity.

WHICH BRINGS US TO HUMOR. To be able to use this mature defense, to be able to find some fun, joke at oneself and create a much more tolerable environment during down times.

PRAGMATISM. To be practical, using common sense, and—together with creativity—to be able to create the fortitude needed to become a more resourceful channel of energy for the management, safety, and treatment of patients in psychiatric crisis.

Approach to Patients in Psychiatric Emergencies

 ## Assurance of a Safe Environment in Which to Interview the Patient

Ideally, the ED should contain an interview room in which the clinician will not be entrapped. There should be at least two exit doors. No wires or tubes should be visible, and the ceiling should not be reachable or it should be constructed with non-removable materials. The room should be large enough to accommodate at least five staff members in case physical restraint is necessary—for example, when patients may hurt themselves or others (see Chapter 3). Ideally, visual monitoring should be available in the interview room.

The furniture should be bolted down, with nothing in the room that could be used as a weapon. An isolation room should be available, and chemical and physical restraints should be accessible (see Chapter 3).

There must be security available when needed, with sufficiently trained staff to survey the ED clinician and patient in the interview room. Screening and searching for weapons by security may be deemed necessary prior to the psychiatric evaluation. A panic button should be available, directly linked to security officers. A coding system should be available to be called overhead, and a team already assembled at every work shift to respond immediately to this type of psychiatric emergency. If there is any possibility that the patient may become violent toward staff members, then security officers should be standing by the door or in the room with the patient and clinician while the evaluation is ongoing.

Interviewing the Patient in the Emergency Psychiatric Setting

The first objective is to assess lethality. If the patient came in voluntarily—for example, asking someone else to bring him or her or just arriving unescorted—the patient is more likely to accept help.

Continue to assess in a calm and methodical manner. Because patients that come to the ED are usually upset about something, it is essential that the ED clinician establish trust and rapport when possible. Paranoid patients may be suspicious, and those that do not want to be there will try to negotiate with the clinician to leave.

The clinician should give a patient who is pacing, with increased psychomotor activities, plenty of room and stay back if possible. Maintain a calm demeanor and avoid direct eye contact with patients who are suspected of being paranoid to avoid the impression of challenging the patient.

The assessment of suicidality is covered in Chapter 6. Only by questioning and assessment will the ED clinician be able to have a dialogue about this subject. Collateral information is invaluable for those patients who are uncooperative or who are set on going through with their suicidal intentions. Box 2-1 lists the more common conditions that may increase the risk of suicidal behavior.

Elements of the Psychiatric Interview

There is no time limit in the emergency psychiatric interview except for constraints imposed by the fact that other patients

---

Box 2–1. Summary of Conditions Associated with an Increased Risk of Suicidal Behavior

- Previous suicide attempt and/or verbalized suicidal ideation
- Psychiatric disorder, including mood disorder, psychosis, and personality disorder; previous psychiatric hospitalization, especially if discharged in the past 3 months
- Family history of completed suicide
- Recent significant losses—in personal relationship, of loved ones, in social status (rejected by peers, unemployed, legal problems); this information should be correlated with cultural acceptability of such losses or shame
- Chronic medical illness that has become more of an incapacitating illness
- Substance abuse, with current intoxication
- Violent rage or acute psychosis (especially patients with persecutory delusions that they believe are directed toward them and patients with command auditory hallucinations)
- Widowed, separated, or divorced; socially isolated; elderly

are waiting to be seen. Take as much time as necessary to gather pertinent information about the patient.

Establish rapport. The ED clinician usually is not familiar with the patient, and suicidal patients may give off (transference) strong feelings of anxiety or anger. Keeping one's internal gauge (countertransference) in check while interviewing the patient in a calm, nonjudgmental manner, the clinician must show and express interest in the patient. Ask general questions first and then proceed to asking about suicidal or homicidal thoughts when the patient appears to have become more familiar with the interview process. From there, proceed to specifics of the situation.

The following general elements should be noted:
- Identification of the patient.
- Chief complaints—the reason why patient has come in or has been brought in.
- History of the present illness—including the present symptoms, the chronology of the present symptoms, medications, adherence to medications, support system, and current stressors. Based on this information, the initial working diagnosis may be established and disposition may be decided.

- Medical history and allergies. Chronic medical illness is found in at least 50% of patients who have completed suicides; thus the contribution of medical illnesses to the present psychiatric emergency is important.
- Current medical illnesses (see Chapter 4 for details). Many medical conditions have symptoms that may be mistaken for psychiatric emergencies rather than medical emergencies—for example, visual hallucinations or psychosis due to delirium. Information regarding medical conditions is especially important for a patient who has no psychiatric history or has the onset of psychiatric symptoms late in life. Medication adverse effects (such as from the induction of alpha interferon for hepatitis C treatment), possibly other toxins, or an overdose could be the culprit. As with all patients, one must first rule out medical conditions.
- Past psychiatric history. This should include current treatment and by whom (to be able to obtain collateral information, how the patient is at baseline, from the treating outpatient psychiatrist is invaluable) and previous psychiatric hospitalizations (to be able to obtain

information regarding hospital treatment and the course of hospitalization is very beneficial).
- Social history. Educational level, support system, family dynamics, and current stressors may be established. When possible, a history of childhood trauma or abuse may be obtained.
- Collateral information. I could not stress how important collateral information is for patients that are in crisis, as during these times they may be unable to contribute to history gathering.

Interview Course

The reason why a patient is currently seeking help now, rather than in a subsequent appointment, is important. What is it that could not wait? This could determine the acuity of the patient's distress.

Continue to use open-ended questions in the beginning of the interview to establish rapport—for example, "How are you feeling when you say you feel depressed?" and "What are the voices telling you to do?".

When you have established the patient's thought process in answering your open-ended questions, it is advisable to then narrow down the questioning in order to obtain chronological history, the when, where, how, why, who, and what—for example, "How long have you been unable to sleep?"; "When the voices started to return, were you taking your medications?"; and "When did you stop taking your lithium?".

Mental Status Examination

A mental status examination (Box 2-2) should be carried out; however, certain aspects of the examination, such as abstraction, may have lower priority. Orientation questions and the establishment of a recent memory recall are important. It may be helpful to find that the patient is capable of attention, using serial 7, digit span testing (naming five numbers consecutively and then backward) which helps in delirium assessment. Thought process and thought content examination are important to diagnose psychosis and mood disorders. Congruency of mood and affect may help the interviewer if a continued course of assessment is necessary. Incongruence of mood and affect may indicate that the interviewer has missed (1) the history;

Box 2–2. Mental Status Examination to Be Obtained in the Psychiatric Emergency Department

Descriptors of appearance may include height, weight, the way patient is dressed, and unusual features such as visible and excessive tattoos and excessive skin piercing. For example, patient demonstrates sufficient self-esteem by attention to grooming and care of self or patient is wearing excessive make-up and is "over-dressed."

Behavior and Attitude

Describe how patient presents self—for example, patient immediately responds and "gets down to business," or patient's response is tentative. Note whether the patient has excessive psychomotor movements, such as pacing and inability to rest, which may imply akathisias.

Orientation

Note whether the patient is aware of surroundings and situation, including the time and date—for example, when the patient is asked if it is morning or night, the response could indicate the patient's attentiveness, or attention level (see "Cognitive Components"). If the patient says that it is 1966, not 2006, this is important information for the next intervention. Orientation to self is rarely affected. When patients say they do not know who they are, a workup for total amnesia may be helpful; however, most likely this is due to some other reason, and malingering should be considered in this case.

Speech

There is generally an overlay of speech with thought process, because thought process often is determined by way of speech. Note the tone, volume, and the rate of speech and whether there is latency (a lag between the time a question is asked and the expected time needed for the patient to process the question and respond to it); this varies, depending on the underlying pathology. For example, manic patients may talk incessantly or interrupt while the question is being asked; depressed patients may take a long time to respond to the question; and psychotic patients, responding to internal auditory hallucinations, may wait until they have "heard" what the voices are directing them to say before responding.

Box 2–2. Mental Status Examination to Be Obtained in the Psychiatric Emergency Department—cont'd

Mood

Mood is the subjective report of how a patient feels. Usually, the patient will express this ("I'm sad"); however, when the patient is vague ("I'm just so-so"), it may be necessary to fine-tune the questions—for example, "How have you been feeling for the past few days?" If there is still no response, be more specific—for example, "Have you felt sad lately?", "angry?", and so on. Some patients may say they are "depressed"; at this point, using a scale of 1 to 10, with 10 representing the most severe depression, the patient can be asked "Where are you now on this scale?" Having this information, one may be able to track the degree of mood once it is established and then determine treatment progress.

Affect

Affect is the subjective aspect of an emotion, considered apart from bodily feeling. Note the presence of congruency or incongruency to the reported mood, abnormal lability in mood (patient cries one minute, laughs another), and inappropriate affect (patient laughs about things that would normally not be funny, such as turning over a piece of paper). The range of affect may also be recorded—for example, blunted or flat (as in schizophrenia), restricted or constricted (as in sadness), or expanded or elated (as in mania).

Thought Process

When patients are goal-oriented, as suggested by their speech, their thought processes are generally organized. However, psychosis may be present even with what seems to be an organized thought process (as in an organized delusion). Patients may have changes in the velocity of their thoughts, such as in mutism or flight of ideas. There may be looseness of association from topic to topic, or the association may be so loose that the words are not understandable, but rather a form of word salad. Other descriptors include circumstantiality (patient goes around a topic but eventually returns to it) and tangentiality (patient has a topic in mind but quickly changes to another, unrelated topic).

Box 2–2. Mental Status Examination to Be Obtained in the Psychiatric Emergency Department—cont'd

Thought Content

Thought content generally refers to significant and occasionally elaborate themes, such as in a delusion (pathologic belief system) and religiosity, or it may be symptomatic, as in auditory hallucinations (hearing voices that aren't real), paranoid ideation (the feeling that someone is out to get you or has devious motives), and suicidal or homicidal ideation.

Insight

In the context of the mental status examination, *insight* is a descriptor of whether patients are aware of their illness and have some concept of the nature of their illness, possible causes, and treatment options. Manic patients often lack insight, because their expansive mood is characterized by the belief that they can do almost anything they can dream of, whereas some insightful patients (depressed patients or substance abusers) are able to give you information regarding their psychosocial stresses ("I lost custody of my children" or "I just couldn't stop drinking once I started").

Judgment

Judgment is best assessed at the end of the interview—for example, if patients come in to get help because they believe that their depression is affecting their work or because they feel suicidal, they exhibit good judgment. Judgment is also assessed by asking standardized questions such as "What should you do when you see smoke coming out of the ceiling while you are sitting in a theater filled with people?"

Cognitive Components

Alertness: It can vary from stupor, drowsy, waxing and waning, sleepy, to alert.

Memory: Cursory and informal screening tests include memorizing three unrelated words. The patient is asked to register them in memory by repeating them to the interviewer and then to repeat them after 5 minutes. If any words are missed, the patient is prompted by supplying a clue to the words that are missed. This helps with identification of ability to recall recent information.

Orientation: See preceding section on "Orientation."

> **Box 2–2. Mental Status Examination to Be Obtained in the Psychiatric Emergency Department—cont'd**
>
> *Attention*: Note the patient's ability to attend to the current situation or attend to the task at hand. This may aid in the diagnosis of delirium and other types of cognitive impairment. Ask the patient to spell a five-letter word such as *world* or *march* and then to spell it backward. If unable to do this, the patient is asked to subtract 7 from 100 and keep subtracting 7 from the answers. This helps determine the patient's attention level. Persons who are illiterate may be asked to repeat five-number digits and then to repeat them backward. If they are unable to do this type of task, there is evidence that attention is impaired. This may help in differentiating dementia from delirium, because patients with dementia may have memory impairment but may have an intact attention span.

(2) the truth about how the patient is presenting, such as in somatization and malingering; or (3) other medical conditions (e.g., multiple sclerosis) that may cause such incongruence. Dangerousness to self and others must always be documented. Again, safety issues for the patient and the staff should be kept in mind.

Assessment of Impulsivity
Due to the dangerousness of impulsivity to violent tendencies, it is important that the emergency clinician establish the presence of impulsivity in the patient.
- Patients who are intoxicated are disinhibited in their behavior and may have increased impulsivity; they may be more dangerous than their baseline functioning indicates. It may be necessary to continue to observe these patients or hold them until intoxication has waned.
- The patient who is reactive, fidgety, and unable to sit still, and who paces or interrupts the clinician, blurting out answers before the question is finished, is also impulsive; this information should be part of the clinician's evaluation for dangerousness.
- Psychotic patients and those at risk of harming themselves or others may require physical or chemical restraint (for details, please see Chapter 3).

Criteria for Hospitalization

There is no standard per se for criteria for hospitalization except for guidelines established by the hospital itself or those used by insurance companies regarding what constitutes payable psychiatric hospitalization.

Because each patient's story is different, the following criteria are general guidelines only and are not meant to be exhaustive.

- Danger to self or others due to a psychiatric crisis. This includes persons with suicidal and homicidal ideation and intention who are unable or unwilling to proceed with treatment or who are unable or unwilling to contract for safety.
- Unable to care for self due to a psychiatric disorder, or due to failure or breakdown of support system. An example is the sudden illness or death of a caregiver mother of a patient who has difficulty controlling schizophrenia.
- Under extreme distress or crisis, even after adequate attempts at crisis intervention, the patient's coping mechanism is completely overwhelmed, with the result that the patient is unable to care for self.
- The exacerbation of a psychiatric illness that is in need of immediate stabilization.
- The requirement for establishing or clarification of a diagnosis in order to render treatment.
- Poor insight and judgment of one's illness, so that the patient is unable to care for self. An example is the manic patient who has delusions of grandeur and believes she owns the airplane that the president is using and wants to go get it back today.
- Intoxication from any substance of abuse or prescribed medication without adequate support.
- Repeated treatment failure as an outpatient.
- A voluntary patient admitted because of lack of beds in a medical floor or upon the request of the treating psychiatrist, or to administer electroconvulsive therapy (ECT) when necessary.

It must be emphasized that crisis intervention is always possible, and hospitalization may not be necessary (see Chapter 1). Persons who are chronically suicidal may not necessarily need hospitalization if they have good family support, are able to contract for safety, and agree to return when suicidal thoughts bother them enough so that they feel they may attempt suicide. Many patients who have had chronic suicidal ideation for years have managed their disorder through clinical treatment and support.

 Hospitalization has a cost to the patient, including financial costs, stigma, time away from work and family, and poor self-esteem and self-perception. Emergency clinicians should do everything in their power to render crisis intervention as much as possible to prevent hospitalization. The reader is referred to Chapter 1 for the application of crisis intervention methods and Chapter 3 for emergency medications.

Further Reading

Carlat D: The Psychiatric Interview: Practical Guides in Psychiatry. Philadelphia, Lippincott Williams & Wilkins. 1999.

Kaplan HI, Sadock BJ: Synopsis of Psychiatry. Behavioral Sciences/Clinical Psychiatry, 8th ed. Baltimore, Lippincott Williams & Wilkins. 1998.

Zealberg J, Santos A, Puckett J: Comprehensive Emergency Mental Health Care. Washington, DC, Beard Books, 1996.

CHAPTER 3

Medications for Psychiatric Emergencies

Doris T. Tan, DO

KEY POINTS

- Emergent administration of medications for sedation and volatility may be required before the patient can be calm enough to be evaluated properly.
- Although psychotropic drugs generally are relatively safe, high doses of these medications or doses given in combination with other medications can result in unique syndromes such as neuroleptic malignant syndrome and serotonin syndrome. These are medical emergencies and must be treated immediately and may require hospitalization.

Overview

This chapter discusses emergent psychotropic medications that are needed at times for patients who are severely psychotic or severely volatile combined with violent tendencies. Chemical restraints commonly used are benzodiazepines such as lorazepam (Ativan), typical antipsychotic agents such as haloperidol (Haldol), and the newer atypical antipsychotic agents, which can be administered singly or combined in an intramuscular form. These medications are discussed in detail later in the chapter.

Many people feel that administering emergent medications with the specific intention of chemical restraint is cruel. I would say that it is not. It is much more cruel to allow a person in a severely psychotic, volatile, and/or violent state to continue to be in that state.

When physical restraint is inadequate—that is, when the patient continues to chafe against soft or leather restraints or continues to show violent behavior with the possibility of self-injury—chemical restraint should be considered.

It should be noted that physical restraint may not be easy to accomplish. At times, patients in a frenzied state of psychosis or fear would fight with all their might and attempt to run away from the evaluating team. A show of force (having numerous staff on hand) may be adequate for the patient to allow a search for contraband, to go into the seclusion room if this is needed, or to take emergent medications.

However, at times, the patient may believe he is fighting for his life and may be extremely strong, with an autonomic sympathetic surge. It may require five people to subdue a patient in this case. Five is the number of staff required, one for each limb and one for the head. If medication is also needed, then a sixth person will need to be at hand to administer the agent, Good staff coordination is important for minimizing injury to the patient and staff, and each member of the team should know beforehand exactly what to do. If the patient continues to resist even after being subdued, then leather restraints may be necessary until the medication takes effect. The patient needs to be constantly checked for possible injuries. It may be necessary to keep a violent and volatile patient in isolation to minimize stimulation.

When the patient is able to contract for safety, negotiations can begin regarding removal of restraints. A lower limb may be freed to see if the patient will conform to the contract provisions. Once this is adequately assessed, and the patient further contracts for safety and nonviolence, other restraints may be removed. Rarely, patients require several cycles before they truly contract for cooperation.

When patients are uncooperative, be it due to psychosis, to medications, or to substance abuse, collateral information becomes extremely important in the history of the present illness, establishing baseline functioning, and the direction of treatment.

 It is imperative that clinicians be very careful of their own safety and avoid being with patients who are violent without other staff members being present. Common sense dictates that space and escape routes are adequate for the clinician if the patient continues to be violent (see Chapter 9). The environment in the emergency department (ED) should ensure the clinician's safety while assessment of violent patients is being carried out. Support staff, technicians, and nurses who are trained in this type of situation should be available. Security personnel are there to help and enable clinicians and other staff members to take care of patients as safely as possible.

Being with a Patient in the Emergency Department with a Psychotic Emergency, One Must Have the Proper Arsenal

The following are medications that should always be available in the ED.

Benzodiazepines

An injectable form of benzodiazepine should be available. Lorazepam (Ativan), 1 or 2 mg, either by mouth (PO) or intramuscularly (IM) is the first choice when sedation with calming effect is desired. Lorazepam is fast-acting, easy to administrate, and has close equivalency when given PO and IM—making it easier to calculate dosages. It is also more reliably and consistently absorbed when given IM than other drugs of the same class. It does not have active metabolites and also does not require glucuronidation. If the reason for the patient's agitation is alcohol withdrawal, then administration of lorazepam is already initiating treatment for it. Caution must be used if the patient has a respiratory ailment (e.g., chronic obstructive pulmonary disease [COPD], sleep apnea), as it may cause respiratory depression.

Antipsychotic Agents

Haloperidol. Haloperidol (Haldol) was widely used before the introduction of injectable atypical antipsychotics (see following section). Haloperidol is a high-potency typical antipsychotic that can be combined with lorazepam in the same syringe. This makes it convenient to give with lorazepam to patients that physically resist medication administration. Due to the side effects of haloperidol, especially the dystonias, often benztropine (Cogentin) or diphenhydramine (Benadryl) is also given. These not only help with the dystonias but also enhance its sedating effects. Side effects include severe torticollis (painful muscle contraction that forces parts of the body to turn to the contracted muscle side), and parkinsonian-type movements. Long-term use of typical antipsychotics such as haloperidol and fluphenazine can lead to tardive dyskinesias (abnormal movements of the facial and jaw muscles and tongue).

Droperidol. Droperidol (Inapsine) is another antipsychotic that is useful in psychiatric emergencies. It is similar in effect to haloperidol, except that the induction of sedation is more rapid. It is used frequently for induction of anesthesia. This would appear to be the medication of choice because of its sedating and quick action; however, it has been found to prolong the QT interval (QTc longer than 440 milliseconds) in a dose-related fashion. Torsades de pointes, cardiac arrest, and death also have been reported. The U.S. Food and Drug Administration (FDA) has not approved droperidol as an emergent medication for acutely agitated patients and carries a black box warning in its product label.

Table 3-1 lists common antipsychotic agents and their routes of administration.

Atypical Antipsychotic Agents

More recently, atypical antipsychotics have become available for intramuscular administration, including olanzapine (Zyprexa) and ziprasidone (Geodon).

Table 3–1
Some Typical Antipsychotic Medications

Generic (Brand) Name	Daily Oral Dose Range	Initial Single IM Dose Range
Chlorpromazine (Thorazine)	50-400 mg	25-50 mg
Fluphenazine (Prolixin)*	2-20 mg	1.25-5 mg (max 10 mg)
Haloperidol (Haldol)*	2.5-100 mg	2.5-10 mg
Mesoridazine (Serentil)[†]	100-400 mg	25-50 mg[†]
Perphenazine (Trilafon)[†]	16-64 mg	5-10 mg[†]
Thiothixene (Navane)[†]	15-60 mg	4-8 mg (max 30 mg)[†]
Trifluoperazine (Stelazine)[†]	4-20 mg	1-2 mg (max 6 mg)[†]

*Available in decanoate form that has an effective time range of 2-4 weeks.
[†]IM preparation is not easily obtainable in the United States.
IM, intramuscular.

OLANZAPINE. Olanzapine may be given IM at doses of 10 mg repeated every 2 hours, with a maximum dosage of 30 mg/24 hours, until the desired effect is achieved. Side effects include sedation and orthostatic hypotension, as well as prolongation of QTc. Weight gain and increased feelings of hunger are also side effects, but this is not of much concern during an emergency, especially as administration is expected to be a one-time event.

ZIPRASIDONE. The recommended dose of ziprasidone is 10 mg IM every 2 hours or 20 mg IM every 4 hours, with a maximum of 40 mg IM/24 hours. Side effects include QTc prolongation; thus its use is contraindicated with concomitant use of Class I and III antiarrhythmics for anyone with recent myocardial infarction.

Administration of Atypical Antipsychotic Agents

Administration of these agents should be switched from intramuscular to oral as early as possible. No long-term study of intramuscular and oral administration of these drugs is available as of this writing. Their advantages include decrease in incidents of acute dystonia, less likely need for concomitant use of other substances such as lorazepam, diphenhydramine, or benztropine. Disadvantages include orthostatic hypotension, severe sedation, and QTc prolongation.

Table 3-2 lists atypical antipsychotics and their routes of administration.

Table 3–2

Atypical Antipsychotic Agents

Generic (Brand) Name	Daily Dose Range	Initial IM Dose
Aripiprazole (Abilify)	10-30 mg	NA
Clozapine (Clozaril)	200-1000 mg	NA
Olanzapine (Zyprexa)	2.5-40 mg	10 mg
Quetiapine (Seroquel)	25-800 mg	NA
Risperidone (Risperdal)*	0.25-8 mg	Long-acting only
Ziprasidone (Geodon)	40-160 mg	20 mg

*Risperidone is only available in long-acting preparation (Risperdal Consta) to be given every other week, starting at 25 mg.
IM, intramuscular; NA, not available.

Severe Adverse Effects of Psychotropic Agents

The most feared adverse effects of medications in psychopharmacology are serotonin syndrome and neuroleptic malignant syndrome.

Serotonin Syndrome

Serotonin syndrome usually occurs due to serotonergic substances such as selective serotonin reuptake inhibitors (SSRIs) and serotonin norepinephrine reuptake inhibitors (SNRIs) (see Tables 11-4 and 11-5). Often it is caused by a combination of several medications, such as benzodiazepines, buspirone (BuSpar), bupropion (Wellbutrin), sertraline (Zoloft), fluoxetine (Prozac), paroxetine (Paxil), citalopram (Celexa), other monoamine oxidase inhibitors (MAOIs), and tricyclic antidepressants. Other substances with serotonergic effects such as dextromethorphan, Saint John's wort, and lithium have been implicated in augmentation that produces serotonin syndrome. When monotherapy is used and serotonin syndrome occurs, it is usually the result of administration of high dosages of these medications or perhaps not having a sufficiently long washout period when switching from MAOIs to SSRIs.

Sternback (1991) has listed three features in his diagnostic criteria for serotonin syndrome—confusion, hypomania or changes of mental status, and agitation. Other symptoms include myoclonus, shivering, tremor, diaphoresis, hyperreflexia, incoordination, fever, and diarrhea. Severe cases of serotonin syndrome may be characterized by rhabdomyolysis, and with increasing muscle damage, a markedly increased serum creatine phosphokinase is seen.

The renal system is unable to keep up with filtration and this may cause renal failure. Respiratory acidosis or respiratory failure could also worsen. Disseminated intravascular coagulation (DIC) and adult respiratory distress syndrome (ARDS) may also develop. Seizures, coma, and death, although rare, may occur.

The differential diagnosis of serotonin syndrome includes neuroleptic malignant syndrome.

Diagnosis

No tests are available to confirm the diagnosis of serotonin syndrome. However, it is recommended that all patients suspected of having serotonin syndrome undergo basic laboratory tests, including assessment of renal and liver function, electrolytes, creatine phosphokinase (CPK), and glucose; electrocardiography (ECG); complete blood count (CBC); and platelet count. Prothrombin time (PT) and partial thromboplastin time (PTT) using the international normalized ratio (INR) may be warranted if there is severe respiratory distress, especially with concomitant hyperthermia or hypotension, which is an indication of a severe and possibly lethal case.

Treatment

There is no known treatment for serotonin syndrome, with the exception of immediately discontinuing the offending serotonergic substance, which is most likely an SSRI or MAOI. If the patient is agitated, than benzodiazepines as a treatment for agitation may be used; respiratory depression must be monitored, and intubation may be necessary.

If the patient's temperature is elevated, muscle activity should be decreased and further loss of fluid from the skin prevented. Intravenous (IV) fluid administration may be necessary. Vigilance and administration of benzodiazepines may slow down this process. Admission to the intensive care unit for monitoring may be necessary in severe cases.

If seizures develop, diazepam, 10 mg, given at rapid IV push, may be repeated every 15 minutes as needed. If this is unsuccessful, other anticonvulsants may be warranted.

Anecdotal treatments include the following:

- Periactin (cycloheptadine)—8 mg PO every 2 hours up to a maximum of 32 mg/24 hours; low dosage does not seem to be effective.
- Chlorpromazine, methysergide, and Remeron (mirtazapine).
- Charcoal administration may be necessary if acute ingestion is suspected. In this case, induction of emesis is not recommended due to possible central nervous system (CNS) suppression.
- Sedation and neural blockade has been used in severe cases.
- Electroconvulsive therapy (ECT) also has been a reported treatment.
- Bromocriptine has its use in the treatment of neuroleptic malignant syndrome but is not recommended in the treatment of serotonin syndrome because of its serotonergic effects.

Neuroleptic Malignant Syndrome

Neuroleptic malignant syndrome is a rare but severe adverse effect of antipsychotic drug administration. It tends to have a more prolonged duration of symptoms and a slower onset of symptoms than serotonin syndrome.

Obviously this syndrome is associated with the use of neuroleptic agents. Symptoms include hyperthermia. and muscle rigidity. Serotonin syndrome, on the other hand, is more likely to be characterized by hyperreflexia and clonus; if fever does develop, it usually is not as high as in neuroleptic malignant syndrome. More information is needed to establish and differentiate these two syndromes. As one can see from Table 3-3, laboratory testing does not aid in distinguishing these two diagnoses.

Symptoms of neuroleptic malignant syndrome include acute autonomic instability, hypertension, diaphoresis, tachycardia, and in severe cases, hypotension. In severe cases hepatocellular injury may occur. Acute renal failure may occur secondary to rhabdomyolysis. In more severe cases, tachypnea may progress to overt respiratory failure.

Musculoskeletal system involvement is reflected in symptoms of myoclonus and hyperreflexia with rhabdomyolysis. Leukocytosis is common, and in very severe cases, DIC may ensue. CNS manifestations initially may include incoordination; confusion and disorientation may occur. Severe cases include seizures, and may progress to severe CNS depression leading to coma. Neuromuscular effects include hyperactivity, ataxia, clonus, tremor, and muscle rigidity of the extremities.

Gastrointestinal system symptoms include diarrhea; abdominal pain does not seem to occur in neuroleptic malignant syndrome, which could be one of the distinguishing factors differentiating it from serotonin syndrome.

Treatment

There are no known guidelines for the effective treatment of neuroleptic malignant syndrome;

Following are reported anecdotal treatment measures:

- Immediate discontinuation of the neuroleptic and any other dopamine antagonists.
- Support of life functions as problems arise (e.g., decrease basal body temperature for hyperthermia).

| Table 3–3 |

Differences between Serotonin Syndrome and Neuroleptic Malignant Syndrome (NMS)

Symptoms	Serotonin Syndrome	NMS
Temperature	elevated	hyperthermia
Abdominal Symptoms		
Diarrhea, nausea	yes	no
Mental State		
Delirium	yes	yes
Confusion	yes	yes
Coma	yes	yes
Euphoria	yes	no
Irritability	yes	no
Anxiety	yes	no
Agitation	yes	yes
Restlessness	yes	yes
Neurologic Symptoms		
Muscle rigidity	yes—may be mild	yes
Hyperreflexia	yes	not common
Tremor	yes	yes
Myoclonus	yes	not common
Incoordination	likely	no
Seizures	yes—in severe cases	yes
Autonomic Nervous System		
Blood pressure	up or down	up or down
Restlessness	yes	yes
Diaphoresis	yes	yes
Tachycardia	yes	yes
Watery mouth	yes	yes
Shivering	yes	no
Laboratory Data		
Hyperkalemia	yes	yes
Hyponatremia	yes	yes
Leukemoid reaction	yes	yes
CPK elevation	yes	yes
LFT elevation	yes	yes
Complications		
Rhabdomyolysis	yes	yes
Renal failure	yes	yes
DIC	yes	yes
Seizures	yes	yes
Death	yes	yes

CPK, creatine phosphokinase; DIC, disseminated intravascular coagulation; LFT, liver function test.

- Medications:
  - Dantrolene (Dantrium)—1 mg/kg by rapid continuous IV push until effective or until a maximum cumulative dose of 8 mg/kg has been achieved during the crisis event; for post-crisis follow up, 4-8 mg/kg/24 hours in four divided doses given PO for 1 to 3 days.
  - Bromocriptine (Parlodel)—1.25-2.5 mg daily; may titrate up to a maximum dose of 100 mg.
  - Amantadine (Symadine)—100-300 mg daily in divided doses.
  - Levodopa (Dopar)—300-1200 mg per day in divided doses.
  - Benztropine (Cogentin)—1-2 mg twice a day
  - Clonazepam (Klonopin)—1-2 mg twice a day
- ECT, especially for cases that are resistant to medication (Ozer et al., 2005).

Hospitalization and support of life functions are absolutely necessary, and the possibility of a stay in the intensive care unit is high with both serotonin syndrome and neuroleptic malignant syndrome.

Further Reading

American Psychiatric Association: Diagnostic and Statistical Manual of Mental Disorders, 4th ed. Text Revision. Washington, DC, American Psychiatric Association, 2000.

Kaplan H, Sadock B: Pocket Handbook of Psychiatric Drug Treatment, 2nd ed. Baltimore, Williams & Wilkins, 1996.

Krause T, Gerbershagen MU, Fiege M, et al: Dantrolene— A review of its pharmacology, therapeutic use and new developments. Anaesthesia 2004;59:1139.

Ozer F, Meral H, Aydin B, et al: Electroconvulsive therapy in drug-induced psychiatric states and neuroleptic malignant syndrome. J ECT 2005;21:125-127. Micromedex Health Care Series Internet web site.

Serotonin Syndrome and Neuroleptic Malignant Syndrome 2002. Clinical Psychopharmacology Seminar. Original 1996 author—Perry P; 2002 revision—Ellingrod V. Virtual Hospital. http://vh.org/adult/provider/psychiatry/CPS/0.9.html.

Sternback H: The serotonin syndrome. Am J Psychiatry 1991;148:705-713.

Torrey, F. 2001. Surviving Schizophrenia, 4th ed. Quill Edition. New York, HarperCollins, 2001.

CHAPTER 4

Emergency Psychiatric Manifestations of Medical Conditions

Hani R. Khouzam, MD, MPH, FAPA

KEY POINTS

- Emergency department (ED) clinicians need to know the common psychiatric manifestations of various medical conditions. It is important to understand that certain medical diseases can present with more than one type of psychiatric presentation.
- The medical assessment of patients presenting with psychiatric symptoms should include a thorough medical assessment with physical examination, including diagnostic laboratory and brain imaging studies if indicated. A thorough medical assessment is extremely important to rule out the presence of treatable and reversible medical conditions.
- The treatment of psychiatric symptoms may take precedence over the treatment of the medical condition, if the psychiatric symptoms interfere with patients' ability to communicate their complaints or when the severity of symptoms prevent the conduction of an accurate medical assessment.
- Most of the psychiatric manifestations of medical conditions will resolve with the treatment of the medical conditions.
- Patients with preexisting psychiatric conditions and patients with residual psychiatric symptoms will need ongoing psychiatric treatment even after their medical conditions are treated and stabilized.
- ED clinicians may need to initiate psychiatric treatment prior to the final ED disposition.

• In certain conditions, consultation with medical, neurologic, surgical, or other specialists may be necessary before the final disposition and/or referral for follow-up care.

Overview

Patients may present to the ED with psychiatric symptoms manifested by alteration in their behavior, mood, thinking, or their perception of reality. Because the assessment of these patients is usually arduous and time-consuming, busy ED clinicians may hastily triage these patients and rush them to be transferred to a psychiatric disposition before conducting a comprehensive medical evaluation.

Because the emergence of psychiatric symptoms may be precipitated or exacerbated by various medical conditions, it is extremely important to perform an appropriate medical evaluation even in patients with preexisting psychiatric conditions. The failure to do so is dangerous and may lead to missed opportunities to reverse medical illness, resulting in prolonged morbidity, inappropriate disposition, catastrophic outcomes, and rarely even death.

The medical evaluation should include a detailed history and physical examination, as well as laboratory, diagnostic, and radiographic tests to rule out any underlying medical causes of the presenting psychiatric symptoms.

This chapter summarizes the psychiatric manifestations of medical and neurologic illness. The psychiatric aspects of delirium are discussed in Chapters 5 and 17; substance abuse in Chapters 14 and 15; the assessment and management of violent patients in Chapter 9; malingering, factitious disorders, and somatoform disorders in Chapter 13; seizure disorders in Chapter 16; and adverse effects of psychopharmacological agents in Chapters 2, 3, and 17.

Definition

The current edition of the *Diagnostic and Statistical Manual of Mental Disorders*, 4th edition, Text Revision (DSM-IV-TR) defines the psychiatric presentation of a medical illness as "mental disorder due to a general medical condition. These disorders are characterized by the presence of mental symptoms that are the direct consequences of an underlying medical condition or are judged to be the direct physiologic consequences of a general medical condition." The definition also states that "the mental disturbances are not better accounted for by another mental disorder."

Epidemiology

Medical illnesses in various organ systems have been reported to cause psychiatric symptoms in up to 10% of cases in the general population, and they may contribute to psychiatric symptoms in up to 50% of patients. This phenomenon may be more frequent in persons with comorbid mental conditions because they have greater health care needs compared to persons of the same age and sex in the general population. An underlying medical problem can be found to explain psychiatric illness in 5% to 60% of the time. The various statistics of the psychiatric manifestations of medical conditions are extensive, and these are just a few examples of such conditions. Approximately 30% to 50% of patients with a seizure disorder have psychiatric symptoms sometime during the course of their illness, and 30% of patients with epilepsy have a history of suicide attempts. Up to 50% of patients with brain tumors reportedly have manifestations of a psychiatric nature. In patients with multiple sclerosis (MS), 30% to 50% have cognitive deficits, and 25% to 50% experience major depression after the onset of MS. Suicide is more common in patients with MS who present with depression. Delusions of grandeur occur in 10% to 20% of patients with neurosyphilis. In patients with Cushing's syndrome, 35% to 50% present with a depressed mood. Neuropsychiatric symptoms occur in 40% to 70% of patients with systemic lupus erythematosus (SLE). Among patients with human immunodeficiency virus (HIV), 4% to 14% will present with symptoms of depression and anxiety even in the absence of clinical signs of HIV infection. Psychiatric symptoms of anxiety and depression may be the first presenting clinical symptoms in 40% to 65% of patients with cardiac and cerebrovascular conditions, in 25% of patients with diabetes, and in one third of patients with substance abuse disorders.

Medical Conditions with Psychiatric Manifestations

Patients who present with psychiatric symptoms may have:
- One or more abnormal vital signs
- Abnormal findings on physical and neurologic examination
- Memory dysfunction, disorientation, and fluctuating level of consciousness

These patients should be regarded as having a possible medical illness. Therefore, it is of paramount importance for ED clinicians to know the common psychiatric manifestations of various medical conditions. It is also important to understand that certain medical diseases can present with more than one psychiatric condition. The common features of medical conditions with psychiatric presentations are summarized in Table 4-1.

Table 4–1

Common Characteristics of Medical Conditions with Psychiatric Symptoms

Characteristic	Description
Onset	Initial presentation at late age; sudden onset
Past medical history	Previously known underlying medical condition
Past psychiatric history	Absence of personal and/or family history of psychiatric conditions
Symptoms presentation	Atypical presentation of a specific psychiatric diagnosis; disproportionate severity of behavioral disturbances compared with what is expected in the psychiatric condition
Mental state	Unstable; waxing and waning mental status
Symptoms progression	Temporal relationship between the onset, progression, exacerbation, or remission of psychiatric symptoms and the treatment of the medical condition

Continued

Table 4–1

Common Characteristics of Medical Conditions with Psychiatric Symptoms—cont'd

Characteristic	Description
Comorbidity	Preexisting systemic diseases; alcohol or illicit substance intoxication/withdrawal; use of prescription medications with psychiatric side effects
Physical examination	Presence of one or more abnormal vital signs; abnormal neurologic findings
Treatment response	Treatment resistance or unusual response to treatment

Adapted from Talbot-Stern JK, Green T, Royle TJ: Psychiatric manifestations of systemic illness. Emerg Med Clin North Am. 2000;18:199-209.

Diagnostic Evaluation of Medical Conditions with Psychiatric Manifestations

Data concerning the use of screening profiles in psychiatric patients have revealed that the widespread use of extensive screening batteries—including a complete blood cell count (CBC), complete blood chemistry analysis, erythrocyte sedimentation rate (ESR), urinalysis, measurement of vitamin B_{12} and folate levels, electroencephalography (EEG), electrocardiography (ECG), and chest x-rays—are not indicated in the majority of psychiatric cases.

 The few tests that have merit as broader screening tests in asymptomatic psychiatric patients include serum glucose, blood urea nitrogen (BUN), creatinine, and urinalysis. Patients on psychotropic medications should be monitored for side effects of that particular therapy. Patients with new psychiatric symptoms may have underlying medical conditions, and their ED medical clearance studies should include a medical history, physical examination, sequential multi-channel analysis with computer-7 (SMA-7), assessment of calcium levels, creatine phosphokinase (CPK) if there is possible myoglobinuria, alcohol and drug screens, computed tomography scan, and lumbar puncture.

The clinical presentation of the various medical conditions that may present with psychiatric symptoms along with laboratory studies are shown in Table 4-2.

Psychiatric Presentation of Specific General Medical Conditions

 The mnemonic **DIVINE MD TEST** described in Table 4-3 can be used as a tool to recall the various medical conditions that can present in the ED with psychiatric manifestations.

D—DRUG ABUSE

The term *drug abuse* is used here as a broad description that includes abuse of alcohol, illicit drugs, prescribed and over-the-counter (OTC) medications, caffeine, nicotine, herbal supplements, and any type of alternative remedies.

Alcohol and Illicit Drugs

Although alcohol and illicit drugs abuse medical and psychiatric presentation are described in detail in Chapters 14 and 15, certain facts related to alcohol and illicit drugs that are pertinent to this discussion are reviewed here.

Alcohol
Alcohol Withdrawal Delirium
Alcohol withdrawal delirium is usually termed delirium tremens (DT). Alcohol withdrawal delirium may present with numerous psychiatric symptoms and these can be fatal if they are not identified and quickly reversed. Clinical features include:
- Hallucinations—most commonly visual and/or auditory
- Acute state of confusion and disorientation
- Autonomic hyperactivity, which can be manifested by tachycardia, fever, sweating, and hypertension
- Agitation and paranoia that prevent the performance of physical examination and comprehensive medical assessment

The tendency of ED clinicians to admit patients to the psychiatric unit before reversing their DT is a grave error of clinical judgment. Even in the absence of a measurable blood alcohol level, untreated DT can lead to a potentially fatal outcome.

Table 4–2

Clinical Presentation of Medical Conditions with Corresponding Laboratory Studies

Medical Condition	Clinical Presentation	Laboratory Studies
Substance abuse (e.g., abuse of illicit drugs, prescription and OTC medications, and herbal remedies)	Clinical symptoms related to specific substance	Urine and blood screen; specific blood levels of suspected substance
General infections	Fever, chills, malaise	CBC with differential count, UA, chest x-ray, ESR
Neurosyphilis	Tremor, ataxia, Argyll-Robertson pupil	Serum FTA-ABS, CSF, VDRL
HIV/AIDS	Weight loss, lymphadenopathy	HIV antibodies, brain imaging, LP
Lyme disease	Tick bite, annular rash	Serum IgG antibody titer
Vascular	Abnormal BP and pulse; cardiovascular signs and symptoms	ECG, Holter monitor, and other studies as indicated
Immunologic/inflammatory	Fever, arthralgia	ESR, ANA, complement levels
Nutritional	Malnutrition, ataxia, ophthalmoplegia	Serum vitamin and folate levels
Hyperthyroidism	Tremor, tachycardia, heat intolerance, exophthalmos	TSH, T_4
Hypothyroidism	Lethargy, bradycardia, cold intolerance	TSH, T_4
Cushing's syndrome (hypercortisolism)	Buffalo hump, moon facies, stria, muscle wasting	Dexamethasone suppression test
Addison's disease (hypocortisolism)	Hypotension, hyperpigmentation	ACTH stimulation test
Pheochromocytoma	Hypertension, bouts of anxiety	Urinary catecholamines and vanillylmandelic acid

Medical Condition	Clinical Presentation	Laboratory Studies
Metabolic		
Fluid and electrolyte imbalance	Skin turgor, dry mucous membrane	Electrolytes and chemistry profile
Liver encephalopathy	Asterixis, lethargy	Ammonia level, liver function tests, prothrombin time
Uremic encephalopathy	Apathy, lethargy, myoclonus, asterixis	Kidney function tests, electrolytes
Wilson's disease	Tremor, rigidity, chorea, Kayser-Fleischer ring	Serum ceruloplasmin
Acute intermittent porphyria	Bouts of abdominal pain, paresthesias	Urinary porphobilinogen
Degenerative/demyelinating disorders	Neurologic signs and symptoms	Special blood tests, brain imaging
Trauma	Signs and symptoms of specific trauma	Radiologic and brain imaging
Epileptic	Aura, ictal, and postictal stages	EEG
Structural disorders	Headache, papilledema	Brain imaging
Toxins/heavy metals	Varies according to the agent; headache, tremor, weakness, lethargy, encephalopathy, coma	Laboratory and diagnostic studies for specific toxin; heavy metal screen

ACTH, adrenocorticotropic hormone; AIDS, acquired immunodeficiency syndrome; ANA, antibody antinuclear test; BP, blood pressure; CBC, complete blood count; CSF, cerebrospinal fluid; ECG, electrocardiogram; EEG, electroencephalogram; ESR, erythrocyte sedimentation rate; HIV, human immunodeficiency virus; LP, lumbar puncture; TSH, thyroid-stimulating hormone test; T_4, thyroxine test; UA, urine analysis; FTA-ABS, fluorescent treponemal antibody absorption test; VDRL, venereal disease research laboratory test.

Adapted from Drooker MA, Byck R: Physical disorders presenting as psychiatric illness: A new view. The Psychiatric Times. Medicine & Behavior 1992;9:19-24.

Table 4–3	

The Mnemonic DIVINE MD TEST

Letter	General Medical Conditions
D	Drug abuse
I	Infectious diseases
V	Vascular disorders
I	Immunologic/inflammatory disorders
N	Nutritional/vitamin deficiencies
E	Endocrine disorders
M	Metabolic disorders
D	Degenerative/demyelinating diseases
T	Trauma
E	Epilepsy/seizures
S	Structural disorders
T	Toxins/heavy metals

Adapted from Brewerton TD: The DIVINE MD TEST. Resident and Staff Physician 1985;31:146-148.

ED Treatment

Supportive therapy is an important component of the treatment of alcohol withdrawal delirium. This includes:

- Environmental measures such as a calm, quiet, well-lit environment
- Reassurance
- Sedation with benzodiazepines as needed
- Ongoing reassessment of fluid and electrolyte imbalance
- Intravenous (IV) line and normal isotonic saline
- Cardiac monitor
- Oxygen per nasal cannula
- IV thiamine administration (100 mg)
- Immediate bedside glucose testing or D50 administration

Commonly, these patients have coexisting medical, surgical, and psychiatric conditions that need ongoing follow-up care, such as emergency assessment and treatment of alcohol-induced complications

Wernicke's Encephalopathy

Wernicke's encephalopathy is a disorder of acute onset that is primarily caused by thiamine deficiency. It is usually found in patients with alcohol dependence, although it is not restricted to this group. Thiamine depletion can occur in other less common conditions, including forced or self-imposed starvation, low-protein diet malnutrition resulting from inadequate diet or malabsorption, conditions associated with protracted vomiting, chronic renal failure, and carbohydrate loading in the presence of marginal thiamine stores (as when feeding after starvation)

    Patients with Wernicke's encephalopathy exhibit the characteristic clinical triad of ocular abnormalities (ophthalmoplegia), global confusional state, and ataxia. Only a third of patients with acute Wernicke's encephalopathy present with this classic clinical triad.

- Ocular abnormalities are manifested by horizontal nystagmus and paralysis of the lateral rectus muscles. Less frequently noted are pupillary abnormalities such as sluggishly reactive pupils, ptosis, and anisocoria.
- Global confusional state is characterized by the following:
  - Apathy
  - Impaired awareness of the immediate situation
  - Spatial disorientation
  - Inattention
  - Inability to concentrate
- Ataxia, the loss of equilibrium, can be seen in the early stages of the disease and is due to vestibular dysfunction; it is uniformly found, yet is often poorly appreciated. The wide-based ataxic gait seen in the subacute and chronic phases of the illness is due to cerebellar dysfunction, either alone or combined with vestibular dysfunction.

Other associated features may include hypothermia, and hypotension, which have been added by some to the traditional triad and are thought to result from hypothalamic involvement. Agitation, aggressive behaviors, hallucinations, and signs of autonomic hyperactivity are also reported.

The diagnosis of Wernicke's encephalopathy is essentially a clinical one. ED clinicians need to differentiate Wernicke's encephalopathy from acute delirium secondary to hypoxia, hypercarbia, central nervous system (CNS) infections, and postictal seizure state. Ataxic gait also can result from cerebellar infarction. Ocular disorders also can result from vasculitis or infarction. ED clinicians need also to be aware that although stupor or frank coma are comparatively rare, they may be the sole manifestations of Wernicke's encephalopathy, and they can be fatal if untreated.

ED Treatment

Due to the frequent subclinical nature of Wernicke's encephalopathy and the difficulty in making the clinical diagnosis, the following course of therapy should be implemented in all ED patients who are alcohol-dependent and who are at high risk for malnutrition:

- IV thiamine (50-100 mg)
- After the initial IV dose, daily doses of thiamine (50-100 mg) as IV, intramuscular, or oral doses, depending on patient status
- Supplementation of electrolytes, particularly magnesium and potassium, if required
- Multivitamin supplements if patient is chronically malnourished

It is extremely important to be aware that the administration of intravenous glucose to patients who are severely malnourished could exhaust their dwindling supply of thiamine and could precipitate Wernicke's encephalopathy. Thus, the administration of thiamine should be initiated before giving glucose infusions.

A balanced diet should be resumed as early as possible. Vitamin and electrolyte supplementation should be adhered to in addition to a well-balanced diet initially; supplementation can be tapered as the patient resumes normal intake and demonstrates symptomatic improvement.

The presence of gait abnormalities requires assisted ambulation during the initial phase of treatment. Patients may require physical therapy evaluation for gait assistance. Gait abnormalities may be permanent, depending on the severity at initial presentation and the timeliness of therapy.

Because long-term alcohol use is the most common cause of Wernicke's encephalopathy, abstinence from alcohol use provides the best treatment outcome. Referral to an alcohol treatment program should be part of the ED final disposition.

Korsakoff's Syndrome

 If persistent learning and memory deficits persist in patients with Wernicke's encephalopathy, then their condition is termed Wernicke-Korsakoff syndrome (the DSM-IV-TR prefers the term *Alcohol-Induced Persisting Amnestic Disorder* as a descriptor of Korsakoff's syndrome). This syndrome usually follows an acute episode of Wernicke's encephalopathy, appearing after the initial confusional state begins to resolve with thiamine administration and persisting to some degree in the most severely affected individuals.

Patients are usually alert and responsive, but they demonstrate the amnestic features of both anterograde and retrograde amnesia. The anterograde amnesia is severe but incomplete; patients are able to repeat a series of numbers or objects as they are stated but not after a recall period. Retrograde amnesia is manifested by gaps in patients' memories of the recent and remote past that antedate the onset of illness. These gaps in memory may lead to confabulation, when patients fill in memory gaps with data they can readily recall. It is unclear whether confabulation represents a deliberate attempt of patients to hide their memory deficits or whether it is a real complication of Korsakoff's syndrome. Up to 20% of patients will achieve long-term recovery if thiamine deficiency is begun immediately. Patients who develop permanent impairment due to Korsakoff's syndrome are often over age 40 years and have many years of heavy alcohol abuse.

ED Treatment

As in the case of Wernicke's encephalopathy, treatment of Korsakoff's syndrome requires immediate administration of thiamine.

Patients with irreversible memory impairment will usually require permanent custodial or institutional care.

Alcohol-Induced Psychosis

Alcohol-induced psychosis is a secondary psychosis with predominant hallucinations or delusions, occurring in many alcohol-related conditions, including acute intoxication and withdrawal. It is often an indication of prolonged exposure and repeated withdrawal and occurs in the setting of recent cessation of alcohol use or significant decrease in the amount of alcohol used. The hallucinations are usually auditory; however, visual and tactile hallucinations may also occur. The psychotic symptoms follow the onset of alcohol use. The symptoms persist for a substantial period of time (e.g., a month) after cessation of use. The psychosis does not occur exclusively during the course of a delirium so the sensorium is clear (differentiating it from DT).

ED Treatment

Most cases of alcohol-induced psychosis are self-limiting, so alcohol abstinence is the most desirable intervention. After medical stabilization, following assessment of respiratory, circulatory, and neurologic systems, alcohol-induced psychosis should be first treated with cautious use of benzodiazepines, such as:

- Lorazepam, 1-2 mg given by mouth (PO) as tablet or liquid, or intramuscularly (IM)
- Chlordiazepoxide 25-50 mg PO as tablet or capsule, or IM
  In cases of persisting psychosis or if the patient is in imminent danger of harming self or others, a high-potency antipsychotic agent should be given, such as:
- Haloperidol (Haldol), 5-10 mg PO or IM
- Olanzapine, 2.5-10 mg PO (oral disintegrated tablet) or IM
- Ziprasidone, 10-20 mg IM

Antipsychotics may lower the seizure threshold and should not be used to treat withdrawal symptoms unless absolutely necessary and used in combination with a benzodiazepine.

Treatment may include thiamine, 100 mg parenterally, followed by supplemental thiamine, 100 mg three times a day, folic acid, 1 mg daily, and a daily multivitamin.

The use of mechanical wrist and leg restraints may be necessary if there is acute danger of assault toward others or self-harm.

Other Alcohol-Induced Psychiatric Disorders

Alcohol-induced mood, anxiety, or sleep disorders are usually considered separately from a symptom cluster if they are excessive and so severe that they warrant independent emergency treatment. ED clinicians need to be aware that more than 50% of patients with alcohol-induced disorders who are monitored for 2 to 4 weeks for alcohol abstinence have full remission of symptoms without additional intervention for these disorders.

Illicit Drug Abuse
Initial ED Assessment

Prior to any psychiatric evaluation or disposition of drug-abusing patients, the ED assessment should determine:

- Vital signs
- Level of consciousness
- Pupil size and reactivity
- The presence of nystagmus or asymmetric gait.

Laboratory studies to confirm the presence or absence of certain drugs and to rule out infections, anemias, hepatic diseases, and other multiple systems involvement may include:

- Blood and urine screening
- Sequential multiple analysis twelve-channel biochemical profile (SMA-12)
- Complete blood count (CBC) with differential
- Hepatitis B surface antigen and surface antibody
- Hepatitis C antibody
- Rapid plasma reagent (RPR) test
- Human immunodeficiency virus (HIV) serum antibody test (performed in two steps, with a screening test such as the enzyme-linked immunosorbent assay [ELISA] and a confirmatory test such as the Western blot)
- Purified protein derivative (PPD) test
  Other tests if warranted by clinical presentation include:
- Electrocardiography (ECG)
- Radiographic studies

The clinical presentation and psychiatric symptoms of illicit drug abuse are summarized in Table 4-4.

ED Treatment

The ED treatment approach to illicit drug abuse, intoxication, and withdrawal is described in detail in Chapters 14 and 15. Pharmacological intervention is only the first phase of the treatment process. The ED clinician needs to impress on the abusing patients the fact that substance abuse is a long-term, possibly lifelong, illness.

The initial ED intervention may be followed by detoxification, followed by inpatient and/or outpatient rehabilitation, and then followed by regular participation in support groups such as Alcoholics Anonymous (AA) and Narcotics Anonymous (NA). Patients need to be directed and encouraged to take responsibility for their ongoing treatment.

Medications That May Cause Psychiatric Symptoms

Side effects of many prescribed medications include psychiatric symptoms; some examples follow.

- Antihypertensives
  - Reserpine—loss of appetite, decreased sexual ability, depression, nightmares
  - Methyldopa—drowsiness, headache, extreme tiredness

Text continues on page 51.

Table 4–4

Clinical Manifestations and Psychiatric Symptoms of Drugs of Abuse

Drug	Clinical Manifestations	Psychiatric Symptoms
Stimulants 1. Amphetamines: methamphetamine, crank, crystal meth, methylphenidate, white dragon, Ciba-19, phenylpropanolamine (Propagest)	Hypertension, dilated pupils; weight loss; dry mouth and nose	Risk for violence; hyperactivity, euphoria; irritability, anxiety; excessive talking followed by depression or excessive sleeping at odd times; may go long periods of time without eating or sleeping; psychosis with prominent paranoid delusions
2. Cocaine	Tachycardia, dilated pupils; weight loss; delirium with autonomic instability	Agitation, hypervigilance; euphoria and increased energy; psychosis
3. Ecstasy (3,4-methylenedioxymethamphetamine [MDMA]); designer drug synthetically derived from amphetamines	Hypertension, dilated pupils Diaphoresis and fever?	Often used in the context of large and energetic parties (raves) at night; initially, causes mild euphoria, increased energy, and increased libido; tolerance develops rapidly; depression, anxiety, and psychosis occur with regular use; some symptoms persist for months after cessation of use

Drug	Clinical Manifestations	Psychiatric Symptoms
Cannabis (Tetrahydrocannabinol [THCl])	Glassy, red eyes; sweet burnt scent; weight gain or loss, increased appetite	Paranoid ideation; increased speech volume, inappropriate laughter, followed by sleepiness, loss of interest and motivation and apathy
Opioids Butorphanol (Stadol), Pentazocine (Talwin), β-endorphin agonists, kappa, heroin, hydromorphone (Dilaudid-Hp), mesipramine, methadone, morphine	Needle marks; characteristic withdrawal symptoms—sweating, vomiting, coughing and sniffling, twitching; loss of appetite; abnormal pupil signs	Lethargy, somnolence with sleeping at odd times; euphoria followed by depressed and despondent mood
Hallucinogens Lysergic acid diethylamide (LSD), mescaline, ketamine (Ketalar), Phenylcyclohexylpyrolidine (PHP), hallucinogenic mushrooms containing psilocybin and psilocin	Tachycardia, tremors, pupillary dilation, slurred speech, clear sensorium; in some cases, intoxication leading to altered consciousness and confusion	Hallucinations, mood swings, bizarre and irrational behavior including delusions, paranoia, aggression, personality change, detachment from people; absorption with self or with objects; LSD-induced hallucinations are usually of relatively short duration, but flashbacks of varying intensity may occur in some users for long periods even after cessation of use

Continued

Table 4–4

Clinical Manifestations and Psychiatric Symptoms of Drugs of Abuse—cont'd

Drug	Clinical Manifestations	Psychiatric Symptoms
Phencyclidine (PCP)	Rotary nystagmus, arrhythmias, hypertension, facial grimacing.	Psychosis with agitated and violent behavior
Sedatives 1. Anxiolytics—GABA agonists, benzodiazepines 2. Hypnotic barbiturates—ethchlorvynol, glutethimide, methaqualone 3. Other hypnotics—zolpidem, zaleplon, esopiclone	Life-threatening withdrawal syndromes; drunk as if from alcohol but without associated odor of alcohol; clumsiness, slurred speech, excessive sleepiness, contracted pupils	Amnestic disorder; difficulty concentrating, impaired judgment, labile mood
Gamma-hydroxybutyrate (GHB)	Life-threatening intoxication and withdrawal syndromes; tremor, nausea, vomiting, respiratory difficulties, seizures, coma	Anxiety, insomnia, excessive sedation, memory and concentration difficulties
Anabolic steroids	Hypertension, weight gain, voice change; acne, hirsutism, premature balding, yellowing of skin; male gynecomastia	Euphoria, hyperactivity, depression, mania, anger, increased arousal, irritability, anxiety, hostility, violence, psychosis

Drug	Clinical Manifestations	Psychiatric Symptoms
Anticholinergics Trihexyphenidyl (Artane), orphenadrine (Disipal), benztropine (Cogentin), procyclidine (Kemadrin), diphenhydramine (Benadryl), ethopropazine	Burning dysuria, dysphagia, constipation, diplopia, miosis, rigidity, fever; life-threatening intoxication, producing delirium, atonic bladder, cardiac arrhythmias, and coma	Atropine-like effects with classical triad of "mad as a hatter, red as a beet, and dry as a bone"; hallucinations, body image distortion, agitation, delusional thought, excitement
Inhalants (solvents, aerosols, and vapors) Glues, paints, cleaning fluids, nail-polish removers, lighter fluids, aerosol propellants, gasoline	Watery eyes, impaired vision; secretions from the nose, rashes around the nose and mouth; headaches, dizziness, nausea; appearance of intoxication, drowsiness, arrhythmias, respiratory depression, poor muscle control; changes in appetite; neurologic impairment, stupor; particularly movement disorders due to cerebellar dysfunction	Euphoria, memory and thought disturbances, anxiety, irritability; impulsiveness; possession of unusual number of spray cans; hallucinations, cognitive impairment, personality change.
"Ts and blues" Talwin (pentazocine), Pyribenzamine (blue-colored 50-mg tripelennamine tablet)	Headaches, vomiting, blurred vision, chest pain, palpitations, generalized seizures	Euphoria, rush similar to that produced by heroin; memory loss

Continued

Table 4–4

Clinical Manifestations and Psychiatric Symptoms of Drugs of Abuse—cont'd

Drug	Clinical Manifestations	Psychiatric Symptoms
Tobacco/nicotine	Smell of tobacco; stained fingers and/or teeth; withdrawal symptoms, restlessness, bradycardia; increased appetite, weight gain	Dysphoria, depressed mood, irritability, frustration, anger, anxiety, insomnia, difficulty concentrating
Caffeine	Flushed face, muscle twitching, diuresis, tachycardia, arrhythmia, GI disturbances	Restlessness, nervousness, excitement, insomnia, psychomotor agitation; rambling thoughts and speech

GABA, gamma-aminobutyric acid; GI, gastrointestinal.

- Beta-blockers—drowsiness or fatigue, trouble sleeping or vivid dreams while asleep, depression, memory loss, confusion, hallucinations, impotence
- Clonidine—depression
- Diuretics—depression
- Digitalis—mood disturbance
- Oral contraceptives—mood changes, including depression
- Steroids—mood changes of either elation or depression, ideas of persecution, delirium, sleep difficulties
- Thyroxine—acute anxiety
- Histamine 2 blockers—fatigue, insomnia, agitation, confusion, hallucinations, depression
- Antiparkinsonian agents—depression
- Antituberculosis therapy—psychosis
- Oronabinol (Beta-9-tetrahydrocannabinol)—anxiety, dysphoria
- Opiates—sedation, confusion
- Zidovudine (AZT)—mania, seizures, anxiety, auditory hallucinations, confusion
- Cancer chemotherapy agents
  - Vinca alkaloids—agitation, confusion, convulsions, hallucinations, loss of appetite, trouble sleeping, unconsciousness
  - Vincristine, vinblastine, and methotrexate—delirium, depressed mood
  - Procarbazine—nervousness, depression, nightmares, fatigue
  - L-Asparaginase—confusion, emotional lability, somnolence
  - Amphotericin—unusual tiredness or weakness, convulsions
  - Interferon and ribavirin (also used to treat hepatitis C)— depression, anxiety, suicidal ideation

The psychiatric symptoms caused by many medications also may be due to delirium. The ED clinician needs to determine whether psychiatric symptoms are a manifestation of a delirious state (see Chapters 5 and 17). Table 4-5 summarizes some common causes of delirium.

Herbal Supplements Associated with Psychiatric Symptoms

Side effects of many herbal supplements also include psychiatric symptoms; some examples follow.

Table 4–5

Some Common Causes of Delirium

Drugs of abuse	Alcohol, amphetamines, cocaine, hallucinogens, inhalants, opioids, phencyclidine (PCP), sedatives, hypnotics
Medications	General anesthetics, analgesics, anti-asthmatic agents, anticonvulsants, antihistamines, antihypertensive cardiovascular medications, antimicrobials, antiparkinsonian medications, corticosteroids, gastrointestinal medications, muscle relaxants, immunosuppressive agents, lithium, psychotropic medications with anticholinergic properties
Toxins	Cholinesterase inhibitors, organophosphate insecticides, carbon monoxide, carbon dioxide, volatile substances such as fuel or organic solvents or glue

- Kava-kava (*Piper methysticum*)—disorientation, somnolence, loss of appetite, sedation, oral and lingual dyskinesia, torticollis, oculogyric crisis, exacerbation of Parkinson's disease, painful twisting movements of the trunk, and rash. Although this herb has potent anxiolytic and muscle relaxation effects, several warnings have been issued in regard to causing fatal liver failure.
- Passionflower (*Passiflora incarnata*); when combined with valerian is used for treating insomnia, anxiety, and irritability—it has been associated with altered consciousness
- Valerian (*Valeriana officinalis*)—restlessness, sleeplessness—mania, restlessness, agitation, insomnia, fatigue, dizziness, confusion
- Ephedra (ma huang)—insomnia, nervousness, tremor, seizures
- *S*-Adenosyl methionine (SAM-e); is widely advertised as a natural cure for several emotional conditions; breaks down into homocysteine, the build-up of which has been correlated with heart disease
- Omega-3 fatty acids; reported to improve depression; may exert a dose-related effect on bleeding time

- Ginkgo (*Ginkgo biloba*); used for memory improvement; can cause vision changes, and anticoagulant activity may cause bleeding
- Ginseng; purported to strengthen normal body functions, increase resistance to stress, and improve sexual function; interaction with warfarin reported to cause nervousness and insomnia

   Given the ongoing increase in the use of herbal and alternative remedies, ED clinicians need to increase their awareness of these compounds. When taking a medical history, they should include questions about the patient's use of these products and involvement with alternative practitioners.

Over-the-Counter (OTC) Medications Associated with Psychiatric Symptoms

Although psychiatric adverse effects of OTC medications are rare, these medications do have the potential to cause psychiatric side effects. It is important to remember that the combination of prescription drugs and OTC medication may be responsible for drug-induced mental symptoms.

   Cough and cold remedies may contain stimulants such as ephedrine, such as the cough remedy Nyquil (pseudoephedrine, doxylamine, dextromethorphan, acetaminophen, alcohol) and the asthma medicine Primatene P (theophylline, ephedrine, phenobarbital). These can cause depression, agitation, psychosis, and sedation.

   OTC medications that contain antihistamines, such as promethazine, can cause psychiatric symptoms of depression, anxiety, insomnia and agitation. Another antihistamine, cyclizine, the active ingredient of the travel sickness pill Marzine (available before February 1987) is still available as Valoid tablets. When cyclizine is injected, it produces an intense "rush," hallucinations, and possibly erratic or violent behavior.

   Dextromethorphan—a common ingredient in many cough preparations such as Cheracol D Cough Liquid, Formula 44D, Naldecon Senior DX Liquid, and Robitussin-DM—can be taken frequently; an accidental overdose can cause dizziness, confusion, slurred speech, excitation, hallucinations, and a number of other side effects. Teenagers abuse dextromethorphan-containing cough medicines, sometimes with tragic results.

   Medications that contain caffeine, such as Anacin, Empirin, Excedrin, and No-Doz, can cause anxiety.

Because of the many anti-inflammatory agents, antacids, asthma treatment medications, vitamins, analgesics, and other OTC medications now available, ED clinicians need to exercise diligence and consistency in asking patients about all classes of OTC medications that they may have been using.

I—INFECTIOUS DISEASES

Infections are commonly associated with fever, malaise, and laboratory abnormalities. These findings may be absent in patients most susceptible to infection, especially the elderly and the chronically medically and mentally ill. It is of paramount importance for ED clinicians to ensure that a complete physical examination and necessary laboratory testing are conducted for all patients presenting with symptoms suggesting the presence of an underlying infectious process.

The psychiatric symptoms associated with infections may be related to pneumonia, urinary tract infection, sepsis, hepatitis, malaria, legionnaires' disease, typhoid, diphtheria, and acute rheumatic fever. These symptoms are usually cleared once these infections are medically controlled. The infections that most commonly present with psychiatric symptoms, along with their recommended treatment, are summarized in this section.

Neurosyphilis

The incidence of neurosyphilis, historically a common cause of mental disturbances (general paresis of the insane), has decreased since the introduction of penicillin. However, its incidence is again increasing due to development of treatment-resistant sexually transmitted diseases (STDs). Also, HIV/AIDS (acquired immunodeficiency syndrome) infections have reintroduced neurosyphilis to certain urban settings.

Syphilis, especially in women, is often undiagnosed due to its initial asymptomatic state, and in later stages it may mimic other conditions. As with other STDs, syphilis is more easily transmitted from men to women. The infection is caused by the spirochete *Treponema pallidum*. Neurosyphilis, or tertiary syphilis, usually becomes clinically apparent only after a latent period of 10 to 20 years after the primary infection; however, HIV infection can lead to an earlier presentation.

Early evidence of neurosyphilis includes tremors, dysarthria, and Argyll Robertson pupils. The diagnosis is confirmed using serologic tests. Cerebrospinal fluid (CSF) analysis shows primary lymphocytosis and increased protein levels.

Manifestations
- Frontal lobes effects result in personality changes, disinhibition, impulsivity.
- Mood effects result in irritability, delusions of grandeur, mania.
- Cognitive effects lead to decreased self-care and progressive dementia.

ED clinicians need to consider neurosyphilis in patients who may have an underlying immunodeficiency disease and present with mental status changes and a progressive dementia that does not coincide with advanced age.

Meningitis

Psychiatric presentation with or without abnormal vital signs can be associated with acute bacterial, fungal, and viral meningitis. These disorders commonly occur in immunocompromised patients who are infected with AIDS or receiving cancer chemotherapy, and in patients with in-dwelling ventriculoperitoneal shunts.

Psychiatric symptoms include acute confusion, memory impairments, and psychosis.

Meningitis, especially bacterial meningitis, is a life-threatening emergency; persons at high risk who have a sudden onset of mental status changes should always undergo a workup that includes a diagnostic lumbar puncture.

Lyme Disease

Lyme disease is a multisystem spirochetal illness that can present with psychiatric symptoms. Its early recognition is important to prevent an acute, treatable illness from becoming a chronic or relapsing one. Because current diagnostic tests are not always reliable, ED clinicians must rely on clinical presentation as the basis for diagnosis.

Medical Presentation
Lyme disease is transmitted by a *Borrelia burgdorferi*–infected nymphal or adult female Ixodes tick. This tick, which is smaller than the dog tick, may easily be missed on casual inspection.

The bite is usually not painful. Transmission of the spirochete appears to require the tick to feed at least 12 to 24 hours. The ticks are most commonly carried by deer and by the white-footed mouse, but other carriers have been described as well. Within the first few weeks after skin infection, *B. burgdorferi* may disseminate to the CNS, where it may remain quiescent for months to years before producing symptoms.

Several similarities exist between Lyme disease and syphilis. Both are caused by a spirochete: syphilis by *Treponema. pallidum* and Lyme disease by *B. burgdorferi*. Both start with skin inoculation and a localized skin reaction, followed by a disseminated multisystemic infection. Both may progress in stages. Both can cause meningitis, encephalitis, cognitive deficits, cranial neuropathy, and vasculitis. Both diseases can, in rare cases, lead to the Tullio phenomenon characterized by nausea and nystagmus in response to sound stimulation.

Unlike *T. pallidum*, which is generally transmitted from host to host, the Lyme disease spirochete is carried by a vector. Furthermore, radiculopathy and peripheral neuropathy are features of Lyme disease that syphilis does not share.

Psychiatric Presentation

Neurosyphilis is associated with memory problems, depression, mania, psychosis, personality changes, irritability, emotional lability, and apathy. Recent evidence suggests that Lyme borreliosis, the "new great imitator," may be associated with a similarly wide spectrum of psychiatric symptoms.

Laboratory Testing

Because *B. burgdorferi* is difficult to culture, indirect methods are used to detect the presence of the spirochete. Currently available serologic tests, such as ELISA and the indirect immunofluorescence assay, rely on the immune response following exposure to *B. burgdorferi*, but they can be unreliable, with both false-positive and false-negative results.

The results of laboratory testing among patients with Lyme disease vary, depending on the stage of the illness. In very early CNS involvement (meningismus) or late-stage infection (encephalopathy), the cerebrospinal fluid (CSF) may appear normal. When clinical signs of meningitis or encephalitis are present, a spinal tap may reveal a mononuclear pleocytosis, mildly increased protein, and, in some cases, an elevated IgG index or oligoclonal immunoglobulins.

ED Treatment

Treatment varies and depends on how early a diagnosis is made and on the various body systems affected by the infection. Long-standing or disseminated Lyme disease responds best to one or several courses of oral or IV antibiotics. The psychiatric treatment of Lyme disease may be geared toward symptomatic relief of depression, anxiety mood swings, and sleep disturbances.

The ED clinician may initiate antidepressants, mood stabilizers, or anxiolytics to decrease the severity of these conditions. Patients should be instructed to abstain from alcohol use and excessive caffeine intake. It is important to initiate referral for ongoing treatment because the disease affects so many aspects of patients' lives, including their physical, emotional, cognitive, familial, sexual, social, and occupational functioning.

Herpes Simplex Encephalitis

Medical Presentation

Herpes simplex virus (HSV) is one of the most common causes of sporadic and severe focal encephalitis. Due to HSV spread along the branches of the trigeminal nerve, the infection is characteristically localized to the temporal and frontal lobes. The diagnosis should be considered in patients with a prodrome of 1 to 7 days of upper respiratory tract infection accompanied by headache, fever, and subsequent bizarre psychiatric symptoms.

Psychiatric Manifestations

HSV encephalitis is associated with bizarre behaviors, waxing and waning mental status due to delirium, seizures, anosmia, olfactory and gustatory hallucinations, personality changes, and psychosis.

Diagnosis

Lumbar puncture, serology studies, neuroimaging, and electroencephalography (EEG) are helpful in confirming the diagnosis.

ED Treatment

Treatment with IV acyclovir usually is effective; however, if herpes simplex encephalitis is not diagnosed and promptly treated, long-term psychiatric and neurologic sequelae are likely to occur.

Rabies Encephalitis

The rabies virus is transmitted from the saliva of an infected animal. The incubation period for rabies is from 10 days to 1 year. It is a fatal encephalitis. It is rare in the U.S. and usually is transmitted by bats.

Clinical Presentation
Symptoms usually develop 1 to 3 months after exposure to the virus, depending on the location of the wound. Pain or numbness occurs in the wound. Initial symptoms are fever, apathy, and headache followed by local twitching and convulsions. Severe laryngeal and diaphragmatic spasms occur, causing profuse salivation. The patient refuses to drink anything due to fear of water (aquaphobia). Once encephalitis develops, it leads to paralysis and coma and is virtually always fatal.

Psychiatric Manifestations
Psychiatric symptoms include hallucinations, overactivity, restlessness, and agitation. Hydrophobia with intense fear of drinking water is due to laryngeal and diaphragmatic body spasms.

ED Treatment
Anyone who is exposed to bats, or is exposed to secretions of an animal suspected of having rabies, should be given the rabies vaccine, whether or not there are indications of rabies. Exposed individuals should also receive immune globulin unless they were previously vaccinated. Veterinarians and animal handlers should be vaccinated.

Vaccination does not eliminate the need for treatment if a person is exposed to rabies, but it reduces the intensity of the treatment. Side effects of vaccination may include pain, redness, headache, stomach pain, nausea, dizziness, muscle aches, and swelling at the injection site. An allergic response can occur after the first shot and as long as 21 days after a booster shot. Rare cases of neurologic side effects have been reported that cause pain and paralysis in the legs and arms, which clear up in about 12 weeks.

 Management of rabies-induced agitation, restlessness, overactivity, and hallucinations should be initiated whenever these symptoms interfere with the overall management of the illness.

HIV/AIDS Infection

Psychiatric presentation in HIV-infected persons can result from preexisting psychiatric conditions or the devastating psychosocial impact of having this life-threatening illness. Psychiatric complications can also be secondary to metabolic derangements, effects of tumors or abscesses, CNS infections, or side effects of antiviral medications. Recognition and proper treatment of AIDS-related complications involving the CNS and its behavioral and neurologic manifestations can be one of the most common challenges faced by ED clinicians.

ED Evaluation
- Consider the possibility of HIV encephalopathy in the evaluation of a patient with a psychiatric disorder and HIV.
- Lumbar puncture and brain imaging are necessary to exclude other causes (e.g., meningitis, malignancy).
- IV drug abusers presenting with first-time psychiatric symptoms and without a positive psychiatric history should undergo HIV testing.
- Awareness of the neuropsychiatric effects of medications used frequently in HIV infection is an essential component of the evaluation process.

Assessment and Treatment
General Treatment Principles
Early therapy with antiretrovirals, particularly zidovudine (AZT), is recommended because it may have a protective effect in delaying or reversing some of the psychiatric and neurologic manifestations of HIV infection.

Symptomatic treatment with psychopharmacological medications is an important aspect of ED intervention. Because patients with HIV infection can be more susceptible to the adverse effects of these medications, lower doses are recommended.

The ED assessment and treatment of various psychiatric manifestation of HIV/AIDS are summarized in the following section.

Depression
The diagnosis of depression in HIV/AIDS patients can be difficult because the clinical indicators of depression are often obscured by the somatic symptoms of medical illness, such as

poor appetite, weight loss, loss of energy, and insomnia. One of the most prevalent differential diagnoses to rule out when assessing depression is the presence of AIDS-related dementia, which may require a specialized neuropsychological assessment and a detailed psychiatric evaluation.

Treatment with antidepressants is effective (see Chapter 7 for details). The choice of antidepressant medication must be individualized, taking into account the patient's physical concerns. Tricyclic antidepressants (TCAs), selective serotonin reuptake inhibitors (SSRIs), serotonin/norepinephrine inhibitors (SNRIs), and, occasionally, psychostimulants are effective.

The key to the successful psychopharmacological treatment of depression in HIV is to identify potentially responsive clusters of symptoms, to use lower starting doses with gradual increases, and to monitor side effects and overall medical status with meticulous care. In severe depression, or for patients unable to tolerate antidepressant medication, electroconvulsive therapy (ECT) can be effective, beneficial, and well tolerated, even in cases of advanced AIDS.

Mania

Although mania is rarely directly associated with HIV infection, it may occur because of the medical complications of HIV or pharmacological treatment. Manic syndromes are most likely to occur during initiation or dose increases of medications such as steroids, AZT, or ganciclovir; however, many cases of medication-induced mania have occurred in patients on chronic and stable dosages.

The treatment of mania is dependent on the identification of the underlying medical precipitants or the discontinuation of the offending agents. If mania persists, then treatment should be initiated, as summarized in Chapter 8, with lithium, other mood stabilizers, or atypical antipsychotics.

Anxiety Disorders

Adjustment disorder with anxious mood-generalized anxiety disorder are prevalent in HIV patients. Other anxiety disorders, such as panic disorder and obsessive-compulsive disorder, do not appear to be markedly elevated above the general population. Some physically healthy patients who engage in high-risk sexual and IV drug-abusing behaviors may develop a preoccupation with the fear of having AIDS despite multiple seronegative HIV results and may subsequently develop AIDS phobia.

The treatment of anxiety disorder is indicated to relieve overt distress, decreased work performance, social dysfunction, interpersonal conflicts, and deterioration in the activities of daily living (ADLs). Psychological support provided by ED clinician referral to specialized group therapy, and self-help groups, in addition to the psychopharmacological treatment, can be extremely effective in limiting the distressing effects of anxiety (see Chapter 11 for detailed discussion of treatment of anxiety disorders). Because some HIV patients with chronic anxiety may require long-term maintenance treatment, especially in cases of advanced HIV infection, the starting dosages of medication may vary between one fourth to one third of the standard dosages.

Psychosis

The presence of depression and anxiety and the development of dementia may complicate the assessment of HIV-induced psychosis. Delirium, drug abuse, iatrogenic sources, and late-stage HIV infection may eventually lead to the development of psychotic symptoms, including delusions, hallucinations, disorganized thought, and looseness of association. Although psychosis is an uncommon complication of HIV infection, its emergence in the ED especially in individuals with AIDS-related dementia may be an indication of an increased risk of death.

Treatment with antipsychotic medications is summarized in Chapter 10. It is important for ED clinicians to know that HIV/AIDS patients may have an increased risk of developing neuroleptic malignant syndrome, extrapyramidal side effects, and tardive dyskinesia. The dose of antipsychotics and the duration of treatment should be kept to a minimum of one tenth to one third of the regular doses given to other patients.

Delirium

Delirium in HIV-infected patients may manifest with a hyperactive-agitated picture or with hypoactive-withdrawn features. The prompt diagnosis of delirium can lead to life-saving treatment; thus a high index of suspicion is required for AIDS patients presenting to the ED who are receiving complicated and advanced medical care. The treatment of delirium is discussed in Chapter 5.

Cognitive Disorders

Some HIV-infected patients will develop cognitive disorders. The most common of these is mild cognitive disorder (MCI). MCI is characterized by defects in two or more cognitive areas and is particularly expressed through reduction in speed of information processing, impairment in attention, and difficulty in learning and recollecting new information. Because depression is a common complication of early cognitive deficits associated with HIV status, it is important for ED clinicians to refer these patients for prompt treatment in addition to referral for ongoing monitoring of MCI.

AIDS Dementia Complex

Because AIDS patients now experience an increase in longevity, AIDS dementia (ADC) may become one of the psychiatric morbidities frequently challenging ED treatment interventions.

ADC is a syndrome of cognitive, motor, and behavior symptoms with no identifiable cause other than HIV infection. The dementia is typically characterized by forgetfulness, poor concentration, slowness, and difficulties with problem solving, and it may be accompanied by apathy and social withdrawal. Psychosis and delirium may also occasionally occur; although relatively rare, arson (fire-setting) may be a dangerous concomitant complication of HIV dementia.

The treatment of ADC is mainly supportive and symptomatic. Symptomatic treatment should depend primarily on patients' complaints. Antipsychotics can help alleviate associated psychosis. Benzodiazepines can be used to alleviate anxiety and agitation. Antidepressants can be used to restore sleep and improve depressed mood.

Although not all cases of ADC are reversible, it is important to identify and treat underlying medical causes such as metabolic disorders, malabsorption syndromes, and vitamin and other nutritional deficiencies. Because dementia is one of the most devastating complications of HIV infection, it is important for ED clinicians to offer reassurance that not all HIV-infected patients will become demented and that asymptomatic patients are usually capable of performing their social, occupational, and personal responsibilities.

⚠ ED clinicians should be aware that other terms for ADC are HIV encephalopathy, HIV encephalitis, and HIV-1 associated cognitive and motor complex.

General ED Interventions for HIV/AIDS

Suicide prevention requires that underlying psychiatric and medical issues be addressed to reestablish bonds and to provide a supportive network of family, loved ones, friends, and caregivers.

Acutely suicidal patients require emergency psychiatric hospitalization and clinically supervised observation during their ED crisis presentation.

Patients who experience a religious conversion report a significant reduction in anxiety associated with the fear of death (see Chapter 24). To improve the coping strategies of patients afflicted with HIV and terminal AIDS, ED clinicians may initiate referral for religious and spiritual counseling, meditation, prayers, and participation in formal religious activities.

V—VASCULAR DISORDERS

Several vascular conditions can precipitate the development of psychiatric symptoms. These are summarized in the following section.

- *Cardiac*—congestive heart failure, endocarditis, mitral valve prolapse, arrhythmias, atherosclerotic heart disease (e.g., angina pectoris, myocardial infarction)
- *Cardiopulmonary*—myocardial infarction, hypoxia, hypercarbia, bronchial asthma, chronic obstructive pulmonary disease (COPD)
- *Blood vessels*—hypertension, hypotension, arteriovenous malformation, thromboangiitis obliterans, polymyalgia rheumatica (giant cell arteritis), temporal arteritis, vasculitis
- *Cerebrovascular*—cerebrovascular accident, syncope, transient ischemic attack, aneurysm
- *Embolism*—pulmonary embolism, fat embolization, nitrogen emboli (bends)

Psychiatric manifestations of vascular conditions are diverse. The majority of patients may present with anxiety (which can be severe to the point of reaching panic proportions), depression, insomnia, agitation (at times accompanied by restlessness), and in rare cases violence, disorientation, and confusion.

ED clinicians need to consider the physical signs of hypertension, tachycardia, diaphoresis, difficulty breathing, chest pain, cyanosis, and body numbness that suggest an underlying vascular cause for the presenting psychiatric symptoms. If vascular causes are identified, their treatment takes precedence over the treatment of the psychiatric symptoms.

I—IMMUNOLOGIC/INFLAMMATORY DISORDERS

Several immunologic and inflammatory conditions can precipitate the development of psychiatric symptoms; the following disorders are discussed in this section:
- Systemic lupus erythematosus (SLE)
- Myasthenia gravis
- Periarteritis nodosa
- Polymyalgia rheumatica (giant cell arteritis)
- Rheumatoid arthritis
- Thrombotic thrombocytopenic purpura
- Bronchial asthma
- Allergies
- Ulcerative colitis
- Peptic ulcer disease

Systemic Lupus Erythematosus (SLE)

The neuropsychiatric manifestations of SLE can occur at any time during the disease course, and most appear in the first few years or before diagnosis of the illness.

SLE psychiatric symptoms include depression, emotional lability, delirium, and psychosis. Treatment, usually with high-dose steroids, can precipitate or exacerbate psychiatric symptoms. However, most instances of psychosis in patients who are on steroid therapy are secondary to lupus cerebritis, and many cases improve with an increase in dosage. It is important to exclude infectious causes of possible brain dysfunction in patients who are on steroid therapy, because steroids may mask fever, resulting in an atypical presentation of infection.

Treatment

Immunologic and inflammatory conditions are commonly associated with repeated vague complaints in addition to the presence of depression, anxiety, sleep and appetite difficulties, low energy, and general fatigue. ED clinicians may wonder about the legitimacy of these complaints. Often these patients will be labeled as "malingerers" or "hypochondriacs" and will not undergo an appropriate medical assessment prior to the final ED disposition (see Chapter 13).

Because of the multiple organ systems involved and the complexities of these disorders, it behooves the ED clinician to consult specialists such as rheumatologists and neurologists as appropriate. The initiation of symptomatic psychiatric treatment may take precedence over treatment of physical symptoms if they interfere with patients' ability to communicate their complaints.

N—NUTRITIONAL/VITAMIN DEFICIENCIES

The following disorders may be associated with psychiatric symptoms ranging from anxiety, depression, agitation, and cognitive deficits to psychosis:
- Vitamin B_1 (thiamine) deficiency
- Vitamin B_{12} (cobalamin) deficiency
- Folate deficiency
- Vitamin B_3 (niacin) deficiency
- Vitamin B_6 (pyridoxine) deficiency
- Hypervitaminosis A
- Hypervitaminosis B_6
- Malnutrition
- Anemia
- Food sensitivity (e.g., gluten)
- Excessive health food supplements (e.g., herbal products, vitamins)

ED treatment of identified nutritional and vitamin deficiencies should be initiated without delay, so as to prevent further progression of psychiatric and medical complications and to reverse the symptoms caused by these deficiencies.

Vitamin B_1 (Thiamine) Deficiency

Chronic and severe deficiency of vitamin B_1 (thiamine) leads to the neuropsychiatric symptoms of asthenia, fatigue, weakness, depressed mood, and confusion. More commonly today, thiamine deficiency manifests as Wernicke's encephalopathy, often but not exclusively in individuals with heavy and prolonged alcohol use.

Immediate treatment with parenteral thiamine reveals that this syndrome is at least partly reversible, because the confusion often resolves within hours. As the confusion improves, impaired cognitive functioning (amnesia) consistent with Korsakoff's syndrome often becomes evident. Long-term treatment with thiamine may result in ongoing improvement over a period of months.

Vitamin B_{12} (Cobalamin) Deficiency

Deficiency of vitamin B_{12} (cobalamin) is the cause of pernicious anemia. The diagnosis of pernicious anemia is made when low serum levels are found on evaluation of patients presenting with megaloblastic anemia and neurologic symptoms due to subacute combined spinal cord degeneration.

Although the direct cause and effect of concomitant psychiatric symptoms are not always clear, depression, fatigue, psychosis, and progressive cognitive impairment usually accompany the neurologic symptoms. These psychiatric symptoms can predate the neurologic symptoms by months to years and may be present in the absence of anemia or macrocytosis.

Vitamin B_{12} early supplementation can reverse the cognitive deficits in some but not all patients with the deficiency, especially in the elderly who may have other dementing illness.

Folate Deficiency

As with vitamin B_{12} deficiency, there is a relationship between folate deficiency and psychiatric symptoms.

Although direct causality is not always clear, evidence suggests that folate deficiency states are observed in patients with depressive and dementing syndromes; and that folate deficiency can exacerbate the psychiatric symptoms. Folate replacement may improve depressive and cognitive symptoms in some but not all patients with the deficiency.

Vitamin B_3 (Niacin) Deficiency

Deficiency in niacin (nicotinic acid) and tryptophan, a precursor from which the body can synthesize niacin, are the principal causes of pellagra. Pellagra is characterized by cutaneous, mucous membrane, and gastrointestinal (GI) symptoms. The complete syndrome of advanced deficiency includes symmetric photosensitive rash, scarlet stomatitis, glossitis, and diarrhea.

Psychiatric symptoms include psychosis, characterized by memory impairment, disorientation, confusion, and confabulation. Depression, mania, and delirium predominate; paranoid ideation also may occur. When encephalopathy occurs, it is characterized by clouding of consciousness, cogwheel rigidity of the extremities, and uncontrollable sucking and grasping reflexes. Differentiating these symptoms from those of thiamine deficiency may be difficult.

Treatment

Supplemental niacinamide, 300 to 1000 mg/day, should be given orally in divided doses. In most cases, 300 to 500 mg is sufficient.

Vitamin B_6 (Pyridoxine) Deficiency

Vitamin B_6 (pyridoxine) deficiency is manifested by general weakness, skin changes such as dermatitis and acne, ridged nails, and inflamed tongue. Osteoporosis, arthritis, and kidney stones also may develop. Vitamin B_6 deficiency can lead to B_3 vitamin deficiency.

Psychiatric symptoms include irritability, nervousness, and insomnia.

Treatment

The recommended dose of vitamin B_6 is 50 mg to 500 mg per day. Neurologic complications and numbness occur at doses that exceed 2000 mg per day. Patients with medication for Parkinson's disease should be careful about taking Vitamin B_6 because it can inactivate levodopa. Patients taking pyridoxine late at night sometimes experience very vivid dreams.

E—ENDOCRINE DISORDERS

Several endocrine disorders may present with psychiatric symptoms, including the following, which are discussed in this section:

- Pancreatic disorders (hypoglycemia)
- Pituitary disorders
- Thyroid disorders (hyperthyroidism, hypothyroidism, autoimmune thyroiditis)
- Parathyroid disorders (hyperparathyroid, hypoparathyroid)
- Adrenal disorders (Addison's disease)
- Cushing's disease
- Pheochromocytoma

Pancreatic Disorders

The most common pancreatic disorders that can have psychiatric presentations are diabetes mellitus, pancreatic tumors, acute pancreatitis, and hypoglycemia. Hypoglycemia and pancreatic tumors are discussed here.

Hypoglycemia
Causes
- Laboratory error—sample sits too long without removal of blood components
- Liver disease (congenital or acquired)—liver mass too small to store glycogen or provide gluconeogenesis
- Storage disease—metabolic pathways are not normal because of enzyme deficiencies
- Sepsis or marked leukocytosis—increased utilization of glucose by white blood cells
- Adrenal disorders (congenital or acquired)—decreased glucocorticoids and catecholamines necessary for normal gluconeogenesis
- Excessive insulin or insulin-like factors
- Drugs—salicylates, ethanol, sulfonylurea compounds
- Pituitary disorders—panhypopituitarism, growth hormone deficiency
- GI disorders—maldigestion, starvation, malabsorption

Symptoms
- Initially there is nausea, sweating, tachycardia, hunger, and apprehension.
- With progression, patients may become disoriented and confused and may hallucinate.
- Eventually, stupor and coma ensue.
- Persistent cognitive impairment can be a serious complication of recurring hypoglycemic states.
- Symptoms of clinical worsening include hyperventilation, headache, nausea, and vomiting; with ketoacidosis, disorientation and confusion can occur, and this state can be fatal if not properly identified and urgently treated.
- With the advent of the new atypical antipsychotics, there seems to be an increased risk of developing non–insulin-dependent type II diabetes, leading to risks of both hypoglycemic and hyperglycemic complications (see Chapters 10 and 17).

• The reversal of hypoglycemia may be associated in certain patients with psychiatric symptoms of anxiety, irritability, and even delirium with psychotic symptoms of visual hallucinations and paranoid delusions. These symptoms can be mistaken for mood or psychiatric disorders.

Pancreatic Tumors
Symptoms
Although uncommon, pancreatic tumors can manifest solely in depression. Despite a broad differential diagnosis, this diagnosis needs to be seriously considered in elderly patients with new-onset depression, especially in the setting of back pain.

Acute Pancreatitis
Symptoms
Acute pancreatitis may present with delirium. Acute exacerbation of recurrent pancreatitis may be accompanied by hallucinations, cognitive impairment, and agitation. Because the majority of patients with pancreatitis are also alcohol-dependent, the symptoms may be mistaken for those of alcohol withdrawal. The presence of abdominal pain, diabetes, and steatorrhea will suggest chronic pancreatitis.

Because it is reversible, ED clinicians need to identify acute pancreatitis-induced delirium. The psychiatric symptoms usually resolve within 7 to 10 days of treatment for the pancreatitis.

Pituitary Disorders

Pituitary disorders are relatively uncommon in the general population. If cases are misdiagnosed or untreated, serious complications, including death, can result. Unfortunately, due to the infrequency of these disorders as well as to their symptomatic diversity, an initial diagnosis is frequently elusive, and the subsequent management of pituitary disease can be complex.

The anterior lobe of the pituitary makes six hormones: prolactin, adrenocorticotropic hormone (ACTH), thyroid-stimulating hormone (TSH), luteinizing hormone (LH), follicle-stimulating hormone (FSH), and growth hormone (GH); the posterior lobe of the pituitary releases vasopressin (antidiuretic hormone [ADH]) and oxytocin. The maintenance of appropriate levels of these hormones constitutes a major control mechanism for virtually all physiologic activities.

For ED clinicians, the nonspecific symptomatology of pituitary disease is a major barrier to even a preliminary diagnosis. To assist in diagnosis, a partial list of common syndromes and clinical presentation of pituitary dysfunctions are summarized in Table 4-6.

Diagnostic Assessment
Although a preliminary diagnosis can be challenging, the initial basic work-up for pituitary disease is straightforward and can

Table 4–6

Common Syndromes and Clinical Presentation of Pituitary Dysfunction

Syndrome	Dysfunction	Clinical Presentation
Pituitary hormone deficiency	ACTH (adrenal insufficiency)	Addison's disease
	TSH abnormality	Hypothyroidism
	LH/FSH (hypogonadism)	Sexual dysfunction, hot flashes, menstrual irregularities
	Adult growth hormone deficiency	Lack of vigor, decreased exercise tolerance, feelings of social isolation
	ADH (diabetes insipidus)	Polydipsia, polyuria, nocturia
Pituitary hormone excess	Prolactin (hyperprolactinemia)	Galactorrhea, sexual dysfunction
	ACTH (Cushing's disease)	Moon face, truncal obesity, purple stria, hirsutism, HTN, DM, proximal muscle weakness
	Growth hormone (acromegaly)	Enlarged hands/feet/jaw/ tongue, carpal tunnel syndrome, oily skin, joint pain

ACTH, adrenocorticotropic hormone; ADH, antidiuretic hormone; FSH, follicle-stimulating hormone; LH, luteinizing hormone; TSH, thyroid-stimulating hormone.

be easily initiated if pituitary disease is suspected, using the laboratory tests listed here:

- Prolactin: 8:00 AM serum cortisol
- TSH and Free T$_4$
- LH and FSH: testosterone (men)
- Insulin-like growth factor-1 (IGF-1)
- 24-hour and urine free cortisol (for Cushing's disease)

Magnetic resonance imaging (MRI) of the head (with and without gadolinium) should be performed if the laboratory evaluation indicates the presence of pituitary disease or if a space-occupying lesion is suspected. The correct interpretation of the laboratory evaluation can sometimes be difficult; assistance in this process is offered through endocrinology consultation.

Thyroid Disorders

Hyperthyroidism

Hyperthyroidism is a common clinical condition, and ED clinicians need be aware of the clinical presentation of this disorder in any patient who presents with psychiatric symptoms.

Causes
Primary Hyperthyroidism

- Graves' disease—the major cause of hyperthyroidism; an autoimmune disorder that accounts for about 70 percent of all cases
- Subacute thyroiditis
- Toxic multinodular goiter—usually develops in older people who may have had hypothyroidism; nodules often produce excess thyroid hormone after the patient is exposed to excess iodine in iodine contrast dyes and imaging tests
- Toxic nodular adenoma—a condition in which the patient has one solitary nodule or has multiple nodules with one of them predominant or larger than the others; usually benign, although in rare instances may invade the thyroid gland and show signs of malignancy
- Thyroid carcinoma (rare)
- Exogenous iodine (jodbasedow)
- Hydatidiform mole
- Ovarian carcinoma (struma ovarii)

- Amiodarone (Cordarone)—adverse effects
- Excessive exogenous thyroid replacement—either iatrogenic or due to self-administration in factitious hyperthyroidism
- Hereditary hyperthyroidism—a genetic mutation similar to Graves' disease except that thyroid antibodies are not present, and patients do not develop the congestive eye disease, pretibial myxedema, acropachy, or vitiligo seen in Graves' disease

Secondary Hyperthyroidism
Hyperthyroidism secondary to pituitary tumors is extremely rare.

Clinical Presentation
- Heat intolerance
- Diaphoresis
- Weight loss despite increased appetite
- Palpitations
- Tachycardia
- Exophthalmos
- Hyperactive tendon reflexes

Psychiatric Manifestations
- Anxiety (most common presentation)
- Agitated depression.
- Hypomania
- Mania
- Psychosis
- Thyroid storm, delirium, and confusion (in cases of extreme toxicity)

Assessment
 Evaluation of TSH (thyrotropin) and free thyroxine (T_4) levels should always be included in the medical workup.

Treatment
In most patients who present with depression or anxiety associated with hyperthyroidism, without other psychiatric history, psychiatric symptoms usually resolve with treatment of the hyperthyroidism. Some patients without prior psychiatric history may need ongoing treatment of the psychiatric symptoms even after the reversal of hyperthyroidism.

Hypothyroidism
Causes
Primary Hypothyroidism
- T_4 dysfunction resulting in an elevated TSH level
- Hashimoto's thyroiditis (autoimmune disorder)
- Subacute thyroiditis
- Surgery for hyperthyroidism; irradiation or iodine-131 treatment
- Drugs (lithium, iodides, thionamides, amiodarone)
- Congenital abnormality
- Biochemical defects
- Iodide deficiency

   In underdeveloped countries, chronic lack of iodine in the diet is a major cause of hypothyroidism because the thyroid needs iodine to produce thyroid hormones. Due to the addition of iodine to table salt and the practice of using iodine-laced disinfectants on cows' udders, this cause of hypothyroidism has disappeared in the United States.

Secondary Hypothyroidism
Secondary hypothyroidism is usually due to complications of a primary pituitary disorder or to hypothalamic disease resulting in low TSH level.

Clinical Features
- Cold intolerance
- Weight gain
- Thin, dry hair
- Facial puffiness
- Constipation
- Menorrhagia
- Muscle cramps
- Slowed and decreased deep tendon reflexes

Psychiatric Manifestations
- Apathy
- Psychomotor retardation
- Depression
- Cognitive decline, especially poor memory
- Mania (rare)

   Acute and rapidly progressive hypothyroidism can lead to myxedema madness manifested by delirium and psychosis.

Treatment

Thyroid hormone (T_4) replacement usually reverses the medical and psychiatric symptoms. The cognitive deficits may persist due to the CNS effects produced by the changes in the central metabolic activity of thyroid hormones.

If psychiatric symptoms persist despite the T_4 replacement, then psychiatric medications for anxiety and depression would be indicated.

Parathyroid Disorders

Dysfunction of the parathyroid glands results in abnormalities in the regulation of electrolytes, especially calcium.

Hyperparathyroidism

Hyperparathyroidism usually occurs in the third to fifth decade of life and is more common in women than in men. It is associated with hypercalcemia. The causes of hypercalcemia include:

- Primary and tertiary hyperparathyroidism
- Sporadic
- Familial
- Malignancy
- Osteolytic changes
- Ectopic production of calcitriol (by lymphoma)
- Granulomatous disease
- Chronic renal failure with aplastic bone disease
- Acute renal failure
- Familial hypocalciuric hypercalcemia
- Lithium
- Vitamin D intoxication
- Increased calcium intake
- Pheochromocytoma
- Congenital lactase deficiency
- Hyperthyroidism
- Vitamin A intoxication
- Thiazides
- Milk-alkali syndrome
- Immobilization
- Theophylline

Psychiatric manifestations associated with hyperparathyroidism can precede other somatic manifestations of the illness and may include:

- Delirium
- Sudden cognitive decline
- Depression
- Anxiety
- Psychosis
- Apathy progressing to stupor and coma

Hypomagnesemia also occurs in association with hyperparathyroidism, usually after surgical removal of a parathyroid adenoma. Common presentation of patients with severe hypomagnesemia include:

- Visual hallucinations
- Paranoid delusions
- Psychosis and delirium

Hypoparathyroidism

Hypoparathyroidism is manifested by low serum levels of calcium (hypocalcemia) and magnesium. Causes of hypocalcemia are summarized in Box 4-1.

The most common psychiatric symptom in patients with hypoparathyroidism is delirium, but psychosis, depression, and anxiety are also seen.

Laboratory Studies

Because imbalances of calcium and magnesium can cause psychiatric symptoms, serum levels of both electrolytes must be ascertained for diagnostic evaluation of any psychiatric presentation. The presence of hypercalcemia requires further evaluation for other causes of hypercalcemia.

ED Management

The management of hyperparathyroidism is focused on the treatment of the hypercalcemia. Specifically, the goal of treatment is to reduce the calcium level to less than 11.5 mg/dL, which is the level at which most patients have resolution of hypercalcemia-induced symptoms. Surgical consultation is mandatory for patients with severe hypercalcemia caused by hyperparathyroidism.

Empirical calcium supplementation may be necessary if severe hypocalcemia is suspected, and if seizures, tetany, life-threatening hypotension, or cardiac arrhythmia are present. Endocrinology consultation may be required.

Box 4–1. Causes of Hypocalcemia

Decreased Entry of Calcium into the Circulation
Hypoparathyroidism (Absence of PTH Secretion)
Postoperative
Autoimmune (isolated or part of polyglandular autoimmune
syndrome)
Congenital (mutations of CaSR, PTH, and parathyroid aplasia)
Pseudohypoparathyroidism, types 1a and 1b, and type 2

Magnesium Depletion
Severe Hypermagnesemia
Deficiency of Vitamin D

Increased Loss of Calcium from the Circulation
Hyperphosphatemia
Renal failure
Rhabdomyolysis
Tumor lysis
Phosphate administration

Acute Pancreatitis
Hungry Bone Syndrome
Chelation
Citrate
EDTA
Lactate
Foscarnet

Widespread Osteoblastic Metastases
Prostate cancer
Breast cancer

Other Causes
Sepsis
Fluoride Administration
Surgery
Chemotherapy
Cisplatin
5-Fluorouracil
Leucovorin

CaSR, calcium-sensing receptor; EDTA, ethylenediaminetetraacetic acid;
PTH, parathyroid hormone.

Adrenal Disorders

Cushing's Syndrome

Cushing's syndrome is due to hypercortisolemia which can result from excessive ACTH secretion from the pituitary or other body organs, adrenocortical excess from the adrenal glands, or secondary to exogenous corticosteroid administration.

Causes

Excessive ACTH Secretion

Pituitary Adenomas. This form of the syndrome is called Cushing's disease and affects women five times more frequently than men. It is the cause of most cases of Cushing's syndrome. Pituitary adenomas are benign tumors of the pituitary gland that secrete increased amounts of ACTH. Most patients have a single adenoma.

Ectopic ACTH Syndrome. Some benign and malignant tumors that arise outside the pituitary can produce ACTH. This condition is known as ectopic ACTH syndrome. Lung tumors make up more than 50% of these cases. Men are affected three times more frequently than women. The most common forms of ACTH-producing tumors are oat cell (or small cell) lung cancer tumors, which account for about 25% of all lung cancer cases, and carcinoid tumors. Other less common types of tumors that can produce ACTH are thymomas, pancreatic islet cell tumors, and medullary carcinomas of the thyroid.

Adrenocortical Excess

Adrenal Tumors. Most of these cases involve noncancerous tumors of adrenal tissue. The average age of onset is about 40 years. Adrenocortical carcinomas, or adrenal cancers, are the least common cause of Cushing's syndrome. Cancer cells secrete excess levels of several adrenal cortical hormones, including cortisol and adrenal androgens. Adrenocortical carcinomas usually cause very high hormone levels and rapid development of symptoms.

Familial Cushing's Syndrome. Most cases of Cushing's syndrome are familial. Rarely, however, some individuals have Cushing's syndrome due to an inherited tendency to develop tumors of one or more endocrine glands. In primary pigmented micronodular adrenal disease, children or young adults develop small cortisol-producing tumors of the adrenal glands. In multiple endocrine neoplasia type I (MEN I), hormone-secreting tumors of the parathyroid glands, pancreas, and pituitary occur. Cushing's syndrome in men may be due to pituitary, ectopic, or adrenal tumors.

Exogenous Corticosteroids
⚠ Factitious, Iatrogenic, or Surreptitious Corticosteroid Administration

Clinical Features
Clinical signs include central obesity, hypertension, striae, easy bruising, buffalo hump, diabetes, and osteoporosis.

Psychiatric Manifestations
Cushing's syndrome is usually associated with moderate to severe depression in up to 50% of patients. Depressive symptoms sometimes are severe enough to precipitate suicide. Decreased concentration and memory deficits may also be present. Some patients present with psychotic symptoms.

Treatment
In patients with depression believed to be etiologically related to the hypercortisolemia of Cushing's syndrome, ED clinicians need to initiate antidepressant treatment while awaiting surgical or medical therapy for Cushing's syndrome. Psychiatric symptoms usually resolve when the cortisol excess is controlled.

Addison's Disease
Addison's disease occurs when the adrenal glands do not produce enough cortisol and, in some cases, aldosterone. Addison's disease is also called adrenal insufficiency and hypocortisolism.

Causes
Addison's disease may be due to a disorder of the adrenal glands themselves (primary adrenal insufficiency), or to inadequate secretion of ACTH by the pituitary gland (secondary adrenal insufficiency).

Primary Adrenal Insufficiency
Addison's disease due to primary adrenal insufficiency is an autoimmune disorder. Tuberculosis (TB) accounts for about 20% of cases of primary adrenal insufficiency. As the treatment for TB improved, however, the incidence of adrenal insufficiency due to TB of the adrenal glands also has decreased.

Less common causes of primary adrenal insufficiency are:
- Chronic infection, mainly fungal
- Cancer cells spreading from other parts of the body to the adrenal glands
- Amyloidosis
- Surgical removal of the adrenal glands

Secondary Adrenal Insufficiency

This form of adrenal insufficiency is much more common than primary adrenal insufficiency and can be traced to a lack of ACTH. It may occur when a person who has been receiving a glucocorticoid hormone such as prednisone for a long time abruptly stops or interrupts taking the medication.

Another cause of secondary adrenal insufficiency is the surgical removal of benign ACTH-producing tumors of the pituitary gland.

Less commonly, adrenal insufficiency occurs when the pituitary gland either decreases in size or stops producing ACTH. These events can result from:
- Tumors or infections of the area
- Loss of blood flow to the pituitary
- Radiation for the treatment of pituitary tumors
- Surgical removal of parts of the hypothalamus
- Surgical removal of the pituitary gland

Clinical Manifestations

The symptoms of Addison's disease usually begin gradually and may include:
- Chronic, worsening fatigue
- Muscle weakness
- Loss of appetite
- Weight loss
- Dark tanning of the skin
- Nausea, vomiting, and diarrhea (in about 50% of cases)

Due to the slow progression of symptoms in Addison's disease, clinical signs may be ignored until a stressful event such as another illness or an accident causes them to become worse. This is called an *addisonian crisis*, or *acute adrenal insufficiency*. In most cases, symptoms are severe enough that patients seek medical treatment before a crisis occurs. However, in about 25% of patients, symptoms are first noticed during an addisonian crisis.

Signs and symptoms of addisonian crisis include:

- Sudden penetrating pain in the lower back, abdomen, or legs
- Severe vomiting and diarrhea
- Dehydration
- Low blood pressure
- loss of consciousness

  Left untreated, an addisonian crisis can be fatal.

Psychiatric Manifestations

Psychiatric symptoms include irritability, apathy, fatigue, and depression. Psychosis and confusion also can develop.

Diagnosis

In its early stages, Addison's disease can be difficult to diagnose. A review of the patient's medical history based on the symptoms, especially the dark tanning of the skin, will lead the clinician to suspect Addison's disease. An ACTH stimulation test, corticotropin-releasing hormone (CRH) stimulation test, and radiographs of the adrenal and pituitary glands are helpful in the diagnosis.

Treatment

Steroid hormones replacement is the treatment of choice for this condition; thus ED clinicians need to monitor the possible psychiatric complications of steroid treatment, which include anxiety, depression, mania, and psychosis.

In patients suspected of having an addisonian crisis, injections of salt, fluids, and glucocorticoid hormones should be given immediately. Measurement of blood ACTH and cortisol during the crisis and before glucocorticoids are given is enough to make the diagnosis.

Pheochromocytoma

Pheochromocytoma is a rare catecholamine-secreting tumor outside the adrenal gland. The clinical manifestations of a pheochromocytoma result from excessive catecholamine secretion by the tumor. Catecholamines typically secreted, either intermittently or continuously, include norepinephrine, epinephrine, and rarely dopamine.

The subsequent stimulation of alpha-adrenergic receptors results in elevated blood pressure, increased cardiac contractility, glycogenolysis, gluconeogenesis, and intestinal relaxation. Stimulation of beta-adrenergic receptors results in an increase in heart rate and contractility.

Clinical Manifestations
- Hypertension (may be paroxysmal in 50% of cases)
- Postural hypotension,
- Tachyarrhythmias
- Cardiomyopathy
- Retinopathy
- Pulmonary edema
- Fever
- Pallor
- Tremor
- Neurofibromas or café au lait spots (patches of cutaneous pigmentation, which vary from 1 to 10 mm in size, can occur any place on the body, and vary from light to dark brown in color)
- Ileus
- Tremor
- Weakness
- Weight loss

Psychiatric Manifestations
- Anxiety
- Sense of doom
- Altered mental status and delirium—if hypertensive encephalopathy

Laboratory Features
- Hyperglycemia
- Hypercalcemia
- Erythrocytosis
- Increased urinary catecholamines and vanillylmandelic acid

General Medical Treatment
Surgical resection of the tumor is the treatment of choice and usually results in cure of the hypertension. Careful treatment with alpha- and beta-blockers is required preoperatively to control blood pressure and prevent intraoperative hypertensive crises.

ED Treatment
 Anxiety in its most severe form can be quite debilitating. ED clinicians should:
- Initiate involuntary hold when an acute anxious state becomes severe or poses a danger to the patient and/or others.

- Provide reassurance.
- Place patient in a calm quiet room where a formal evaluation can begin to identify the various manifestations of the anxiety.
- Use rhythmic breathing imagery techniques and hypnotic suggestion if appropriate.
- Begin treatment with a short course of fast-acting anxiolytics, preferably a benzodiazepine.

Treatment of chronic anxiety requires a comprehensive referral to psychotherapy, social intervention agencies, and a wider spectrum of pharmacological intervention, which may include benzodiazepines, buspirone, and antidepressants.

M—METABOLIC DISORDERS

Several metabolic disturbances may present with psychiatric symptoms; among these are:
- Fluid/electrolyte disorders
- Acid/base disorders
- Respiratory disorders of O_2/CO_2 exchange (e.g., hyperventilation syndrome, asthma, acute respiratory distress syndrome, dyspnea, COPD, hypoxia, sleep apnea/pickwickian syndrome)
- Hepatic encephalopathy
- Uremic encephalopathy
- Porphyria
- Wilson's disease (hepatolenticular degeneration)
- Lesch-Nyhan syndrome
- Homocystinuria
- Mucopolysaccharidoses
- Sphingolipidoses
- Glycolytic pathway disorders
- Amino acid transport disorders
- Phenylketonuria
- Urea cycle disorders
- Maple syrup urine disease
- Metachromatic leukodystrophy
- Glucose-6-phosphate dehydrogenase (G-6-PD) deficiency

The treatment of these metabolic conditions is beyond the scope of this chapter; however, a review of some ED evaluations and interventions are summarized in the next section.

Electrolyte Imbalance

Sodium Imbalance
Hyponatremia

Hyponatremia occurs in various conditions and can be divided into isotonic hyponatremia and hypotonic (hypo-osmolar) hyponatremia.

Causes of Isotonic Hyponatremia

The serum osmolality ranges between 280 and 295 mOsm/Kg. This condition is termed pseudohypernatremia. The main causes are hyperlipidemia and hyperproteinemia (as immunoglobulins in multiple myeloma). Lipids and proteins occupy a disproportionately large portion of plasma volume, but the serum osmolality and sodium concentration are normal.

Causes of Hypotonic (Hypo-osmolar) Hyponatremia

In such cases, the plasma osmolality is usually less then 280 mOsm/Kg. The differential diagnosis of hypo-osmolar hyponatremia is summarized in Table 4-7. One of the major causes is syndrome of inappropriate antidiuretic hormone (SIADH). The causes of SIADH are summarized in Table 4-8.

Clinical and Psychiatric Manifestations

ED clinicians need to consider hyponatremic disorders in patients experiencing acute mental status changes.

Classic symptoms of hyponatremia include nausea, anorexia, and muscle weakness.

As the serum sodium level continues to drop, patients may become:

- Irritable
- Depressed
- Intensely anxious
- Psychotic with delusions and hallucinations
- Confused

At this stage, without correction and treatment of hyponatremia, seizures, stupor, and coma ultimately ensue.

Treatment

Treatment consists of correcting the serum sodium level at a slow but adequate rate. Overly rapid correction of hyponatremia can lead to central pontine myelinolysis.

Table 4–7

Differential Diagnosis of Hypo-osmolar Hyponatremia

Volume State	Possible Causes
Hypovolemic	Renal loss through diuretic use, salt-wasting nephropathy
	Hypoaldosteronism
	GI loss through vomiting, diarrhea, and tube drainage
	Skin loss through sweating, burns, cystic fibrosis
	Peritonitis
Euvolemic	ADH excess through SIADH
	Use of thiazide diuretics or oral hypoglycemic agents
	Pain
	Postoperative state including transurethral prostatic resection syndrome
	Cortisol deficiency
	Hypothyroidism
	Decreased solute intake
	Psychiatric disorders in cases of psychogenic polydipsia
	Resetting of osmostat through pregnancy
Hypervolemic	Congestive heart failure
	Cirrhosis
	Nephrotic syndrome
	Acute and chronic renal failure

ADH, antidiuretic hormone; GI, gastrointestinal; SIADH, syndrome of inappropriate antidiuretic hormone.

Hypernatremia

Hypernatremia usually results from inadequate ingestion of water leading to dehydration particularly in the elderly population or from kidney dysfunctions.

Causes
- Water loss
- Insensible losses
- Increased sweating
- Fever
- Exposure to high temperatures

Table 4–8

Causes of SIADH

Cause	Specific Conditions
Pulmonary	Pneumonias, tuberculosis, pulmonary abscess, ventilators with positive pressure
CNS disorders	Trauma, infection (encephalitis, meningitis), thrombosis, abscesses, hemorrhage, hematoma
Malignancy	Bronchogenic (e.g., small cell lung carcinoma), pancreatic, urethral, prostatic, lymphoma, leukemia, thymoma, mesothelioma
Drugs leading to increased ADH production	Antidepressants (amitriptyline, clomipramine, desipramine, imipramine, MAO inhibitors, fluoxetine)
	Antineoplastics (cyclophosphamide, vincristine, vinblastine)
	Carbamazepine
	Clofibrate
	Antipsychotics (thiothixene, thioridazine, fluphenazine, haloperidol, trifluoperazine)
Drugs leading to potentiated ADH action	Carbamazepine
	Chlorpropamide
	Tolbutamide
	Cyclophosphamide
	NSAIDs
	Somatostatin and analogues
Postoperative hyponatremia	Severe postoperative hyponatremia can develop in 2 days or less after elective surgery in healthy patients who have received excessive postoperative hypotonic fluid in the setting of elevated ADH levels related to pain, surgery, or anesthesia

CNS, central nervous system; MAO, monoamine oxidase; NSAIDs, nonsteroidal anti-inflammatory drugs; SIADH, syndrome of inappropriate antidiuretic hormone.

- Respiratory infections
- Burns
- Renal losses
- Central diabetes insipidus
- Nephrogenic diabetes insipidus
- Osmotic diuresis (due to glucose, mannitol, urea)
- Hypothalamic disorders
- Hypodipsia
- Resetting of osmostat (primary aldosteronism)
- Sodium retention
- Administration of hypertonic NaCl or sodium bicarbonate
- Ingestion of sodium with no absolute change in total body salt or water
- Water loss into cells (seizures, severe exercise, rhabdomyolysis)

Treatment

As with hyponatremia, the rate of correction of hypernatremia is important. Overly rapid correction can lead to cerebral edema.

ED clinicians should always consider cerebral edema if the patient has worsened mental status when hypernatremia has been corrected.

Potassium Imbalance

Potassium imbalance can be due to hypokalemia or hyperkalemia.

Hypokalemia
Causes

Hypokalemia may be due to a total body deficit of potassium, which may occur chronically with the following conditions:
- Prolonged diuretic use
- Inadequate potassium intake
- Laxative use
- Diarrhea
- Hyperhidrosis
- Hypomagnesemia
  Acute causes include:
- Diabetic ketoacidosis
- Severe GI losses from vomiting and diarrhea
- Dialysis and diuretic therapy

Hypokalemia also may be due to excessive potassium shifts from the extracellular to the intracellular space, as seen with:

- Alkalosis
- Insulin use
- Catecholamine use
- Sympathomimetic use
- Hypothermia
  Other recognizable causes of hypokalemia include:
- Renal tubular disorders, such as Bartter and Gitelman syndromes
- Type I or classic distal tubular acidosis
- Periodic hypokalemic paralysis
- Hyperaldosteronism
- Cystic fibrosis with hyperaldosteronism from severe chloride and volume depletion
- Cushing's syndrome
- Exogenous steroid administration
- Acute myelogenous, monomyeloblastic, or lymphoblastic leukemia.
- Medication effects
  - Diuretics (most common cause)
  - Beta-adrenergic agonists
  - Steroids
  - Theophylline
  - Aminoglycosides
  - Verapamil (with overdose)
  - High-dose penicillin
  - Ampicillin
  - Carbenicillin
  - Drugs associated with magnesium depletion, such as aminoglycosides, amphotericin B, and cisplatin
- Renal losses
  - Renal tubular acidosis
  - Hyperaldosteronism
  - Magnesium depletion
  - Leukemia (mechanism uncertain)
- GI losses
  - Vomiting, nasogastric suctioning
  - Diarrhea
  - Enemas, laxative use
  - Ileal loop
- Transcellular shift
  - Insulin
  - Alkalosis
- Malnutrition or decreased dietary intake; parenteral nutrition

Clinical Manifestations

Hypokalemia can present with muscular weakness, cramping, tetany, paresthesias, and cardiac arrhythmias.

Psychiatric Manifestations

Psychiatric symptoms include apathy, weakness, and confusion.

Diagnosis

Useful laboratory studies include measurement of serum potassium, other electrolytes, blood urea nitrogen (BUN), creatinine, and, if indicated, arterial blood gases.

ED Treatment

Close monitoring is important. Treatment includes repletion of potassium and correction of any pH abnormalities.

Hyperkalemia

Causes

- Laboratory error
- Metabolic acidosis—shift of K^+ to extracellular space in exchange for H^+
- Acute and chronic renal failure—electrolyte shift as result of metabolic acidosis and because of a failure to excrete the K^+
- Disruption of excretory pathway—rupture of both ureters, urinary bladder, urethra
- Obstruction of excretory pathway—urolithiasis, neoplasia, foreign bodies

Clinical Manifestations

The main symptoms include weakness and paresthesias. Hyperkalemia rarely presents with psychiatric manifestations.

Hepatic Encephalopathy

 Hepatic encephalopathy is a complex neuropsychiatric syndrome that complicates advanced liver disease. In acute hepatic encephalopathy, fulminant hepatic failure is usually present.

Precipitants

Some patients with a history of hepatic encephalopathy may have normal mental status while under treatment. Others have chronic memory impairment in spite of medical management.

Both groups of patients are subject to episodes of worsened encephalopathy. Common precipitating factors are described here.

Renal Failure. Renal failure leads to decreased clearance of urea, ammonia, and other nitrogenous compounds.

GI Bleeding. The presence of blood in the upper GI tract results in increased ammonia and nitrogen absorption from the gut. Bleeding may predispose to kidney hypoperfusion and impaired renal function. Blood transfusions may result in mild hemolysis, with resulting elevated blood ammonia levels.

Infection. Infection may predispose to impaired renal function and to increased tissue catabolism, both of which increase blood ammonia levels.

Constipation. Constipation increases intestinal production and absorption of ammonia.

Medications. Drugs that act upon the CNS, such as opiates, benzodiazepines, antidepressants, and antipsychotic agents, may worsen hepatic encephalopathy.

Diuretic Therapy. Decreased serum potassium levels and alkalosis may facilitate the conversion of NH_4^+ to NH_3.

Dietary Protein Overload. This is an infrequent cause of hepatic encephalopathy.

Clinical Manifestations

Following is a list of the clinical manifestations and stages of hepatic encephalopathy.

- Stage I
  - Apathy
  - Restlessness
  - Impaired cognition
  - Impaired handwriting
  - Reversal of sleep rhythm
- Stage II
  - Lethargy
  - Drowsiness
  - Disorientation
  - Asterixis
  - Beginning of mood swings
  - Beginning of behavioral disinhibition
- Stage III
  - Arousable stupor
  - Hyperactive reflexes
  - Short episodes of psychiatric symptoms

- Stage IV
  - Coma (responsive only to pain)

Psychiatric Manifestations

In acute exacerbations, impairment of consciousness is prominent. Rapid changes in consciousness may be accompanied by hallucinations, mainly visual. Hypersomnia also occurs early in the course of the illness. Before the development of coma, patients can also experience abrupt mood swings and behavioral disinhibition. Patients also may experience short episodes of depression, hypomania, anxiety, and obsessive-compulsive symptoms. At this stage, patients usually have neurologic signs such as asterixis, myoclonus, constructional apraxia, and hyperreflexia.

The mental status changes associated with hepatic encephalopathy are believed to be related to inadequate hepatic removal of mostly nitrogenous compounds or other toxins formed in the GI tract. Inadequate removal of these toxins results from both impaired hepatocyte function and shunting of portal blood into the systemic circulation.

Treatment

Treatment consists of identification of precipitating factors, correcting underlying causes, dietary protein restrictions, and removal of ammonia from the bowel by the use of lactulose.

Uremic Encephalopathy

Uremia results from impairment in kidney functioning.
  Early symptoms include:
- Anorexia
- Nausea
- Restlessness
- Drowsiness
- Diminished ability to concentrate
- Slowed cognitive functions
  More severe symptoms include:
- Vomiting
- Emotional volatility
- Decreased cognitive function
- Disorientation
- Confusion
- Bizarre behavior

As uremic encephalopathy progresses, symptoms may include:
- Cranial nerve signs (nystagmus)
- Papilledema
- Hyperreflexia, clonus, asterixis
- Stupor
- Coma—occurs only if uremia remains untreated and progresses

Causes
The exact cause of uremic encephalopathy is unknown. It may occur in patients affected with acute or chronic renal failure of any etiology. Accumulation of metabolites and imbalance in excitatory and inhibitory neurotransmitters are possible etiologies. Parathyroid hormones and abnormal calcium control also have been identified as possible contributing factors.

Treatment
Adequate dialysis can reverse some of the psychiatric and mental abnormalities, but subtle deficits in mentation may remain.

Psychopharmacological treatment of uremic encephalopathy should target the individual symptoms, but with a lower starting dosage of medication and small, cautious dosage adjustments.

Acute Intermittent Porphyria

Porphyria is a disorder of heme biosynthesis that leads to buildup of excessive porphyrins. In the classic form, patients have a triad of symptoms, including colicky abdominal pain, motor polyneuropathy, and psychosis. Acute intermittent porphyria is an autosomal dominant disorder, and onset usually occurs in persons 20 to 50 years of age. Some studies have shown that 0.2% to 0.5% of psychiatric patients have undiagnosed porphyrias.

Treatment
ED clinicians should promptly refer patients with acute intermittent porphyria for hospitalization, because of the possibility of acute attacks. Close observation as well as medications for pain, nausea, and vomiting are generally required. A high intake of glucose or other carbohydrates can help suppress disease activity and can be given by IV or oral administration.

IV heme therapy with Panhematin is effective in suppressing disease activity. It can be started after a trial of glucose therapy.

However, the response to heme therapy is best if started early
in an attack. Therefore, delaying heme therapy until it has
been determined that glucose therapy has not been effective
may not be warranted unless an attack is mild. Barbiturates
precipitate attacks of acute porphyria and therefore are
absolutely contraindicated.

Wilson's Disease

Wilson's disease is a rare autosomal recessive disorder of
copper transport resulting in copper accumulation and toxicity
in the liver and brain. Liver disease is the most common symptom in children; neurologic disease is the most common in
young adults. Symptoms may include jaundice, abdominal
swelling, vomiting blood, and abdominal pain. Acute liver
failure or fulminant hepatitis may also occur.

The cornea of the eye can also be affected. The "Kayser-
Fleischer ring" is a deep copper-colored ring at the periphery
of the cornea and is thought to represent copper deposits.

Clinical Manifestations
Neurologic symptoms include:
- Tremors or shaking.
- Poor coordination.
- Difficulty with speech, eating, or walking.

Patients may resemble older persons with manifestations
of Parkinson's disease, with rather fixed and rigid postures
and little spontaneous movement.

Psychiatric Manifestations
These include personality changes, mood disturbances, depression, anxiety, phobias, or just poor memory.

Treatment
Following any needed emergency psychiatric treatment for
anxiety and mood disturbances, ED clinicians should refer
patients for special dietary consult and for special treatment of
Wilson's disease with any number of different medications, such
as zinc acetate, penicillamine, and trientine. Although the
specific treatment prescribed will vary from patient to patient,
Wilson's disease requires lifelong treatment. With an early
diagnosis and proper treatment, patients with Wilson's disease
can have a good prognostic outcome.

D—DEGENERATIVE/DEMYELINATING

Central and peripheral nervous system disorders that can present with psychiatric symptoms include:

- Alzheimer's disease
- Pick's disease
- Huntington's disease
- Parkinson's disease
- Friedreich's ataxia
- Amyotrophic lateral sclerosis (Lou Gehrig's disease)
- Multiple sclerosis
- Muscular and myotonic dystrophies
- Creutzfeldt-Jacob disease

Although description of all these conditions is beyond the scope of this chapter, ED interventions for some of these conditions are described here (see Chapter 17 for discussion of other conditions).

Parkinson's Disease

Parkinson's disease (PD) is a disorder characterized by movement abnormalities with the classic triad of the following motor signs:

1. Tremor—usually a resting tremor involving the hands, described as pill rolling
2. Rigidity
3. Bradykinesia/akinesia.

The classic motor signs may not be obvious early in the disease, and patients may initially present with only clinical signs of depression. Thus, PD may be misdiagnosed as a primary depressive illness, and concomitant depression may remain undiagnosed in the patient. Similarities in the symptoms common to major depression and PD include impaired memory/concentration, slowed psychomotor activity, restricted affect, and fatigue or decreased energy.

  Depression can precede development of motor symptoms, suggesting that the depression itself may be a neurologic sign of PD. In addition to mood disturbances, patients commonly present with symptoms of anxiety, including general anxiety disorder, social phobia, and panic disorder.

The anxiety syndromes of PD may develop before or after the onset of motor symptoms. Psychosis in the form of hallucinations and delusions can develop spontaneously or in association with mood disturbance but usually develops either late in the disease process when significant cognitive impairment is also evident or is due to the use of antiparkinsonian dopaminergically active medications.

Treatment

Most treatments are aimed at the patient's specific symptoms. PD must be considered in the differential diagnosis of an elderly person presenting with first-time depression/anxiety symptoms, especially when the patient appears depressed but denies experiencing a depressed mood. In addition, treatment of symptoms can be complicated in patients with PD because antiparkinsonian medications may exacerbate psychiatric symptoms, and vice versa.

ED clinicians may need to refer PD patients for neurologic consultation prior to the initiation of psychiatric treatments.

Multiple Sclerosis

Multiple sclerosis (MS) is a demyelinating disorder characterized by multiple episodes of physical and neuropsychiatric symptoms. MS is more frequent in colder and temperate climates than in tropical locales, which may suggest a viral etiology. MS is more common in women than in men and usually manifests in persons 20 to 40 years of age. This disorder is a highly variable illness, with differences among patients and changes in a single patient over time.

Cognitive and Psychiatric Symptoms

Symptoms can be categorized as cognitive and psychiatric. Of the cognitive deficits, memory loss is the most common. Abstract reasoning, planning, and organizational skills are impaired. Dementia also may develop.

Psychiatric symptoms in MS include personality changes and feelings of euphoria and/or depression. The euphoria differs from that of hypomania and is characterized by an unusually cheerful mood. MS patients have an increased risk of bipolar disorder. Major depression is also very common. Suicide attempts are common in patients with MS who are depressed. Personality changes and emotional dyscontrol can also occur. Patients sometimes laugh without cause or weep suddenly.

Such emotional lability can be disturbing for patients and their families and can make assessment of psychiatric symptoms more difficult.

Treatment

ED clinicians may initiate treatment for depression or bipolar disorder in patients presenting with these conditions even during times when there is partial remission of the neurologic symptoms of MS.

Creutzfeldt-Jakob Disease

Creutzfeldt-Jakob disease (CJD) is a rare disorder caused by a slow virus infection and mutation of the prion protein gene. It can occur sporadically as a result of exposure to contaminated products. Rarely, it can be genetically inherited. It usually first appears in midlife, beginning between ages 20 and 70, with average age at onset of symptoms when the patient is in the late 50s. Some cases have occurred in adolescents who have received growth hormone derived from the pituitary glands of cadavers. Other cases have occurred when patients were given corneal transplants from infected donors. More recently, a type of disease called new-variant Creutzfeldt-Jakob disease has emerged. It was first reported in the UK in people who had eaten meat from cows who were fed infected bone meal. This version of the disease, when found in cows, has come to be known as "mad cow disease," and new-variant CJD is sometimes called "the human form of mad cow disease"; it tends to affect younger people and has early psychiatric manifestations. No cases of human mad cow disease have been reported in the United States.

Clinical Manifestations

Clinical symptoms include muscle stiffness, nervousness, jumpy feelings, changes in gait, lack of coordination, stumbling, falls, speech impairment, and excessive sleepiness.

Psychiatric Manifestations

Psychiatric symptoms include personality changes, hallucinations, deterioration in all aspects of human function, profound confusion, and disorientation. Delirium or dementia may develop rapidly.

Diagnosis

Examination of visual fields shows areas of blindness. There is loss of coordination related to visual-spatial perception changes.

An electroencephalogram will show characteristic changes indicating CJD if the symptoms have been present for at least 3 months.

Although not diagnostic, presence of the 14-3-3 protein in the spinal fluid obtained by lumbar puncture is highly suggestive of CJD when this finding is accompanied by other characteristic symptoms.

Ultimately, the disease can only be confirmed by brain biopsy or by a postmortem examination showing the characteristic spongiform (sponge-like) changes in the brain.

Treatment

There is no known cure for CJD. Custodial care may be required early in the course of the disease. Medications such as sedatives and antipsychotics may be needed to control aggressive behavior.

The need to provide a safe environment, control aggressive or agitated behavior, and aid the patient in performing ADLs may require monitoring and assistance in the home or in an institutionalized setting. Family counseling may help in coping with the changes required for home care.

Visiting nurses and aides, volunteer services, homemakers, adult protection services, and other community resources may also be helpful in caring for these patients.

Behavior modification may be helpful, in some cases, for controlling unacceptable or dangerous behaviors. Reality orientation, with repeated reinforcement of environmental and other cues, may help reduce disorientation.

T—TRAUMA

The following traumatic events may present with psychiatric symptoms:

- Dementia pugilistica
- Postconcussion syndrome
- Brain contusion/hemorrhage
- Penetrating brain trauma
- Epidural hematomas
- Subdural hematoma

Psychiatric symptoms may include sleep disturbances, inattention, difficulty concentrating, impaired memory, poor judgment, depression, irritability, emotional outbursts, diminished libido, difficulty switching between two tasks, and slowed thinking. These symptoms need to be treated only if they interfere with the diagnostic evaluations of the trauma.

In general, these disorders require immediate medical and surgical interventions before any ED psychiatric treatment.

E—EPILEPSY/SEIZURES

The following seizure disorders may be associated with psychiatric symptoms:
- Generalized (grand mal) seizures
- Absence (petit mal) seizure
- Myoclonus
- Simple partial seizures (motor, sensory, affective)
- Complex partial seizures
- Episodic dyscontrol
- Kindling phenomena
- Narcolepsy/cataplexy
- Postelectroconvulsive therapy delirium or confusion

Epilepsy is one of the most common chronic neurologic diseases, affecting approximately 1% of the U.S. population. Approximately 30% to 50% of patients with a seizure disorder have psychiatric symptoms at some time during the course of their illness. Psychiatric symptoms of seizures can be viewed in the context of their time relationship as being preictal, ictal, postictal, or interictal, with each phase presenting with different psychiatric symptoms. The two major categories of seizures are partial and generalized.

Generalized seizures simultaneously involve both cerebral hemispheres, with classic symptoms of loss of consciousness, tonic-clonic movements or limbs, tongue biting, and incontinence. Although the diagnosis is relatively straightforward, the postictal state is characterized by a gradual clearing of delirium lasting a few minutes to many hours.

Partial seizures have focal signs and symptoms resulting from electrical discharge in a limited site in one brain hemisphere.

Simple partial seizures occur without any impairment of consciousness and usually stem from primary motor, sensory, or visual cortical regions.

Complex partial seizures (temporal lobe epilepsy) are associated with impairment of consciousness and usually originate from a focus in the temporal lobe. In such seizures, psychiatric signs abound, including memory dysfunction, affective auras, perceptual changes (e.g., hallucinations), and depersonalization.

 In *temporal lobe epilepsy,* the most common psychiatric abnormality is personality change. Hyperreligiosity, hypergraphia, and hyposexuality are reportedly more commonly associated with temporal lobe epilepsy. Development of psychosis has also been reported.

For details related to the psychiatric aspects of seizures and a review of their treatment, see Chapter 16.

S—STRUCTURAL DISORDERS

The following structural abnormalities may be associated with psychiatric symptoms:
- Brain tumor
- Infection
- Infarction
- Hematoma
- Normal pressure hydrocephalus
- Rachischisis (e.g., Arnold-Chiari malformation, basilar impression, microcephaly)
- Paget's disease
- Spinal cord/vertebral disorders (e.g., radiculopathy)
- Tuberous sclerosis
- Aneurysm
- Arteriovenous malformation
- Developmental disorders or delays (e.g., cerebral palsy, dyslexia, stuttering, chromosomal abnormalities)

Discussion of the psychiatric and neurologic manifestations of all these structural disturbances is beyond the scope of this chapter. Brain tumors and normal pressure hydrocephalus are described here.

Brain Tumors

Brain tumors are important causes of psychiatric symptoms, and patients with these diseases can present with virtually any symptom.

Psychiatric Manifestations

In general, meningiomas are likely to cause focal symptoms because they compress a limited region in the cortex, whereas gliomas can cause more diffuse symptoms. Delirium is most often secondary to a large, fast-growing, or metastatic tumor. Specific psychiatric symptoms largely depend on the location of the tumor within the brain and the structures affected by direct invasion or pressure.

Approximately 88% of patients with brain tumors and psychiatric symptoms have frontal lobe tumors. These tumors elicit presenting signs such as cognitive impairment, personality change, and motor and language dysfunction. Patients frequently also have bowel or bladder incontinence.

Patients with dominant temporal lesions may present with memory and speech abnormalities. Nondominant tumors can cause auditory agnosia. Bilateral lesions can lead to global amnesia. Occipital lesions can cause visual hallucinations, agnosia, and Anton's syndrome (denial of blindness). Visual hallucinations can occur with lesions in the temporal, parietal, and occipital lobes. Auditory hallucinations can also occur with temporal lobe lesions but are apparently less common.

Limbic and hypothalamic tumors can cause symptoms of rage, mania, emotional lability, and altered sexual behavior. They may also produce delusions related to complicated plots.

Hallucinations, which are often considered the hallmarks of psychiatric illness, can be caused by focal neurologic pathology.

Diagnosis

The diagnostic procedure of choice is brain imaging with contrast computed tomography (CT) or MRI. In many cases when a CNS tumor is considered likely, the initial CT scan may be normal, and MRI may be required to confirm the diagnosis.

ED Treatment

 ED interventions are only initiated if the psychiatric manifestations of brain tumors interfere with the diagnostic procedures that are deemed necessary in an emergency situation.

Normal Pressure Hydrocephalus

Idiopathic normal pressure hydrocephalus (NPH) is a potentially reversible dementia, most commonly affecting patients in their

60s or 70s. Patients with a known cause of hydrocephalus (e.g. intracranial hemorrhage, meningitis, traumatic brain injury, brain tumor, previous intracranial surgery) do not meet the criteria for idiopathic NPH, and their management differs according to their primary disease. The clinical deterioration in NPH is probably due to slow, progressive impairment of the periventricular blood.

Clinical Manifestations

 Clinical signs include gait disturbance, cognitive impairment, and urinary incontinence.

Psychiatric Manifestations

In addition to the cognitive impairment that includes slowing of mental processing, there is difficulty in planning and mental shifting and impaired memory; an under-recognized symptom common in the setting of NPH is the high rate of depression in this population.

Diagnosis

Head CT shows a moderate to severe ventricular enlargement out of proportion to cerebral atrophy and includes ballooned frontal horns and enlarged temporal horns without evidence of hippocampal atrophy.

Neuropsychological testing can determine the degree of cognitive decline, and formal screening for depression should be performed.

General Medical Treatment

NPH is commonly treated with implantation of a shunt to divert excess CSF from the ventricles into another body cavity such as the abdomen. However, the procedure historically has the potential for seizures, infections, and other complications from multiple shunt revisions.

Given the burden of dementia on patients, families, and society, it is extremely important that patients with a reversible dementia such as NPH are effectively treated. At the same time, it is important to avoid neurosurgical procedures on patients for whom the risks outweigh the benefits.

The recent development of a programmable valve for use in a CSF shunt has greatly increased neurosurgical flexibility of management of NPH and decreased the incidence of shunt-related adverse effects.

ED Treatment

The ED treatment of patients with NPH may require neurologic and surgical consultation.

Although antidepressant medications have not been extensively studied for the treatment of NPH-associated depression, it can be used in certain patients in whom the depression has caused worsening of cognition and performance ADLs.

T—TOXINS/HEAVY METALS

Toxins include medications, drugs of abuse, solvents, pesticides, and heavy metals. Some toxins associated with psychiatric symptoms include:

- Heavy metals such as mercury, manganese, lead, bismuth, arsenic, thallium, lead, carbon disulfide, methyl bromide, bromides, and organic mercury compounds
- Industrial chemicals such as organophosphates and dioxin

Heavy metals exposure is usually industrial or environmental and should be considered in the appropriate settings. The role of exogenous toxins in inducing various medical and neuropsychiatric conditions is a very broad subject and is beyond the scope of this chapter.

ED clinicians need to know that separating causal factors is arduous and not always evident. A high index of clinical awareness is helpful in considering underlying causes of conditions that can appear as primary idiopathic psychiatric illness. Knowledge of the time course can also be helpful in comparing the onset of symptoms with the initiation of or change in dosage of the putative offending agent.

The psychiatric manifestations of toxins are usually reversible if these toxins are properly identified and removed. In certain cases the psychiatric symptoms may persist, requiring appropriate ongoing psychiatric treatment.

Treatment Follow-up

Interventions for patients with psychiatric manifestation of medical conditions should be accompanied by careful follow-up. The response to the psychiatric ED treatment plan should receive careful scrutiny. Patients discharged from the ED with psychiatric medication may require periodic screening for drug levels, side effects, and behavioral changes depending upon the medication used. In addition, the diagnosis may need to be reconsidered in light of the response to implemented ED treatment.

Further Reading

American College of Emergency Physicians: Clinical policy for the initial approach to patients presenting with altered mental status. Ann Emerg Med 1999;33:251-280.

American Psychiatric Association: Diagnostic and Statistical Manual of Mental Disorders, 4th ed. Text Revision. Washington, DC, American Psychiatric Association; 2000, pp 135-296.

Barr WG, Merchut MP: Systemic lupus erythematosus with central nervous system involvement. Psychiatr Clin North Am 1992;15:439-454.

Benseler SM, Silverman ED: Systemic lupus erythematosus. Pediatr Clin North Am 2005;52:443-467.

Brewerton TD: The DIVINE MD TEST. Resident and Staff Physician 1985;31:146-148.

Casey DE: Metabolic issues and cardiovascular disease in patients with psychiatric disorders. Am J Med 2005;118 (Suppl 2):S15-S22.

Citrome L, Blonde L, Damatarca C: Metabolic issues in patients with severe mental illness. South Med J 2005; 98:714-720.

Cryer P, Slone R, Whyte M: Depression and hypercalcemia. Clinicopathologic Conference. Am J Med 1996;101: 111-117.

Dieperink E, Ho SB, Thuras P, Willenbring ML: A prospective study of neuropsychiatric symptoms associated with interferon-alpha-2b and ribavirin therapy for patients with chronic hepatitis C. Psychosomatics 2003;44:104-112.

Drooker MA, Byck R: Physical disorders presenting as psychiatric illness: A new view. The Psychiatric Times. Medicine & Behavior 1992;9:19-24.

Estrada AL: Epidemiology of HIV/AIDS, hepatitis B, hepatitis C, and tuberculosis among minority injection drug users. Public Health Rep 2002;117(Suppl 1):S126-S134.

Fennell EB, Smith MC: Neuropsychological assessment. In Rao SM (ed): Neurobehavioral Aspects of Multiple Sclerosis. New York, Oxford University Press, 1990, pp 63-81.

Folstein MF, Folstein SE, McHugh PR: "Mini-mental state."
A practical method for grading the cognitive state of
patients for the clinician. J Psychiatr Res 1975;12:189-198.

Fukunishi I, Hosokawa K, Ozaki S: Depression antedating
the onset of Parkinson's disease. Jpn J Psychiatry Neurol
1991;45:7-11.

Glassman AH, Shapiro PA: Depression and the course of
coronary artery disease. Am J Psychiatry 1998;155:4-11.

Gonera EG, van't Hof M, Berger HJ, et al: Symptoms and
duration of the prodromal phase in Parkinson's disease.
Mov Disord 1997;12:871-876.

Grafman J, Rao SM, Litvan I: Disorders of memory. In Rao
SM (ed): Neurobehavioral Aspects of Multiple Sclerosis.
New York, Oxford University Press, 1990, pp 102-117.

Grossman J: Disulfiram—one tool of recovery. Psychiatric
Times 2001;18:1, 6-12.

Guido ME, Brady W, DeBehnke D: Reversible neurological
deficits in a chronic alcohol abuser: A case report of
Wernicke's encephalopathy. Am J Emerg Med
1994;12:238-240.

Huff JS: Altered mental status and coma. In Tintinalli JE,
Kelen GD, Stapczynski JS (eds): Emergency Medicine: A
Comprehensive Study Guide, 5th ed. New York, McGraw-
Hill, 2000, pp 1440-1449.

Hutto B: Subtle psychiatric presentations of endocrine
diseases. Psychiatr Clin North Am 1998;21:905-916.

Hutto BR: Folate and cobalamin in psychiatric illness.
Compr Psychiatry 1997;38:305-314.

Irani DN: The classic and variant forms of Creutzfeldt-Jakob
disease. Semin Clin Neuropsychiatry 2003;8:71-79:

Khouzam HR, Donnelly NJ, Ibrahim NF: Psychiatric
morbidity in HIV patients. Can J Psychiatry
1998;43:51-56.

Khouzam HR, Emery PE, Reaves B: Secondary mania in
late life. J Am Geriatr Soc 1994;42:85-87.

Khouzam HR, Weiser PM, Emes R, Gill T: Thyroid
hormones therapy: A review of their effects in the
treatment of psychiatric and medical conditions. Compr
Ther 2004;30:148-154.

Marsh L: Neuropsychiatric aspects of Parkinson's disease.
Psychosomatics 2000;41:15-23.

Miller NS, Gold MS: A neurochemical basis for alcohol and other addictions. J Psychoactive Drugs 1993;25:121-128.

Modai I, Rabinowitz J: Why and how to establish a computerized system for psychiatric case records. Hosp Community Psychiatry 1993;44:1091-1095.

Morgan MJ: Ecstasy (MDMA): A review of its possible persistent psychological effects. Psychopharmacology (Berl) 2000;152:230-248.

Musselman DL, Evans DL, Nemeroff CB: The relationship of depression to cardiovascular disease: Epidemiology, biology, and treatment. Arch Gen Psychiatry 1998;55:580-592.

National Institute on Alcoholism Abuse and Alcoholism: 6000 Executive Boulevard, Willco Building, Bethesda, MD 20892-7003. http://www.niaaa.nih.gov

Olanow CW, Koller WC: An algorithm (decision tree) for the management of Parkinson's disease: Treatment guidelines. American Academy of Neurology. Neurology 1998;50(Suppl 3):S1-S57.

Pajeau AK, Roman GC: HIV encephalopathy and dementia. Psychiatr Clin North Am 1992;15:455-466.

Reeves RR, Robbins RA, Carter OS: Psychiatric presentations of medical problems. Fed Pract 1998;15:38-50.

Reeves RR, Pendarvis EJ, Kimble R: Unrecognized medical emergencies admitted to psychiatric units. Am J Emerg Med 2000;18:390-393.

Rummans TA, Evans JM, Krahn LE, Fleming KC: Delirium in elderly patients: Evaluation and management. Mayo Clin Proc 1995;70:989-998.

Sadock BJ, Sadock VA (eds): Kaplan & Sadock's Synopsis of Psychiatry, 9th ed. Philadelphia, Lippincott Williams & Wilkins, 2003, pp 250-370.

Schmidt T: An overview of psychiatric emergencies. In: Rosen P, Barkin RM, Braen CR, et al (eds): Emergency Medicine: Concepts and Clinical Practice. St Louis, Mosby–Year Book, 1992, pp 2014-2020.

Skuster DZ, Digre KB, Corbett JJ: Neurologic conditions presenting as psychiatric disorders. Psychiatr Clin North Am 1992;15:311-333.

Stein MB, Heuser IJ, Juncos JL, Uhde TW: Anxiety disorders in patients with Parkinson's disease. Am J Psychiatry 1990;147:217-220.

Talbot-Stern JK, Green T, Royle TJ: Psychiatric
   manifestations of systemic illness. Emerg Med Clin North
   Am 2000;18:199-209.

Trenton AJ, Currier GW: Behavioural manifestations of
   anabolic steroid use. CNS Drugs 2005;19:571-595.

Whittier WL, Rutecki GW: Primer on clinical acid-base
   problem solving. Dis Mon 2004;50:122-162.

Williams ER, Shepherd SM: Medical clearance of
   psychiatric patients. Emerg Med Clin North Am
   2000;18:185-198.

POSTSCRIPT

*If patients do not respond to the suggested treatment,
we have either made a wrong diagnosis, or the patients
have a wrong illness. Since it is not possible to have a
wrong illness, most probably we made the wrong
diagnosis.*

Anonymous, Egyptian papyrus—800 BC

CHAPTER 5

The Delirious Patient

Tirath S. Gill, MD

KEY POINTS

- Delirium is a frequent complication in residents of nursing homes and hospitals.
- It is under-recognized and undertreated, leading to increased health care costs, longer hospital stays, and increased human suffering.
- Preventive measures to assess adequate hydration and nutrition, review of medications, and adequate rest can almost halve the incidence of postoperative delirium.
- To be most effective, treatment should be cause-specific. Inadequate treatment of the underlying causes of delirium can result in a significant increase in 1-year mortality.

Overview (Fig. 5-1)

Delirium is a psychiatric and medical emergency. It is one of the most common problems resulting in agitation in patients over age 65. The frequency of delirium is noted to be quite high among hospitalized patients. The presence of delirium often indicates an underlying metabolic disturbance affecting functioning of the brain. Many factors, alone or in combination, can lead to delirium.

The emergency department (ED) clinician assessing a patient suspected to be in delirium should always aspire to identify the underlying medical causes and focus on treatment directed toward the resolution of these causes. The immediate agitation may require control with medications and sometimes restraints in order to avoid injury during this period of impaired cognition and judgment.

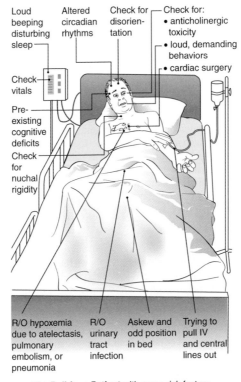

Loud beeping disturbing sleep

Check vitals

Pre-existing cognitive deficits

Check for nuchal rigidity

Altered circadian rhythms

Check for disorientation

Check for:
- anticholinergic toxicity
- loud, demanding behaviors
- cardiac surgery

R/O hypoxemia due to atelectasis, pulmonary embolism, or pneumonia

R/O urinary tract infection

Askew and odd position in bed

Trying to pull IV and central lines out

The Delirious Patient with some risk factors

Postoperative recovery room
Fluid shifts
Arrhythmias
Dehydration
Infection
Prolonged anesthesia
Unrecognized alcohol/sedative withdrawal
Fat embolism from severe trauma
Toxins, drugs, heavy metals

FIGURE 5–1

The delirious patient.

Definition

Delirium is defined in the American Psychiatric Association's *Diagnostic and Statistical Manual of Mental Disorders, 4th edition, Text Revision* (DSM-IV-TR) as a clinically significant deficit in cognition or memory that represents a significant change from a previous level of functioning. Other features of delirium include impaired or altered perceptions, illusions, and disturbances of circadian rhythms. Thus the patient may often be up and agitated during the night and somnolent during the day. There is also a reduced ability to focus and sustain attention. The clinical picture may vary, as patients can have lucid intervals, and the intensity of the delirium can fluctuate during the day. Such worsening may be related to personnel shift change or may occur at dawn and dusk when different stimuli overwhelm the impaired brain.

Epidemiology

Several epidemiologic studies have shown that delirium is quite common among hospitalized patients. The elderly and patients undergoing operative procedures appear to be particularly at risk; 15% to 18% of patients on medical and surgical wards have delirium, 30% or more of cardiac surgery patients have delirium, and 50% of patients undergoing hip repair are delirious at some point in the course of their hospitalization.

Importance of Recognizing Delirium

 Delirium generally carries a grave prognosis for the patient. It is reported that 25% to 70% of the elderly who develop delirium in the hospital die during that hospitalization; 25% to 33% or more are likely to die within 6 months to a year following discharge from the hospital.

A good way to grasp the gravity of the situation is to compare delirium, as brain failure, with heart failure. The state of delirium indicates a physiologic disturbance that has been precipitated by disturbance in the body's ability to maintain a milieu of interior or internal homeostasis. It is often an indicator of serious illness and systemic disease. For the best possible outcome for these patients, such illnesses should be identified and treated. Risk factors for developing delirium are listed in Box 5-1.

Box 5–1. Risk Factors for Developing Delirium

Orthopedic surgery
Cardiac surgery
Cognitive deficits related to any disorder
Impaired vision
Impaired hearing
Dehydration
Malnutrition
Metastatic lesions to the brain
Metastatic lesions to the liver
Duration of anesthesia and surgery
Exposure to benzodiazepines, opioids, or corticosteroids
Presence of Foley catheter

Initial ED Clinical Assessment

The patient in delirium should have a thorough history and physical examination, including basic laboratory studies. Sometimes the patient is not able to provide an adequate history, and in such cases prior records and information from collateral sources may be very helpful.

Basic Laboratory Studies

The following laboratory studies are indicated to rule out medical causes of delirium (Box 5-2).

A basic metabolic panel includes electrolytes, blood urea nitrogen (BUN), creatinine, blood glucose, urinalysis, urine toxicology screen, and a complete blood count (CBC). If pneumonia is suspected, a chest x-ray should be obtained. Computed tomography (CT) or magnetic resonance imaging (MRI) may be considered for ruling out intracranial pathology such as bleeding and strokes. Laboratory tests for drug levels, blood gases, ammonia levels, and other tests specific to a medical illness may be revelatory if the cause is not immediately clear.

Electroencephalography (EEG) may be useful. The usual pattern in delirium is a diffuse, slow wave pattern, except in delirium tremens (DT), in which the wave pattern is one of fast amplitude. EEG is a relatively inexpensive and simple procedure and can yield useful information to confirm the diagnosis if there is some clinical doubt. At times EEG findings can

---

Box 5–2. Laboratory Studies Indicated for Assessment of Delirium

CBC
Urinalysis with culture and sensitivity if indicated
Basic and, if indicated, comprehensive metabolic panel
Specific studies as indicated, such as:
- Ammonia level
- Chest radiograph
- CT scan or MRI if indicated by neurologic or atypical psychiatric findings
EEG if indicated

CBC, complete blood count; CT, computed tomography;
EEG, electroencephalogram; MRI, magnetic resonance imaging.

---

indicate a specific disease such as Creutzfeldt-Jakob disease, narcolepsy, a focal intracranial pathology, or an unrecognized epileptic disorder.

Some Medical Conditions That May Cause Delirium

Many medical conditions can cause delirium (Box 5-3). Those most commonly seen are discussed here.

Urinary Tract Infection

Urinary tract infection is a common cause of altered mental status and delirium among elderly residents in nursing homes and patients in hospitals. The infection often may be silent, without the usual symptoms of burning and tenderness during voiding. The development of incontinence in a person who was previously continent may be a clue that a urinary tract infection is causing the altered mental status.

Alcohol Withdrawal

Alcohol withdrawal and delirium can occur on the medical or surgical ward when the patient is admitted for an emergent illness; the history of alcohol use may not have been explored

Box 5–3. Medical Conditions Associated with Delirium

Urinary tract infection
Dehydration
Constipation
Unidentified source of pain
Acute intermittent porphyria
Aspiration pneumonia
Sepsis
Alcohol withdrawal
Sedative hypnotic withdrawal
Alcohol intoxication
Electrolyte imbalance
Uremia
Hepatic failure
Hyperammonemia
Hypoxemia
Congestive heart failure
Acute exacerbation of COPD
Cardiac arrhythmias
Intracranial bleeding
Intracranial mass with increased intracranial pressure
CNS infections

CNS, central nervous system;
COPD, chronic obstructive pulmonary disease.

by the clinician and may have been minimized by the patient. An alert clinician may notice an unexplained tachycardia and tremulousness and detect the withdrawal phenomenon in the early phase before delirium ensues. There may be other tell-tale signs such as ruddy complexion of the cheeks and dilated capillaries over a red nose (rhinophyma). Seborrhea, palmar erythema, and various scrapes and bruises from prior falls related to intoxication may be other clues. More obvious signs such as ascites and jaundice are usually evident in the physical examination at the time of admission.

When withdrawal in this setting is noted, it is imperative that the patient receives thiamine, 100 mg parenterally, either by the intramuscular (IM) or intravenous (IV) route, to prevent the Wernicke-Korsakoff syndrome. Prudence dictates the use of benzodiazepines to manage the dependence related to alcohol and to initially produce a mild sedation. It is better to treat the withdrawal assertively than to try to manage the DT, which can be a risk in these patients. Underlying malnutrition and medical causes and head injuries related to falls should be investigated and treated as indicated.

Drug-Related Intoxication

Drug-related intoxication may cause delirium. This is well evidenced by acute intoxication from amphetamines, cocaine, PCP (phencyclidine), LSD (lysergic acid diethylamide), and other psychedelics. The patient may manifest symptoms of panic and fear or extreme agitation and may respond to verbal reassurance and use of low-dose benzodiazepines.

Other Disorders

Pneumonia in the elderly in the context of a compromised respiratory system or a failing heart can easily lead to hypoxemia and delirium. Heart failure exacerbation due to any cause may lead to delirium. Acute electrolyte disturbances caused by diarrhea or vomiting or other causes may also induce this state of delirium.

Hypothyroidism and hyperthyroidism can induce states of delirium when these are extreme. Hyperglycemia and hypoglycemia can alter brain functioning and induce delirium.

Opioid overdose can induce respiratory depression and subsequent hypoxemia and delirium. This can be easily reversed with naloxone. Repeat doses may be needed due to the short-acting nature of the opiate antagonist.

An overdose of benzodiazepines in their potent short-acting form, such as alprazolam (Xanax) and triazolam (Halcion), can induce a state of delirium. If the patient does not regularly use benzodiazepines, this delirium may be treated by the use of flumazenil (Romazicon), 0.2 mg given over 15 seconds and repeated every minute to the maximum dose of 1 to 2 mg. Adequate precautions should be taken to avoid the emergence of seizures due to unstated problems of dependence on sedative hypnotics.

Epilepsy (postictal state) can induce delirium. A history of epilepsy is usually present, and there may be signs of injury related to the fall and accompanying features such as incontinence. When the patient is in the postictal state the airway should be protected and precautions should be taken against aspiration of gastric contents.

Concussion can sometimes cause a short-lived delirium. Infections of the central nervous system (CNS) may cause an altered mental status or delirium. Short-acting episodes of ischemia known as transient ischemic attacks (TIAs) may induce a confusional state akin to delirium as well. Intracranial masses can increase intracranial pressure and also lead to delirium and mood changes.

Heavy metal and carbon monoxide poisoning can induce delirium by interfering with oxygenation and cerebral metabolism. Lithium in toxic doses can induce a delirium that can last for several days to a week even after lithium levels have returned to normal.

Endocrine dysfunction of the pituitary, pancreas, adrenal, parathyroid, and thyroid glands can induce delirium by altering the metabolic milieu of the body. Liver disease in the context of constipation, a high-protein diet, and certain medications such as valproic acid and topiramate given independently or in combination can cause hyperammonemia and related hepatic encephalopathy and delirium. Kidney failure and compromised renal function can result in uremia and secondary delirium in many patients. The elderly patient with decreased sensation of thirst and poor liquid intake may be particularly at risk.

Respiratory failure and cardiac failure are other causes of an *altered mental status* (a common rubric for delirium). Arrhythmias such as atrial fibrillation may induce delirium; it may be episodic, as the nature of the arrhythmia varies.

Deficiencies of vitamin B_{12}, folic acid, thiamine, and nicotinic acid can include delirium as part of the deficiency syndrome.

High fever and sepsis in postoperative states are susceptible conditions for the emergence of delirium. The common postoperative delirium may be related to shifts of fluid and electrolytes, loss of blood, and effects of general anesthesia.

Medications Associated with Delirium

Many medications have the potential to cause delirium (Box 5-4). Any medication that causes anticholinergic side effects such as dry mouth, blurred vision, and constipation may induce delirium if given in high doses or if inadvertently combined with other anticholinergic agents. Medications with anticholinergic effects include anti-parkinsonian agents, such

---

Box 5–4. Medications Associated with Delirium

Anticholinergics
Antihistamines in high doses
Stimulants in high doses
Short-acting sedative hypnotics in high doses
OTC sleep agents containing scopolamine
Some antiarrhythmics
Digoxin
Diuretics
Tricyclic agents at high doses
Lithium at high doses
SSRIs at high doses
Low-potency antipsychotic agents at high doses
Corticosteroids at high doses
Anti-infective agents and antiviral agents

OTC, over-the-counter; SSRIs, selective serotonin reuptake inhibitors.

---

as benztropine (Cogentin), and low-potency antipsychotic drugs, such as chlorpromazine (Thorazine).

Insulin can cause delirium. Antihypertensive agents may cause delirium by inducing an electrolyte imbalance or hypotension. Cardiac glycosides such as digoxin can induce delirium even at normal levels in the elderly. Psychedelics such as PCP are well-known causes of agitated delirium and psychosis.

Other agents that have on rare occasions been implicated in causing delirium include disulfiram and H_2 blockers such as famotidine, ranitidine, and cimetidine. Nonsteroidal agents such as diclofenac and indomethacin have also on occasion been implicated.

Differential Diagnoses

The presence of delirium requires a thorough workup for any treatable medical cause.

Differentiation from Dementia

See Table 5-1.

Differentiation from Schizophrenia

This differentiation usually is not difficult because schizophrenia is a lifelong illness that begins in early adulthood, whereas delirium often occurs the first time in the setting of an acute hospitalization due to severe medical illness. In addition, delusions, if present in delirium, are often transient and nonbizarre compared with those of schizophrenia, in which they are entrenched and long-term in nature.

Differentiation from Mania

Differentiation from mania is possible by focusing on the mood of the patient. Although attention problems may exist in both conditions, the mood state in delirium is clearly dysphoric and not grandiose, as is often noted in states of mania. Extreme states of mania may at times present with coexisting delirium due to metabolic exhaustion if the mania is left untreated. Unlike patients in delirium, a colorful history of spending sprees, sexual indiscretions, grandiosity, impulsivity, is often a part of the life story of patients with mania.

Differentiation from Depression

An apathetic delirium may look like depression, but there are certain distinguishing features. The clinically depressed person may show disinterest or apathy but retains the ability to sustain attention and does not exhibit the wandering state of attention and alertness that is noted in delirium. The delirious patient does not have the hallmark features of clinical depression such as feelings of hopelessness, worthlessness, and thoughts of suicide. This is not to imply that the delirious individuals are not a potential danger to themselves; they may be frightened and prone to accidents or misjudgments because of their fright—for example, jumping out of a window while trying to escape from caregivers. Concentration is much more severely impaired in the delirious patient compared with depressed persons, and circadian rhythm disturbance with reversal of the sleep cycle may be noted. Such disturbances in circadian rhythm are less likely in mood disorders such as depression. A prior history of depression may be present in a person who is apathetic due to depression, as opposed to a patient in delirium. There are rare

Table 5–1

Comparison of the Characteristics of Delirium and Dementia

Delirium	Dementia
Onset of cognitive dysfunction is more acute, with changes in altered mental functioning occurring over hours and days	Onset of dysfunction is more gradual, occurring over months to years; strokes however, may cause sudden changes in stepwise patterns
Usually related to reversible causes	Usually a progressive illness with gradual worsening and decline; exceptions are dementias related to hypothyroidism, vitamin B_{12} deficiency, normal pressure hydrocephalus, neurosyphilis, and to some extent dementia related to alcoholism; complete recovery may not occur
Illusions and hallucinations common	Hallucinations uncommon except for Lewy body dementia
Vital signs usually abnormal	Vital signs tend to remain stable
Circadian cycle disturbed, with alteration of sleep cycle	Disturbance of circadian rhythm is unusual
Patient may exhibit significant anxiety, fear, and dysphoria	Patient may be unaware of deficits and may present a placid and calm appearance
Increased morbidity and mortality at 1-year follow-up	Dementias follow a progressive course over a number of years particular to the specific nature of the disorder
Short-term use of antipsychotics may be useful	Long-term use of antipsychotics in demented patients may be associated with increased risk of mortality and morbidity
May occur at any age	Onset usually late in life

occasions when a depressed patient may also have delirium due to medical causes.

Management

Management has several different components, including identification and treatment of the underlying medical cause and reassurance of the family and the patient, who are often quite distressed by the sudden change in the patient's behaviors. Measures for management of the patient with delirium in the emergency department are listed in Box 5-5.

All nonessential medications should be withdrawn if possible. Vital signs should be monitored. The patient should be protected from falls and from physical harm that may result from pulling

---

Box 5–5. ED Management of the Patient with Delirium

- Ensure adequate hydration and nutrition.
- Check if vital signs are elevated, perform physical examination and appropriate laboratory studies to determine etiology, treat as indicated.
- Explain the events that are happening to patients at their level of understanding.
- Provide pictures of familiar faces and familiar objects.
- Try to maintain one set of nurses and aides for the patient so that staff changes are minimized.
- Orient to time, date, place, and person at least twice a day.
- Encourage ambulation and visiting outside the hospital when feasible.
- Monitor electrolytes and fluid shifts during postoperative periods and take prophylactic steps to prevent imbalances when possible.
- If possible, reduce the number of medications and their dosages.
- Monitor the patient's bowel and bladder functions to detect problems early and correct if possible.
- Provide adequate control of fever and its underlying cause in children; encourage the presence of parents and others when possible.
- Avoid sensory overload and sensory isolation.

ED, emergency department.

out IV lines and catheters. A one-to-one sitter may be required during the acute phase of confusion and agitation. Frequent reorientation of the patient is reassuring. The presence of a family member may help to calm the anxious delirious patient.

Medications

The main focus of management of delirium is correction of the metabolic or underlying disturbance. In addition, IV or IM administration of haloperidol, 2 to 5 mg, every 30 minutes as needed, along with low doses of benzodiazepine, may help to calm the agitated delirious patient. One must be careful, however, with benzodiazepines. The use of IV haloperidol is relatively free of the side effects of extrapyramidal symptoms (EPS), but there is some risk of cardiac conduction delay at high doses, and the patient should be monitored by ECG for QTc prolongation.

There are reports of increased mortality in the demented elderly from agitation and long-term atypical antipsychotic use; however, short-term administration of these agents may be beneficial. Olanzapine (Zyprexa) is available in a rapidly dissolving formulation in strengths of 5 mg and 10 mg (Zydis). A liquid form of risperidone (Risperdal), 0.5 mg to 1 mg, used every hour up to a maximum dose of 4 mg, is also available. Higher doses are rarely needed, but if they are used, one must monitor for EPS and orthostatic hypotension. Experience using these agents for delirium is limited.

Quetiapine also may be useful for delirium. However, possible side effects include somnolence, dizziness due to fall of blood pressure, occasional problems with swallowing, and EPS symptoms. The starting dose of quetiapine usually is 12.5 mg to 50 mg per day.

A modality that is effective for delirium associated with catatonia, neuroleptic malignant syndrome, and mania is electroconvulsive therapy (ECT). This is a safe procedure that may abort a lethal delirious state with great efficacy.

A useful mnemonic MINTWINE may help the reader recapitulate the causes of delirium (Box 5-6).

Postdelirium Intervention

Patients may feel embarrassed and sensitive about their behavior during delirium. Supportive therapy should be provided

Box 5–6. Medical Causes of Delirium

M—Metabolic disturbances related to hepatic failure, renal failure, uncontrolled diabetes, impaired pulmonary or cardiac function

I—Infections such as urinary tract infection, pneumonia, intoxication with stimulant drugs, iatrogenic infection due to dopaminergic agent

N—Neoplasms of central nervous system, paraneoplastic syndromes

T—Traumatic brain injuries, subdural or extradural hemorrhages, fat embolism from trauma of the long bones

W—Wernicke's encephalopathy, alcohol and sedative hypnotic withdrawal

I—Impaired circulation to the brain, strokes, impaired oxygenation due to cardiorespiratory failure or other causes

N—Neuroleptic malignant syndrome, other treatment emergent syndromes such as serotonin syndrome

E—Epileptic, interictal, and postictal states; endocrinopathy such as hyperthyroidism and thyroid storm, rarely hypothyroidism, hypoadrenalism, hyperadrenalism, hypoparathyroidism, hyperparathyroidism

and education of the family should be undertaken to ameliorate any ill feelings caused by any agitated and disorganized behavior directed toward family members. Families should also be educated about the risk for delirium in the elderly patient who is unable to perform self-care and may fail to take medications, and is prone to dehydration.

It is often difficult for the patient and the family to accept the need for placement of the patient in a supervised setting. Referrals to social services and the psychiatry department to assess the social situation and cognitive functioning are recommended.

Further Reading

Adamis D, Morrison C, Treloar A, et al: The performance of the Clock Drawing Test in elderly medical inpatients: Does it have utility in the identification of delirium? J Geriatr Psychiatry Neurol 2005;18:129-133.

Bourgeois JA: The incidence of delirium in older people with a mood disorder is similar with lithium and valproate. Evid Based Mental Health 2005;8:95.

Cavaliere F, D'Ambrosio F, Volpe C, Masieri S: Postoperative delirium. Curr Drug Targets 2005;6:807-814.

Cobb JL, Glantz MJ, Nicholas PK, et al: Delirium in patients with cancer at the end of life. Cancer Pract 2000;8:172-177.

Fayers PM, Hjermstad MJ, Ranhoff AH, et al: Which mini-mental status exam items can be used to screen for delirium and cognitive impairment? J Pain Symptom Manage 2005;30:41-50.

Gaudreau JD, Gagnon P, Harel F, et al: Psychoactive medications and risk of delirium in hospitalized cancer patients. J Clin Oncol 2005;23:6712-6718.

Inouye SK: Prevention of delirium in hospitalized older patients: Risk factors and targeted intervention strategies. Ann Med 2000;32:257-263.

Inouye SK, Bogardus ST Jr., Charpentier PA, et al: A multicomponent intervention to prevent delirium in hospitalized older patients. N Engl J Med 1999 Mar 4;240:669-676.

Leslie DL, Zhang Y, Holford TR, et al: Premature death associated with delirium at 1 year follow-up. Arch Intern Med 2005;165:1657-1662.

Mercantonio ER, Flacker JM, Wright RJ, Resnick NM: Reducing delirium after hip fracture: A randomized trial. J Am Geriatr Soc 2001;49:516-522.

Milisen K, Lemiengre J, Braes T, Foreman MD: Multicomponent intervention strategies for managing delirium in hospitalized older people: Systematic review. J Adv Nurs 2005;52:79-90.

Pepersack T: The prevention of delirium. Rev Med Brux 2005;26:S301-S305. Review. [French.]

Plonk WM Jr, Arnold RM: Terminal care: The last weeks of life. J Palliat Med 2005;8:1042-1054.

Sharma PT, Sieber FE, Zakariya KJ, et al: Recovery room delirium predicts postoperative delirium after hip-fracture repair. Anesth Analg 2005;101:1215-1220.

Weber JB, Coverdale JH, Kunik ME: Delirium: Current trends in prevention and treatment. Intern Med 2004;34:115-121.

CHAPTER 6

The Suicidal Patient

Hani R. Khouzam, MD, MPH, FAPA, Tirath S. Gill, MD, and Doris T. Tan, DO

KEY POINTS

- The difference between suicidal ideation, intention, and suicidal gesture needs to be clarified during the initial assessment of the suicidal patient.
- In the United States, suicide accounts for more than 31,000 deaths annually, or 80 each day.
- The emergency department (ED) clinician needs to ask specific questions in the clinical assessment to determine suicidal imminence.
- Knowledge of the various risk factors for suicide is necessary to determine the appropriate disposition of the suicidal patient.
- The ED clinician may initiate certain psychopharmacological medications for the suicidal patient with comorbid psychiatric conditions.
- Referral for psychotherapy and spiritual interventions may be helpful.
- No-suicide contracts ("safety contracts") are rarely useful except for certain patients with nonlethal self-destructive behaviors.

PRELUDE

As people approach suicide, they become very constricted in their awareness, as if the world had begun to close in on them. A kind of tunnel vision develops in which the individual loses the ability to contemplate his own set of motivations. As people near the moment of their own self-destruction, they begin to feel as if they

no longer have a choice. . . . described as if in a theatre
suddenly filled with smoke, with only the EXIT sign
in sight."*

Robert Litman, MD—1981

Epidemiology

Following are some general statistics about suicide:
- In the United States, suicide accounts for more than
  31,000 deaths annually, or 80 each day.
- Up to 33% of persons in the general population
  contemplate suicide at some point in their lives.
- Although suicide is a public health problem for all
  segments of the population, suicide disproportionately
  impacts people of certain ages, ethnic/racial backgrounds,
  and geographic locations.
- Overall, suicide is the eleventh leading cause of death
  for all Americans (it has been as high as the ninth
  leading cause).
- Suicide is the third leading cause of death among
  Americans ages 15 to 24 and the second leading cause of
  self-inflicted injury.
- Males are more than four times likely to die from suicide
  than are females. However, females are more likely to
  attempt suicide than are males.
- The use of firearms is the most common method of suicide
  in men; in women, it is overdosing on medications.
  Following are some facts about suicide attempts:
- In addition to completed suicides there are over half a
  million unsuccessful attempts each year—1300 each day,
  or 1 each minute.
- In the United States, there were an average of 775,000
  suicide attempts and 30,900 completions each year over
  the last 10 years.
- Five million living Americans have attempted to kill
  themselves.

---

*From keynote address by Robert Litman, MD; Proceedings of a National
Symposium presented by the University of Arkansas for Medical Services
(UAMS), Little Rock, Arkansas; Monogram, *The Physician and the
Depressed Patient*, Roche Laboratory & UAMS, Nutley, NJ, 1981.

- Most people who complete suicide have previously attempted to do so up to four times.
- There is an estimated ratio of 8 to 25 attempted suicides to one completion; the ratio is higher in women and youth and lower in men and the elderly.
- The vast majority of completed suicides—more than 90%—occur among persons with diagnosable psychiatric disorders such as substance abuse, depression, anxiety, schizophrenia, and personality disorders, or a combination of other disorders with substance abuse.

Clinical Presentation

Suicidal patients may present on their own volition to the emergency department (ED), or they may be brought in by family, friends, or law enforcement personnel or by an ambulance that may have responded to a psychiatric emergency.

Interviewing and Assessment

Asking patients about suicide will not give them the idea or the motive to commit suicide. Most patients who consider suicide are ambivalent about the act and will feel relieved that the ED clinician is interested and willing to talk with them about their ideas and plans.

Some patients are not so forthcoming about psychiatric symptoms or thoughts of suicide. In these cases, the ED clinician may make introductory statements followed by specific questions—for example, "Sometimes when people feel sad or depressed or have problems in their lives they think about suicide. Have you ever thought about suicide?"

Patients may make indirect statements suggesting suicidal thoughts—for example, "I've had enough," "I'm a burden," or "It's not worth it." These statements mandate follow-up with specific questions about suicidal intentions. In addition to questions about the duration and onset of suicidal ideation, questions should also be asked about the lethality of patients' intentions and plans.

Specific questions to ask patients with suicidal intentions are listed in Box 6-1.

Box 6–1. Examples of Questions to Ask Patients with Suicidal Ideation

Questions Related to Suicidal Intention

When did you experience suicidal thoughts?
Were there any recent events that brought these thoughts?
How often do these thoughts cross your mind?
Have you felt that you were being a burden?
Have you felt that life isn't worth living?
What in life makes you feel better?
What in life makes you feel worse?
Do you have a plan to end your life?
How much control of your suicidal ideas do you have?
Can you suppress them or call someone for help?
What stops you from killing yourself (e.g., family, religious beliefs)?

Questions Related to Suicidal Plan

Do you own a gun or have access to firearms?
Do you have access to potentially harmful medications?
Have you imagined your funeral and how people will react to your death?
Have you "practiced" your suicide?
Have you changed your will or life insurance policy or given away your possessions?

Reproduced by permission from Gliatto MF, Rai AK: Evaluation and treatment of patients with suicidal ideation. Am Fam Physician 1999;59:1500-1506.

Stressors Assessment

Open-ended questions are useful to assess stressors. Examples are "How are things going in your relationship with your family?" (at home, at work) and "How is your health?" (or name other stressors, such as financial, marital, family, legal, and occupational stressors).

The *Diagnostic and Statistical Manual of Mental Disorders, Fourth Edition, Text Revision* (DSM-IV-TR) suggests asking the following questions to identify underlying stressors related to depression and anxiety:

• Have you experienced sad, blue, or empty feelings and at least two of the following in the past two weeks?

- Trouble falling or staying asleep
- Feeling tired or having little energy
- Poor appetite or overeating
- Little interest or pleasure in doing things
- Feeling bad about yourself
- Trouble concentrating
- Feeling fidgety, restless, or unable to sit still
- Have you felt nervous, anxious, or on edge?
- Have you had anxiety or panic attacks recently?

Assessment for Substance and Alcohol Abuse

See assessment details in Chapters 14 and 15.

Risk Factors Assessment

The ED clinician can use the acronym SAD PILLS to identify the conditions that are associated with increased suicide risks (see later).

Assessment of suicide risk factors is an essential element of the ED evaluation; these risk factors are described in Box 6-2.

The acronym SAD PILLS:

S —Schizophrenia and other psychotic disorders

A —Affective (mood) disorders, whether unipolar depression or bipolar disorder

D —Despair/hopelessness; high-risk demographic group

P —Plan: passive suicidal ideations, vague suicidal plans, specific plans with suicide notes, active suicidal ideation or active suicidal plans

I —Impulsivity associated with personality disorders

L —Lethality of the suicide attempt or suicide plan

L —Losses or setbacks that are significant

S —Substance abuse: alcohol and/or illicit drug abuse

The first evidence-based list of suicide warning signs has been fashinoned in the mnemonic IS PATH WARM (American Association of Suicidology, 2006):

I —Ideation

S —Substance abuse

P —Purposelessness

A —Anxiety

T —Trapped

H —Hopelessness

Box 6–2. Suicide Risk Factors

Gender
Females attempt suicide three times more often than males.
Males are three times more successful at completing suicides than females.
Males usually use firearms; females tend to use medication overdose.

Age
The risk for suicide increases with age; however, younger patients make more suicide attempts.
Older patients are more apt to succeed in their first attempt.

Race/Ethnic Background
There is a higher suicide rate in the United States in Caucasians, Native Americans, and the foreign-born than in the general population.

Sexual Orientation
There is a higher suicide rate in homosexuals than in heterosexuals.

Religious Affiliations
Moslems (Muslims) have the lowest suicide rate, followed by Catholics, Jews, and Protestants.

Marital Status
There is a higher suicide rate in single, divorced, separated, and widowed (especially in the absence of children) persons than in married persons. Single persons commit twice as many suicides as married persons.

Vocational Status
There is a higher suicide rate in unemployed than in employed persons.

Family History
There is an increased risk of suicide if other family members have attempted or completed suicide (40% to 80% of successful suicides had a history of suicide attempts by family members).

Day of the Week
More suicides occur on Wednesdays and Saturdays, and fewest occur on Sundays.

Box 6–2. Suicide Risk Factors—cont'd

Psychiatric History
Past suicidal attempts, prior inpatient treatment, and the presence of comorbid psychiatric conditions, especially depression, anxiety disorders, psychosis with command hallucinations, and substance abuse.

Medical History
Terminal illness, recent onset of a severe medical illness.

Personal History
Recent stressful life events.

Mental Status
Anhedonia; feelings of hopelessness, helplessness, guilt, and low self-esteem.

Plan and Access
Presence of a suicidal plan with availability of lethal means.

W—Withdrawal
A —Anger
R —Recklessness
M—Mood changes

Schizophrenia
Although patients with schizophrenia, particularly the young, are at high risk for suicide, it is often difficult to predict their suicidal ideations or intentions. Patients with command hallucinations telling them to kill themselves are at the highest risk. When evaluating the presence of depression in patients with schizophrenia who are not currently psychotic, it is important to rule out the presence of "postpsychotic depression," which is associated with an increased risk for suicide.

Personality Disorder
Patients with borderline personality disorder may make repeated suicide attempts or gestures and will frequently present to the ED demanding hospitalization. The ED clinician should never assume that these are merely manipulative threats aimed at getting attention. Before discharging these patients, questions such as the following should be asked:
• Have you had thoughts about death or about killing yourself?

- Do you have a plan for how you would do this?
- Are there means available (e.g., a gun and bullets or poison)?
- Have you actually rehearsed or practiced how you would kill yourself?
- Do you tend to be impulsive?
- How strong is your intent to do this?
- Can you resist the impulse to do this?
- Have you heard voices telling you to hurt or kill yourself?

The presence of concomitant substance abuse and mood disorder increases the risk of suicide in borderline patients.

Verbal as well as nonverbal clues that may be observed in suicidal patients are reviewed in Table 6-1.

Table 6–1

Assessment of Suicidal Clues

Verbal Clues	Behavioral Clues	Situational Clues
It won't matter soon	Giving away possessions	Prior suicide attempts dismissed as accidents; accident proneness
They're better off without me	Suicidal note	Serious illness
The world would be a better place without me	May present with physical symptoms for which no medical cause can be determined; new purchases of weapons, poisons, or ropes	History of being physically or sexually abused or of being threatened with abuse
I can't take it any more	Noncompliance with treatment; accumulates medications or drugs that could be used for overdose	Recent important losses
I am no good anyway	Repeated relapses of substance or alcohol abuse	Rapid decline in vocational, interpersonal, and social functioning

Table 6–1

Assessment of Suicidal Clues—cont'd

Verbal Clues	Behavioral Clues	Situational Clues
I'll show them	Risk-taking behaviors such as driving at high speed, traveling in dangerous parts of town without purpose; visiting isolated or dangerous places such as high-rise buildings, bridges, and mountain cliffs	Perceives personal experiences as being shameful or unaccepted by the prevailing culture
I don't know how I feel	Mood changes with irritability or angry outbursts	Social isolation and withdrawal

Management

Once a patient is considered to be at risk for suicide, the clinician must decide whether the risk is imminent (48 hours or less), short-term (within days or weeks), or long-term. The approach to management is dictated by the immediacy of the threat. The management and disposition of suicidal imminence is summarized in Table 6-2.

The risk of suicide is imminent if the patient expresses the intent to die, has a plan in mind, and has lethal means available. Expressions of deep despair or signs of psychosis (such as "command" hallucinations telling the patient to kill himself) clearly are ominous. In this setting, immediate action—generally, psychiatric hospitalization—is required. A staff member should remain with the patient in a secure room while arrangements are made for hospital admission. The patient should not be left alone, even briefly. If an acutely suicidal patient refuses intervention or has a weapon, security or the police should be called in.

 Availability of firearms, potentially lethal medication, and other potential means of suicide should be identified and documented, and steps taken to remove them.

Table 6–2

The Management and Disposition of Suicidal Imminence

Imminence	Management Approach	Disposition
Imminent risk (48 hours or less)	1. Recommend inpatient hospitalization. 2. Need one-to-one observation until disposition is arranged	Voluntary hospitalization if accepted by the patient; involuntary hospitalization if the patient refuses.
Short-term risk (days to weeks)	1. Limit access to weapons and lethal means to commit suicide. 2. Mobilize patient's social and interpersonal support network, including spouse, close family members, friends, extended family, etc. 3. Evaluate for co-existing medical and psychiatric conditions, especially depression, anxiety disorder, and substance abuse.	If medical conditions are identified, refer for treatment; if depression or anxiety disorders are present, initiate treatment with nonlethal medications; if substance abuse is present, initiate referral to substance abuse treatment programs.
Long-term risk (weeks to months)	1. Mobilize patient's social and interpersonal support network, including spouse, close family members, friends, extended family, etc. 2. Evaluate for co-existing medical and psychiatric conditions, especially depression and substance abuse.	If medical conditions are identified, refer for treatment; if depression is present, initiate treatment with nonlethal medications; if substance abuse is present, initiate referral to substance abuse treatment programs.

Table 6–2

The Management and Disposition of Suicidal Imminence—cont'd

Imminence	Management Approach	Disposition
	3. Identify underlying psychosocial stressors.	Apply psychosocial interventions to reduce identified stressors as described in Chapter 1.

Adapted from Hirschfeld RM: The suicidal patient. Hosp Pract (Minneap) 1998;33:119-123.

Patients with short-term risk of suicide may have coexisting depression and alcohol abuse, or depression accompanied by panic attacks or other signs of anxiety. Although immediate hospitalization usually is not necessary, immediate intervention is warranted. The ED clinician may seek the patient's permission to involve a family member or close friend as collaborator in dealing with the crisis. Telephone calls and appointments should be encouraged so that patients are in regular contact with their treatment providers.

The presence of one or more risk factors in relatively mild form in the absence of overt suicidal ideation or intention may indicate a long-term risk of suicide. Pharmacological and psychosocial treatment are indicated to reduce underlying psychosocial stressors.

Pharmacological Management

Pharmacological treatment of depression or other psychiatric disorders should be initiated or continued as needed. If alcohol or other substance abuse is present, referral to a substance abuse treatment program is advisable.

When choosing medication for patients who express suicidal ideation, the risk of an overdose should always be considered. Tricyclic antidepressants (TCAs), such as imipramine and amitriptyline, and monoamine oxidase inhibitors (MAOIs), such as phenelzine, although effective, are toxic in high doses and can be lethal. The newer agents, including selective serotonin

Table 6–3

Antidepressant Agents

Medications	Average Daily Oral Dose
SSRIs	
Fluoxetine (Prozac)	20-40 mg
Sertraline (Zoloft)	50-200 mg
Paroxetine (Paxil)	20-40 mg
Fluvoxamine (Luvox)	150-250 mg
Citalopram (Celexa)	20-60 mg
Escitalopram (Lexapro)	10-40 mg
SNRIs	
Venlafaxine (Effexor)	75-300 mg
Duloxetine (Cymbalta)	10-40 mg
Other	
Mirtazapine	15-45 mg

SSRIs, selective serotonin reuptake inhibitors; SNRIs, serotonin/norepinephrine reuptake inhibitors.

reuptake inhibitors (SSRIs) and serotonin/norepinephrine reuptake inhibitors (SNRIs) (Table 6-3) can be as effective and safer than TCAs. Patients with comorbid anxiety or insomnia may benefit from concomitant use of a benzodiazepine. Antipsychotic medications can be administered to treat psychotic symptoms.

Long-term use of SSRIs can result in sexual difficulties such as delayed orgasm and loss of libido in both men and women. Because depression also dampens libido, the source of the problem may not always be due to the medication.

All antidepressants need time (usually several weeks) to show their effects. For an agitated patient, the interval can seem endless. Until relief is apparent, it may be advisable for the patient's spouse, another family member, or professional caregivers to keep all medications (including over-the-counter (OTC) agents such as acetaminophen) in a secure place and to monitor medication intake.

Suicidal patients should be closely monitored during follow-up for medication side effects. To prevent non-compliance, the ED clinician should educate patients about these side effects and about the duration of time needed to experience relief of symptoms. Patients should be assured that side effects are common and generally subside with continued use.

For more detailed discussion of antidepressants, see Chapters 3, 4, 7, 8, 10, and 22.

Intervening in Anxiety and Insomnia

Because anxiety and insomnia have been associated with increased suicidal attempts, these symptoms should be treated promptly, and often concomitantly with antidepressant therapy. Benzodiazepines are rarely fatal in an overdose, unless they are taken in conjunction with another central nervous system depressant and/or alcohol. Assuming close follow-up, a 2- or 3-day supply of a benzodiazepine or other anxiolytic or hypnotic agent may be dispensed. Table 6-4 lists some benzodiazepines and hypnotic medications.

Patients with a history of nonresponse to antidepressant therapy who exhibit symptoms of major depression with psychotic features should be considered for ECT and referred for immediate and intense psychiatric treatment.

Electroconvulsive Therapy (ECT)

Misunderstanding continues to persist about the contemporary role of ECT. This is a potentially lifesaving option for patients with severe depression or depression with psychotic features, as

Table 6–4

Antianxiety and Hypnotic Medications

Medications	Average Daily Oral Dose
Benzodiazepines*	
Lorazepam (Ativan)	0.5-4 mg
Oxazepam (Serax)	15-45 mg
Temazepam (Restoril)	15-30 mg
Hypnotics†	
Zolpidem (Ambien)	5-10 mg
Zaleplon (Sonata)	5-0 mg
Eszopiclone (Lunesta)	1-3 mg
Ramelteon (Rozerem)	8 mg

*Can be taken every evening and at bedtime or during the daytime if not sedating.
†Can be taken before bedtime.

well as for those who cannot tolerate or have been nonresponsive to other treatments. However, the effects are not permanent,
and cases that respond favorably may revert to depression.
Therefore it is recommended and advisable that after ECT is
completed, patients who can later tolerate antidepressants should
be treated with these medications. Certain patients will also
require long-term ECT maintenance treatment.

Antipsychotic Medications

Antipsychotic medications can be used to treat overt psychotic
symptoms in suicidal patients. A detailed description of these
medications is given elsewhere in this book (see Chapters 3, 10,
and 17). Table 6-5 describes certain antipsychotics that are
useful in the ED.

Although most medications are effective in treating underlying psychiatric conditions, antidepressant, antianxiety, and
the majority of antipsychotic medications do not prevent suicide.
The only exception is the atypical antipsychotic clozapine
(Clozaril), which is approved by the Food and Drug Administration (FDA) for treatment-resistant schizophrenia and for the
prevention of suicide in patients with schizophrenia. Although
not approved for the treatment of schizoaffective disorder,
clozapine has been reported to prevent suicide in patients with
this condition. Because clozapine carries the risk of agranulocytosis, weekly monitoring of the white blood cell (WBC)
count is advisable during the first 6 months of treatment and
every 2 weeks thereafter.

Nonpharmacological Management

Crisis Intervention

See Chapters 1 and 2.

Psychotherapy

Treatment of severe depression in the suicidal patient should
include, in addition to antidepressant therapy, psychotherapy
to address some of the underlying issues that have been sustaining the depression. The emphasis should be practical and
targeted to solving current problems. Patients are encouraged

Table 6–5

Antipsychotics That Can Be Used in the Emergency Department

Agent	FDA-Approved Indications	Dose, PO or IM (mg)	Half-life (hr)	Advantages	Disadvantages
Haloperidol (Haldol)	Psychotic disorders	0.5–7.5	12–36	Antipsychotic effect over time	Akathisia; dystonia; can lower seizure threshold
Ziprasidone mesylate (Geodon)	Control of agitation in patients with schizophrenia, using oral form	10–20	2.2–3.4	No akathisia or dystonia; antipsychotic effect over time; also available in intramuscular form	Prolongation of QTc interval
Olanzapine (Zyprexa)	Control of agitation associated with schizophrenia, bipolar mania; oral form indicated for psychotic disorders and bipolar mania	10 (2.5 for patients with dementia)	34–38	No akathisia or dystonia; antipsychotic effect over time; available in disintegrating tablet form (Zydis) and intramuscular form	Weight gain over time

Adapted from Citrome L: Atypical antipsychotics for acute agitation. New intramuscular options offer advantages. Postgrad Med 2002;112:85-88, 94-96.

to bring their spouses or other family members into the process because their insights are often useful in promoting recovery. It is not unusual for the families of patients receiving antidepressants to notice improvement before the patient does. Depressed patients become so focused on their internal pain that they may not notice gradual improvement in their relationship with others. Hearing good news from an outside source provides reassurance that therapy is having an effect and reinforces antidepressant compliance.

Addressing Substance Abuse

Intoxicated or psychotic patients who express suicidal ideations or intentions should be transported securely to a private, supervised room with one-to-one constant observation. If a patient is considered dangerous, agitated, aggressive, or impulsive, security officers or the police may be called in to assist (also see Chapters 2-4, 9, 10, 12, and 19). Often, intoxicated patients require prolonged evaluation, which is done more effectively in the ED than in a triage office. The ED clinician needs to be aware that in most patients who present with substance abuse and suicidal ideations or intentions and who are newly diagnosed with depression, commitment to sobriety and abstinence from alcohol and substance abuse is necessary before the initiation of antidepressants for depression. However, concurrent treatment of depression and substance abuse increases the chance of success in patients with preexisting comorbid depression and substance abuse.

Medical Disorders and Risk of Suicide

Some evidence indicates an increased risk of suicide in patients with cancer, head injury, and peptic ulcer disease. Persons with illnesses related to acquired immune deficiency syndrome (AIDS) are 16 to 36 times more likely to die by suicide than persons in the general population. Suicide among medically ill patients, including those with AIDS, rarely occurs in the absence of a comorbid psychiatric disorder, such as major depression, substance abuse, and dementia.

The ED clinician needs to carefully assess patients with medical conditions and suicidal ideations and should plan for follow-up medical and psychiatric care following discharge from the ED.

Terminal Illness and the Risk of Suicide

The assessment and treatment of depression and other mental disorders and the management of pain in terminally ill patients can increase the chance that such patients will choose life over death. The ED clinician should offer empathy and initiate vigorous palliative and pharmacological treatments to reduce pain and improve the quality of life.

Twelve-Step Programs

Spiritually centered twelve-step programs such as Alcoholics Anonymous formerly recommended against medication treatment for fear that mood stabilizers and antidepressants might themselves become drugs of abuse. Some physicians may not be aware of the effectiveness of these programs. There now is a greater mutual appreciation of the benefit of such programs and medical therapy.

A very positive development in recent years has been the increasing collaboration between treatment programs for depression and substance abuse, arising from the growing perception that, for many patients, these represent two sides of one coin. Often, heavy drinkers find that much of their depression clears away after sustained sobriety while other patients with comorbid depression may need antidepressant therapy in order to stop drinking.

The ED clinician needs to consider the importance of the religious and spiritual beliefs of patients and incorporate this dimension of intervention in management plans when considering the disposition of the suicidal patient (see Chapter 24).

The "Safety Contract"

Suicidal patients may avoid hospitalization if they promise via a safety, or no-suicide, contract, that they will contact an ED clinician if the inclination to commit suicide becomes overwhelming. Clinicians may assume that these contracts have clinical utility; however, they should not take excessive comfort from the fact that their suicidal patients agree to contract for safety. No medicolegal protection is conferred by a no-suicide contract.

Safety contracts, however, may be effective in dealing with nonlethal self-destructive behaviors, which are interpreted as a covert plea for help. In these instances it is therapeutically helpful to outline an intervention plan with the patient to explore alternative ways of asking for help that do not involve real or potential self-harm.

The Denial of Suicidality

The ED clinician should be aware patients may retract previously expressed suicidal ideation and intentions when they are brought for an evaluation. A history of "suicidal tendencies" should guide the necessary emergency intervention even if the patient denies current suicidal intention.

Hospitalization

The patient with a plan for suicide, access to lethal means, and/or recent social stressors and symptoms suggestive of a psychiatric disorder should be hospitalized immediately. The spouse or another family member should be informed of the decision to proceed with hospitalization.

If an imminent danger of suicide is ascertained and the patient refuses to allow the ED clinician to contact a family member, then confidentiality may be breached. Legal consultation may be advisable if there are any questions about infringing on a patient's autonomy.

If the patient refuses to be hospitalized, involuntary commitment may be necessary. Grounds for involuntary commitment include one or more of the following conditions:

- Imminent danger to self
- Imminent danger to others
- Inability to care for self

In most states, procedures are in place to allow involuntary hospitalization for 48 to 120 hours before a hearing is held to extend the hospitalization.

Medicolegal Aspects of Suicide

Most state and federal laws acknowledge that there are no standards for the prediction of suicide and that suicide results from several complex and often unidentifiable factors. The standard of care for suicidal patients is based not on "predictability" but rather on "foreseeability," which includes the reasonable physician's professional ability and clinical experiences, including taking a thorough history, recognizing relevant risk factors, and designing and implementing a treatment plan that provides preventive measures and precautions against the completion of suicide. The ED clinician needs to document accurately and clearly all encounters with suicidal patients. The documentation should include the entire examination, discussions with family members and consultants, and treatment recommendations, in addition to a summary of implementation of the recommended actions.

Summary

Most patients who express or admit to having suicidal ideation do not complete the act. However, because some patients will eventually commit suicide, all patients who present in the ED with suicidal ideation and intention require thorough evaluation. The assessment of suicidal patients should be made at the time suicidality is expressed as well as periodically thereafter during ongoing follow-up care.

Psychiatric disorders are present in most patients who express suicidal ideation or those who attempt to complete suicide. These patients should be asked specific questions about recent stressors and thoughts of suicide, and appropriate treatment strategies should be initiated to prevent suicide.

Families, friends, and significant others should be invited to be an integral part of treatment planning. Medication and psychosocial and spiritual interventions are necessary components of the ED management of suicidal patients.

Further Reading

Beautrais AL: A case control study of suicide and attempted suicide in older adults. Suicide Life Threat Behav 2002;32:1-9.

Berman AL, Cohen-Sandler R: Suicide and the standard of care: Optimal vs. acceptable. Suicide Life Threat Behav 1982;12:114-122.

Citrome L: Atypical antipsychotics for acute agitation. New intramuscular options offer advantages. Postgrad Med 2002;112:85-88, 94-96.

Fawcett J, Scheftner WA, Fogg L, et al: Time-related predictors of suicide in major affective disorder. Am J Psychiatry 1990;147:1189-1194.

McIntosh JL: U.S.A. Suicide: 2001 Official Final Data. Available at www.suicidology.org/associations/1045/files/2001datapg.pdf. Accessed Oct. 28, 2003.

Pompili M, Girardi P, Ruberto A, et al: Emergency staff reactions to suicidal and self-harming patients. Eur J Emerg Med 2005;12:169-178.

Theodoulou M, Harriss L, Hawton K, Bass C: Pain and deliberate self-harm: An important association. J Psychosom Res 2005;58:317-320.

Rubenowitz E, Waern M, Wilhelmson K, Allebeck P: Life events and psychosocial factors in elderly suicides—a case-control study. Psychol Med 2001;31:1193-1202.

Sakuraba S, Kubo M, Komoda T, Yamana J: Suicidal ideation and alexithymia in patients with alcoholism: A pilot study. Subst Use Misuse 2005;40:823-830.

Simon RI: Psychiatry and Law for Clinicians. Washington, DC, American Psychiatric Press, 1992.

Stanford EJ, Goetz RR, Bloom JD: The no-harm contract in the emergency assessment of suicidal risk. J Clin Psychiatry 1994;55:344-348.

Swartz M: Malpractice liability for suicide: Clinical, legal, and rhetorical dimensions. Psychiatr Forum 1988;14:45-53.

Szanto K, Mulsant BH, Houck P, et al: Occurrence and course of suicidality during short-term treatment of late-life depression. Arch Gen Psychiatry 2003;60:610-617.

POSTSCRIPT

Human nature has its limits. It can endure a certain degree of joy, sorrow, and pain, but collapses as soon as this is exceeded. The question, therefore, is not whether he is able to endure the measure of his suffering, moral or physical; and in my opinion it is just as absurd to call a man a coward who kills himself as to call a man a coward who dies of a malignant fever.

From *The Sorrows of Young Werther*
by Johann Wolfgang von Goethe—1774

There are two kinds of psychiatrists out there: those who have had a patient commit suicide and those who will.

Paraphrased by A. A. Howsepian, MD, PhD—2005

CHAPTER 7

The Severely Depressed Patient

Tirath S. Gill, MD

KEY POINTS

- Depression is a common debilitating illness equal in its burden on society to heart disease in terms of morbidity, mortality, and financial costs.
- It is important for the emergency department (ED) clinician to inquire about depressive symptoms because many patients present with related complications such as injuries, alcoholism, and unexplained somatic symptoms.
- Once recognized, the depressive syndrome is eminently treatable with a number of effective medications and psychotherapies.

Overview (Figs. 7-1 and 7-2)

Depression is a common and under-recognized illness. Its emotional and economic impact is second only to that of cardiovascular disease in the number of productive days lost and the overall impact on society. Depressed patients are not always readily recognized because they may present with different types of physical complaints for which no medical cause can be found. They may describe their depression in terms that are unique to their cultural background—for example, having problem of "nerves" or an imbalance of spiritual life, suffering from "stress," or just being "down in the dumps."

Some depressed patients are averse to admitting that they have an illness that is severely debilitating and that has begun to interfere with their ability to maintain social and occupational functioning. In addition, patients with depression often may have other comorbid psychiatric issues such as alcohol addiction and substance abuse that further confound recognition of the disease.

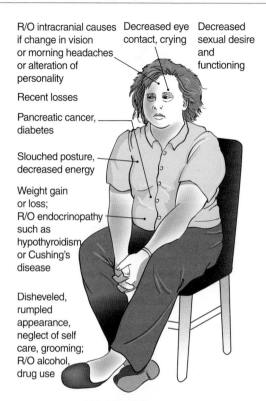

R/O intracranial causes if change in vision or morning headaches or alteration of personality

Recent losses

Pancreatic cancer, diabetes

Slouched posture, decreased energy

Weight gain or loss; R/O endocrinopathy such as hypothyroidism or Cushing's disease

Disheveled, rumpled appearance, neglect of self care, grooming; R/O alcohol, drug use

Decreased eye contact, crying

Decreased sexual desire and functioning

The Depressed Patient—Part 1
Clinical features and some risk factors

Slouched posture
Downcast gaze
Rumpled appearance
Weight gain
Apathetic look and feelings of hopelessness*
Decreased occupational performance
Decreased performance of social roles

*Important to explore thoughts of suicide

FIGURE 7–1

The depressed adult patient.

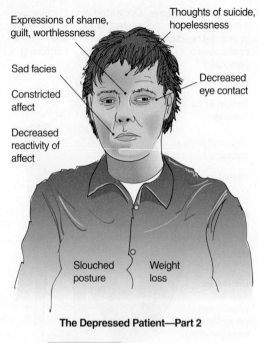

Expressions of shame, guilt, worthlessness

Thoughts of suicide, hopelessness

Sad facies

Decreased eye contact

Constricted affect

Decreased reactivity of affect

Slouched posture

Weight loss

The Depressed Patient—Part 2

FIGURE 7–2

The depressed young adult patient.

If it is determined at any time that the patient is at high risk for suicide, hospitalization—involuntary if necessary—is mandatory.

Definition

Depression has been defined by different individuals in different ways dating back to the early period of written history. The *Diagnostic and Statistical Manual of Mental Disorders, 4th Edition, Text Revision* (DSM-IV-TR) definition of major depression states that the patient must have a depressive episode for at least 2 weeks that is marked by depressed mood or loss of interest in most activities. In addition, the depressed individual must experience at least four symptoms that indicate a disturbance in biologic functioning and thinking such as disturbance of appetite; changes in sleep habits and energy level; decreased libido; feelings of worthlessness, hopelessness, and guilt; and recurring thoughts of death or suicide. Depressive syndromes other than major depression are listed in Table 7-1.

Epidemiology

The incidence of depression in the general population has been reported to range from 2% to 25% in various studies. It tends to be more prevalent among certain demographic groups (e.g., female, single, unemployed, minorities, immigrants, and the terminally ill).

The likelihood that a patient will have a primary affective disorder increases if there is a family history of depression.

Causes of Depression

The exact cause of depression is not fully understood. However, it is apparent that biologic and social factors can combine to produce an episode of clinical depression meeting the criteria for major depression in certain vulnerable individuals. Thus depression may be the result of a combination of genetic vulnerability and certain psychosocial stressors. Various neurochemical causes have been hypothesized, including dopamine, norepinephrine, and serotonin, but none of these can fully explain how depression is precipitated or how it resolves with the use of medications that target these neurotransmitters. Some newer theories suggest a role for neuroactive steroids that modulate the receptors of gamma-aminobutyric acid (GABA).

Importance of Recognizing the Depressed Patient

Depression is an eminently treatable illness. ED clinicians have at their disposal a number of options for treatment of depression that are relatively safe and have a good likelihood of improving the patient's condition. It is, however, important to

Table 7-1

Various Depressive Syndromes

Mood Disorder	Features*
Major depression	A persistent state of depressed mood and anhedonia (or irritability in children) for a period of at least 2 weeks, accompanied by at least four other symptoms such as decreased or increased sleep, increased or decreased appetite, decreased energy, decreased libido, decreased interest in usual activities of pleasure, feelings of worthlessness, difficulty with concentration, and in severe cases feelings of hopelessness and thoughts of suicide. The median onset of an episode of major depression is at about 30 years of age. Prevalence is reported to be 5% to 25%. The depressed mood is not caused by an organic factor such as a medical problem or substance abuse but may be complicated by it.
Dysthymic disorder: 1. Primary dysthymic disorder—onset before age 18, duration of at least 1 year; 2. Secondary dysthymic disorder—onset after age 18	Chronic state of mild depression lasting at least 2 years in adults and 1 year in those less than age 18; the criteria for major depression are not met but there are significant problems with decreased self-esteem, low energy, difficulty concentrating, and distractibility. Prevalence is 5% to 6%.
Bipolar disorder	Depressed phase of the disorder. Prevalence is 1% to 2%.
Cyclothymic disorder	Periods of cyclic mood swings lasting less than 2 weeks that do not meet criteria for mania or major depression. Prevalence is 0.4% to 1%.

Mood Disorder	Features*
Depressed mood related to medical conditions	A number of endocrinopathies and medical conditions such as pancreatic cancer may lead to distinct syndromes of depression.
Depressed mood related to alcohol	Usually tends to resolve within 3 to 4 weeks of abstinence; some residual effects such as sleep disturbance may linger for months, increasing the risk of relapse.
Depressed mood related to illicit drugs	A number of stimulant drugs such as amphetamines and cocaine have withdrawal symptoms, such as lassitude and decreased energy, that are the opposite of the intoxication symptoms. The depressive syndrome is usually of short duration and tends to resolve in 2 to 4 days.
Depressed mood related to medications	A panoply of different medications have been implicated as a cause of depressive symptoms. Some of the more notable ones have been the antihypertensive medications that deplete or block norepinephrine or dopamine.
Situational depression	This term can be grouped under the rubric of "adjustment disorders" and is caused by psychological or social stress that the individual finds overwhelming. This type of depression usually responds to social support, supportive therapy, and short-term adjunctive medication, as needed for insomnia.

*Prevalence in this context refers to the general population.

rule out medical and organic causes that may be manifesting or exacerbating the depressed state.

Differential Diagnosis

Medications That May Cause or Exacerbate Depression

Some commonly used medications that may precipitate depression are listed in Box 7-1. These include reserpine, which is no longer used for the treatment of hypertension because of the high risk of induction of a major depressive episode. Other antihypertensive medications such as alpha-methyldopa, propranolol, prazosin, clonidine, and guanethidine may also contribute to clinical depression. Withdrawal of these agents is sometimes associated with the resolution of the depressed state.

Digitalis glycosides have been used in patients with congestive heart failure and atrial fibrillation to increase myocardial contractility and suppress sinoatrial activity and AV nodal conduction. These medications, however, have been associated with the onset of a mildly depressed state in older individuals. Substitution, when possible, may help to lessen depression.

Disopyramide phosphate, used to correct ventricular dysrhythmia, has been reported to cause depression in some individuals.

Box 7–1. Medications Associated with Depression

Corticosteroids (also associated with inducing manic states)
Digitoxin
Digoxin
Disopyramide
Metoprolol
Pegylated interferon
Propranolol
Reserpine
Vinblastine
Vincristine

Corticosteroids administered for rheumatoid arthritis, systemic lupus erythematosus (SLE), and other chronic inflammatory diseases may contribute to depression. At times corticosteroid use may be associated with a mild hypomanic to manic state. Production of excessive endogenous cortisol in cushingoid syndrome may be associated with depression.

Oral contraceptives with a high progestin content may cause depression. Newer contraceptives that contain less progestin may be substituted. Certain H_2 blockers such as cimetidine have been associated with depression as well. Data on the association of depression with proton pump inhibitors is limited. Timolol maleate, used for glaucoma, has been associated with delirium and depression. Indomethacin and certain antimicrobial agents such as isoniazid (INH), cycloserine, and nalidixic acid have been associated with depression.

Disulfiram and antineoplastic drugs such as vincristine sulfate and vinblastine sulfate, organophosphate insecticides, and anti-parkinsonian drugs such as levodopa have been associated with depression. It is to be noted that anti-parkinsonian drugs such as D_2 agonist agents have also been associated with the induction of euphoric or hypomanic states.

Symptoms of withdrawal from caffeine, nicotine, amphetamine, cocaine, and other stimulants may be associated with depression. The use of sedative hypnotics such as barbiturates and benzodiazepines on a chronic basis may lead to depression. Psychotropic drugs with significant extrapyramidal symptoms (EPS) side effects have been associated with "deficit symptoms" that are at times difficult to differentiate from depression.

Anesthetic agents such as halothane and phenylephrine, anticonvulsants such as baclofen and pentazocine, and certain opiates have been associated with depressed mood.

Revision of the pharmacological regimen should be considered if the depressed patient is taking any of these agents.

Medical Conditions That May Cause or Exacerbate Depression

Many medical conditions may cause or exacerbate depression (Box 7-2). These should be considered in the differential diagnoses of the depressed patient. Included are infections such as influenza, hepatitis, viral encephalitis, viral pneumonia, and—in some adolescents—infectious mononucleosis. Other illnesses associated with depression are brucellosis, typhoid, malaria,

Box 7–2. Medical Conditions Associated with Depression

Addison's disease
Brain tumors
Bronchogenic carcinoma
Pancreatic carcinoma
Cerebrovascular accidents/strokes affecting left frontotemporal area
Chronic electrolyte disturbances
Chronic inflammatory diseases
Cushing's syndrome
Diabetes mellitus
Huntington's disease
Hyperparathyroidism
Hyperthyroidism
Hypogonadism
Hypoparathyroidism
Hypopituitarism
Hypothyroidism
Infectious mononucleosis
Influenza
Mesenteric artery occlusion
Parkinsonism
Systemic lupus erythematosus
Viral hepatitis
Rosacea
Sleep apnea
Folate deficiency
Vitamin B_{12} deficiency

tuberculosis, syphilis, amebiasis, giardiasis, strongyloidiasis, pancreatic carcinoma, carcinoma of the lung, lymphoma, and brain tumors.

Sleep apnea, hypoxia due to any cause, and mesenteric artery occlusion have been reported to be associated with depression, as well as endocrine disorders such as hypothyroidism, hyperthyroidism, and Addison's disease. Crohn's disease, menopause, postpartum depression, diabetes mellitus, hyperinsulinism, hypoparathyroidism, hyperparathyroidism, hypopituitarism, and acromegaly are also associated with depressed mood states.

Other medical causes of depression include metabolic disturbances such as uremia, hyponatremia, hypokalemia, elevated serum bicarbonate, and gout. Nutritional deficiencies such as pellagra, scurvy, and deficiencies in thiamine, vitamin B_{12}, folate, pyridoxine, iron, and protein may also be implicated. Gastrointestinal disorders such as cirrhosis, inflammatory bowel disease, celiac disease, Whipple's disease, pancreatitis, and pancreatic cancer have well-known associations with depression.

Chronic inflammatory illnesses such as SLE, rheumatoid arthritis, polyarteritis nodosa, and giant cell arteritis have been implicated in depression as well. Central nervous system (CNS) diseases in this category, including parkinsonism, strokes, multiple sclerosis, Huntington's disease, chronic subdural hematoma, and temporal lobe seizures, may induce depressive states through direct effects on certain parts of the brain. Various autoimmune illnesses often have depression as a secondary clinical feature.

Clinical Presentation and Assessment of the Depressed Patient

Depressed patients may appear tired and haggard due to lack of sleep and may be thin, with loose clothing because of loss of weight due to decreased appetite. Eye contact is usually minimal, and patients may slouch or sit with drooping shoulders, staring at the floor. Psychomotor activity may be decreased, and patients may appear anxious and fidgety, wringing their hands, with a tense facial expression (i.e., furrowed brow and creased forehead; see Figs 7-1 and 7-2).

Patients should be approached in a respectful manner. Their reason(s) for coming to the ED should be explored, and they should be allowed to tell their story. If they wish to focus on their somatic symptoms, this should be allowed, and the clinician should avoid interruption.

Questions should be asked about sleep habits, appetite, sense of hopelessness, and thoughts of suicide. If patients admit having thoughts of suicide, one may inquire about any specific plans for suicide (see Chapter 6 for detailed discussion about the suicidal patient).

 A history of depression and responses to any medications should be noted. The clinician should ask about antidepressant medications that have worked for other family members; the same agent may work for the patient.

It is important to ask about the use of alcohol or substance abuse and to determine whether the patient has experienced a recent setback, such as a job lay-off, death of a loved one, or diagnosis of a serious illness. The clinician should also ask about methods used by the patient to cope with depressive symptoms and physical complaints.

Collateral information, if available, from spouse or other family members and friends is often quite helpful

On completion of the clinical assessment, patients should be reassured that their concerns are understood and that the clinician has been attentive to their complaints.

The presence of any medical illness should be ruled out and a thorough medication history should be obtained to rule out any offending agents that could be contributing to the depressed state. If such medications are found, consultation with the primary care physician or internist who is prescribing these medications may be necessary to substitute alternative medications, such as a less lipophilic beta-blocker in place of propranolol or an angiotensin-converting enzyme (ACE) inhibitor in place of an antihypertensive agent that may be contributing to the depression.

Studies to determine endocrinologic abnormalities and tests for deficiencies in vitamin B_{12}, folic acid, and micronutrients deficiency may be indicated, because these conditions are sometimes subtle in their manifestations and difficult to recognize.

Management of the Depressed Patient

Management of the depressed patient requires a multifaceted approach, because the etiology of depression usually is multifactorial.

The treatment of depression is often dictated by the symptom pattern that appears to be the most predominant problem. If insomnia and appetite disturbance are noted, a frequent choice may be mirtazapine, 15 mg, titrated every 3 to 4 weeks as needed up to 30 to 60 mg. For the patient with significant comorbid anxiety, paroxetine, 20 to 30 mg, may be a good choice. There is some evidence that dual-agent antidepressants such as serotonin/norepinephrine reuptake inhibitors (SNRIs) such as venlafaxine and duloxetine may be more effective in treating psychiatric symptoms of depression, especially depression accompanied by somatic complaints and symptoms of peripheral neuropathy related to diabetes.

Tricyclic agents are quite effective in treating major depression, and some studies suggest that they may be especially effective therapy for the more severe types of depression. There is, however, a risk of fatal overdose with these agents.

Selegiline (L-deprenyl), a selective reversible monoamide oxidase-A (MAO-A) inhibitor, is now available as a patch. At a dose of 10 mg, it is relatively selective, but at higher doses it may be nonselective, with the risk of interaction with other serotonergic agents.

Bupropion (Wellbutrin) has shown some efficacy as an augmenting agent for patients who do not respond to selective serotonin reuptake inhibitors (SSRIs) such as fluoxetine, paroxetine, and sertraline. Bupropion has also been reported to help with the sexual dysfunction attributed to certain SSRIs.

Control of underlying medical conditions often is crucial to a lasting remission of depressive episodes. Any comorbid substance or alcohol abuse issues must be addressed. Depression that is induced by alcohol tends to improve in 2 to 4 weeks. If the patient is significantly depressed after this period of time, he may suffer from a primary affective disorder and may require treatment with antidepressant medications.

Antidepressant medications may be used to promote sleep and stimulate appetite, depending on the side effect profile of the agent. Insomnia and lack of appetite usually respond first to antidepressant agents, especially mirtazapine. Energy levels begin to improve over the next 2 to 4 weeks.

There may be a paradoxical increase in the risk of suicide at this stage, when there is an increase in energy level and concentration with continuing depressive symptoms. If discharged at this point in time without adequate supervision, patients may act out their suicidal intentions.

Patients should be educated about the time course of the response to antidepressants so that they do not become disheartened by the apparent lack of improvement in symptoms. If there is no improvement by 4 weeks, the dosage may be increased; another 4 weeks should be allowed for a response. If no response is seen after this time, augmentation strategies include addition of lithium to achieve a therapeutic plasma level of at least 0.6 mmol/L.

With lithium, improvement of mood usually is seen within a week to 10 days, in which case the patient may be maintained on lithium for as long as 6 to 9 months. While the patient is on lithium therapy, the usual precautions must be observed, including monitoring of thyroid function, blood urea nitrogen (BUN), creatinine, and electrocardiograms (ECGs).

If no response to lithium is seen, other augmentation strategies include buspirone (BuSpar), 10 to 15 mg three times daily, titrated up; atypical antipsychotics such as olanzapine; and the beta-blocker pindolol. Occasionally, triiodothyronine (T_3) augmentation is used for depressive states if they are refractory to standard pharmacological regimens. If the depression is life-threatening, the use of electroconvulsive therapy (ECT) may be a viable and suitable option.

Some Words of Caution

- Educate the patient about the time course of the response to medications so that lack of an immediate and early response does not add to the patient's feelings of hopelessness.
- If no response is seen by 3 to 4 weeks, consider increasing the dose of the medications.
- SNRIs such as venlafaxine and SSRIs are first-choice agents because they are not lethal in overdose.
- Treat coexisting anxiety symptoms with anxiolytics because anxiety has been noted to be an independent risk factor for suicide.
- Referral to appropriate support groups can yield long-term dividends.
- Make telephone contact with the patient and family if visits cannot be scheduled every week.
- Discuss cognitive distortions and encourage patients to analyze their assumptions about their life.
- Inquire about suicide risk and monitor the patient carefully during the early phase of mood recovery when energy levels improve but significant depression remains.
- Monitor for signs of suicidal intent such as giving away of gifts and pets; consider hospitalization.
- SSRIs have been noted to increase suicidal ideations in some patients during the first few weeks of treatment. Arrange for weekly follow-ups if patient is being treated with an SSRI on an outpatient basis. It is also prudent to inform the family of the risk period and to tell them to call if they or the patient notices a worsening of depression or irritability.

- If the patient is indeed suicidal, refer to the guidelines provided in Chapter 6 and consider hospitalization on a voluntary or involuntary basis.
- Offer and discuss the option of ECT early in the course of treatment of seriously depressed patients, including those at risk for suicide.
- It is always wiser to err on the side of safety when considering hospitalization for the severely depressed patient.

Further Reading

American Psychiatric Association: Diagnostic and Statistical Manual of Mental Disorders, 4th ed. Text Revision. Washington, DC, American Psychiatric Association, 2000.

Bettinger TL, Crismon ML, Trivedi MH, et al: Clinicians' adherence to an algorithm for pharmacotherapy for treatment of depression in the Texas public mental health sector. Psychiatr Serv 2004;55:703-705.

Dombrovski AY, Mulsant BH, Haskett RF, et al: Predictors of remission after electroconvulsive therapy in unipolar major depression. J Clin Psychiatry 2005;66:1043-1049.

Eser D, Romeo E, Baghai TC, et al: Neuroactive steroids as modulators of depression and anxiety. Neuroscience 2006;138:1041-1048.

Gleason OC, Yates WR, Philipsen MA: Major depressive disorder in hepatitis C: An open-label trial of escitalopram. Prim Care Companion J Clin Psychiatry 2005;7:225-230.

Gupta MA, Gupta AK, Chen SJ, Johnson AM: Comorbidity of rosacea and depression: An analysis of the National Ambulatory Medical Care Survey and National Hospital Ambulatory Care Survey—Outpatient Department data collected by US National Center for Health Statistics from 1995 to 2002. Br J Dermatol 2005;153:1176-1181.

Jiang W, Davidson JR: Antidepressant therapy in patients with ischaemic heart disease. Am Heart J 2005;150:871-881.

Jorge RE, Sarkstein SE: Pathophysiologic aspects of major depression following traumatic brain injury. J Head Trauma Rehabil 2005;20:475-487.

Ranjkesh F, Barekatain M, Akuchakian S: Bifrontal versus right unilateral and bitemporal electroconvulsive therapy in major depressive disorder. J ECT 2005;21:207-210.

Reichenberg A, Gorman JM, Dieterich DT: Interferon-induced depression and impairment in hepatitis C virus patients: A 72-week prospective study. AIDS 2005;19(Suppl 3):S174-S178.

Ros S, Aguera L, de la Gandara J, et al: Potentiation strategies for treatment of resistant depression. Acta Psychiatr Scand Suppl 2005;428:14-24.

Rossini D, Lucca A, Zanardi R, et al: Transcranial magnetic stimulation in treatment-resistant depressed patients: A double-blinded placebo-controlled trial. Psychiatry Res 2005;137:1-10.

Seidman SN, Miyazaki M, Roose SP: Intramuscular testosterone supplementation to selective serotonin reuptake inhibition treatment of resistant depressed men: Randomized placebo controlled clinical trial. J Clin Psychopharmacol 2005;25:584-588.

Walsh SP, Kling MA: VNS and depression: Current status and future directions. Expert Rev Med Devices 2004;1:155-160.

CHAPTER 8

The Acutely Manic Patient

Hani R. Khouzam, MD, MPH, FAPA

KEY POINTS

- Patients may present with different symptoms depending on the type and phase of their illness.
- Patients who express suicidal ideation or intention may require emergency psychiatric hospitalization.
- Newly diagnosed patients should have a comprehensive medical and psychiatric assessment to rule out the presence of underlying medical and psychiatric conditions.
- The use of mood stabilizers, atypical antipsychotics, and other pharmacological agents may be initiated by the Emergency Department (ED) clinician if urgent emergency needs arise during the initial assessment of the patient with bipolar disorder.
- Contemporary treatment of bipolar disorder focuses almost exclusively on psychopharmacological treatment. Nonetheless, psychotherapy is a useful adjunctive treatment to maintain stability and to prevent relapse.

Definition (Fig. 8-1)

There are two primary types of bipolar disorder—bipolar I disorder and bipolar II disorder. Patients with bipolar I disorder have had at least one full manic episode with periods of major depression. Patients with bipolar II disorder seldom experience full-blown mania. Instead, they experience periods of hypomania (elevated levels of energy and impulsiveness that are not as extreme as the symptoms of mania). These hypomanic periods alternate with episodes of major depression.

A mild form of bipolar disorder called cyclothymic disorder (cyclothymia) is characterized by periods of hypomania and mild depression, with less severe mood swings. Patients with

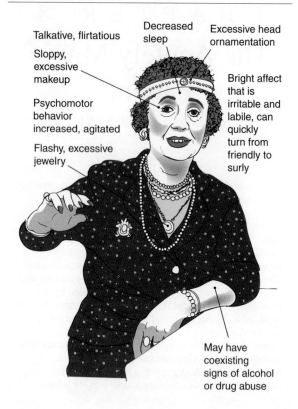

Talkative, flirtatious

Decreased sleep

Excessive head ornamentation

Sloppy, excessive makeup

Psychomotor behavior increased, agitated

Flashy, excessive jewelry

Bright affect that is irritable and labile, can quickly turn from friendly to surly

May have coexisting signs of alcohol or drug abuse

FIGURE 8–1

The manic patient.

bipolar II disorder or cyclothymic disorder may be misdiagnosed as having depression alone.

During the manic phase of the illness, mood is elated and judgment is impaired, and patients are likely to deny that they are ill or that they need treatment. During the depressive phase, patients may feel so hopeless that they are incapable of seeking or accepting treatment, and they may at times believe that they are beyond any effective treatment. Mixed episodes involve the simultaneous occurrence of depressive and manic symptoms.

Patients with bipolar I disorder may also experience psychotic symptoms, including hallucinations and paranoid delusions. The duration of the different mood episodes ranges from a few days to many months.

Epidemiology

Bipolar disorder is estimated to affect 4% of the U.S. population, with an annual cost of over $45 billion. The lifetime prevalence of bipolar disorder is 1%, compared to a lifetime prevalence of 6% for unipolar depression. The prevalence of bipolar disorder type I does not differ in males and females. The prevalence of bipolar disorder type II is higher in females than males.

Bipolar disorder affects persons of all ages. An epidemiologic catchment area study revealed the highest prevalence in the 18- to 24-year age group. However, bipolar disorder does not become manifest in some patients until they are older.

The incidence of bipolar disorder is increased in first-degree relatives of persons with the disorder, as is the incidence of other mood disorders. The mode of inheritance remains unclear, and no algorithm exists to predict the risk of bipolar disorder.

Bipolar disorder causes significant morbidity and mortality, including suicide, and has a deleterious impact on social and occupational functioning, which increases the risk of divorce and unemployment. Completed suicide occurs in approximately 10% to 15% of patients with bipolar I disorder. Over half of patients diagnosed with bipolar disorder have a history of substance abuse. There is a high rate of association of cocaine abuse and bipolar disorder. Some studies have shown that up to 30% of alcohol and drug abusers meet the criteria for bipolar disorder.

Risk Factors

Seasonal Variables. A higher incidence of bipolar disorder occurs in persons born in the winter. The time of the year also appears to play a role in increasing the risk for certain episodes. Manic episodes are more likely to occur in the summer, whereas depressive episodes usually occur from October through May; this seems to differ from seasonal affective disorder (SAD), in which depression occurs during the darker months of the year.

Socioeconomic Variables. Bipolar disorder is more prevalent among individuals with a higher socioeconomic status. The rate of the disorder is estimated to be 10 to 20 times higher among individuals with creative and artistic talents than in the general population.

Other Variables. A higher incidence of bipolar disorder occurs in persons who had experienced complications around the time of their birth. Children who lose a parent early in life appear to be more likely to develop bipolar disorder in their adult years. A family history of depressive disorder or bipolar disorder increases the risk of bipolar disorder.

Clinical Presentation and Assessment

Bipolar disorder can be difficult to recognize if symptoms of mania or depression are not evident during the initial phases of the patient's assessment. Because much of bipolar disorder consists of the depressive phase, it can be difficult to distinguish bipolar depression from unipolar depression (see Chapter 7).

Bipolar disorder is associated with a high rate of suicide, substance abuse, and other comorbidities. Early recognition and appropriate management can improve patient outcome. Clues that can lead to a diagnosis of bipolar disorder include a positive family history, early age at onset, the presence of symptoms such as irritability and rapid cycling (see later in chapter), and poor or unusual response to antidepressant therapy in the absence of a mood-stabilizing agent.

Because of frequent patient noncompliance it is often extremely challenging for the ED clinician to maintain ongoing treatment.

Types of Bipolar Disorder

Clinical presentation varies, depending on the type of bipolar disorder. Following is a brief description of some of the different types.

Bipolar I Disorder—Manic Phase
This phase may last from days to months and may include:
- Elevated mood
- Racing thoughts
- Hyperactivity
- Increased energy
- Lack of self-control
- Inflated self-esteem with delusions of grandeur and beliefs in superhuman special abilities

- Overinvolvement in goal-directed activities, either socially, at work or school, or sexually
- Reckless behavior and excessive involvement in pleasurable activities that have a high potential for painful consequences (e.g., unrestrained buying sprees, sexual indiscretions, foolish business investments)
- Binge eating, drinking, drug use
- Easy distractibility
- Decreased or little need for sleep
- Agitated or irritable and labile mood

Mood disturbance may be sufficiently severe to cause marked impairment in occupational functioning or in usual social activities or relationships with others or to necessitate hospitalization to prevent harm to self or others. Psychotic features of hallucinations and delusions may be prominent.

Bipolar II Disorder—Hypomanic Phase

This phase may last for as long as 4 days. Symptoms are similar to those seen in the manic phase of bipolar I disorder but are less intense; they include:

- Inflated self-esteem or grandiosity
- Decreased need for sleep
- Excessive talkativeness
- Flight of ideas or subjective experience that thoughts are racing
- Distractibility
- Increased goal-directed activity or psychomotor agitation

Mood disturbance is not severe enough to cause marked impairment in social or occupational functioning or to necessitate hospitalization, and there are no psychotic features. Compared with bipolar I disorder, bipolar II disorder is less intense, less severe, lacks psychotic symptoms, and does not cause marked impairment.

Bipolar I and Bipolar II Disorder—Depressed Phase

In both types of bipolar disorder, depression has very serious symptoms, including:

- Persistent sadness
- Fatigue or listlessness
- Abnormal sleep patterns such as excessive sleepiness and inability to sleep
- Eating disturbances
- Loss of appetite and weight loss

- Overeating and weight gain
- Loss of self-esteem
- Feelings of worthlessness, hopelessness, and guilt
- Difficulty concentrating, remembering, and making decisions
- Withdrawal from friends
- Withdrawal from activities that were once enjoyed
- Persistent thoughts of death

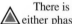 There is a high risk of suicide with bipolar disorder. While in either phase, patients may abuse alcohol or other substances, which can worsen the symptoms.

Mixed Type of Bipolar Disorder

In the mixed type of bipolar disorder, there is an overlap of the manic and depressed phases. The manic and depressive symptoms may occur simultaneously or in quick succession to each other.

Rapid-Cycling Bipolar Disorder

Rapid cycling occurs in up to 20% of cases of bipolar disorder. Manic and depressive episodes alternate frequently; this occurs at least four times in a 12-month period. In some cases of "ultra-rapid cycling," patients may bounce between manic and depressive states several times within a 24-hour period. It may be difficult to distinguish this type from the mixed type of bipolar disorder.

Cyclothymic Disorder

Cyclothymic disorder is characterized by cycling of hypomanic episodes with depression that does not reach major depressive proportions. One third of patients with cyclothymic disorder may develop bipolar I or II disorder later in life.

Bipolar Disorder Not Otherwise Specified (NOS)

This category includes bipolar states that do not clearly fit the description of bipolar I, bipolar II, or cyclothymic disorder.

Bipolar Disorder Due to Medical Conditions and Medications

 Numerous medical conditions can lead to the development of mania, depression, and psychotic symptoms. The mnemonic MANIC in Table 8-1 summarizes some of these conditions.

Table 8–1

The Mnemonic MANIC Classification of Bipolar Disorder due to Medical Conditions/Diseases

Mnemonic Category	Condition/Disease
M = Metabolic	Electrolyte imbalance, uremia, vitamin deficiencies (B_{12}, folate, niacin, thiamine)
A = Alcoholic and substance abuse	Intoxication or withdrawal from alcohol and/or prescribed, OTC, or illicit drugs (amphetamines, cocaine, hallucinogens, opiates)
N = Neurologic	Multiple sclerosis
	Huntington's disease
	Wilson's disease
	Head trauma
	Partial complex seizures
	Cerebrovascular accidents
	Migraine headache
	Neoplasms (primary, especially diencephalic or third ventricle, and secondary metastasis)
	Cerebrovascular accident
	Subdural hematoma
	Parkinson's disease
I = Infections	Neurosyphilis
	Herpes encephalitis
	St. Louis encephalitis
	HIV
	Influenza
C = Conditions not mentioned elsewhere	Toxicity
	Heavy-metal poisoning
	Carbon monoxide poisoning
	Collagen vascular disease
	Systemic lupus erythematosus
	Endocrinologic disorders, including thyroid disease (hypothyroidism, hyperthyroidism)
	Adrenal disease

HIV, human immunodeficiency virus; OTC, over-the-counter.
Compiled from Citrome L, Goldberg JF: The many faces of bipolar disorder. How to tell them apart. Postgrad Med 2005;117:15-16, 19-23.

Features of medical conditions such as altered state of consciousness, impaired memory, disorientation, endocrine abnormalities, and a positive toxicology screening test suggest the presence of bipolar disorder.

Certain medications are associated with the development of bipolar disorder. Box 8-1 lists some of these.

Psychiatric Evaluation

As part of the initial evaluation of the patient with bipolar disorder, the clinician should:
- Observe behavior and affect
- Obtain a detailed medical history, including any medical problems and any medications

---

Box 8–1. Medications Associated with Bipolar Disorder

Neuropsychiatric
Monoamine oxidase inhibitors (MAOIs)
Antidepressants (TCAs, SSRIs, SNRIs, and others)
Methylphenidate
Disulfiram (Antabuse)
Levodopa
Bromocriptine
Entacapone

Cardiovascular
Captopril
Hydralazine

Endocrinologic
Corticosteroids
Thyroid hormones

Miscellaneous
Baclofen
Bromide
Procarbazine
Yohimbine
Cimetidine
Isoniazid
Modafinil

- Ask about recent mood swings and their duration
- Ask about family medical history, particularly whether anyone has or had bipolar disorder
- Ask family members (after obtaining authorization of information release) for information that can complement the history

 Patients with mania, bipolar depression, or a mixed episode should be evaluated thoroughly for evidence of suicidal intent.

Medical Evaluation

Patients with newly diagnosed bipolar disorder require a medical evaluation as well as a psychiatric evaluation. The following assessment is recommended.
- Complete physical examination
- Serum levels of lithium, valproic acid, carbamazepine and other selected medications (if relevant)
- Thyroid function tests
- Complete blood count (CBC) and general chemistry screening
- Urinalysis if lithium therapy is initiated
- Pregnancy test (if relevant)
- Urine toxicology for substance abuse (if relevant)

Computed tomography (CT), magnetic resonance imaging (MRI) and electroencephalography (EEG) are second-line options in the evaluation of treatment-resistant patients. These studies are not routinely required without specific clinical reasons. Similarly, the need for electrocardiography (ECG) in patients younger than 40 years depends on the clinician's judgment and pre-existing cardiac conditions.

Diagnosis

Comorbid Psychiatric Conditions

Psychiatric comorbidities can complicate accurate diagnosis of bipolar disorder and make clinical management difficult. Such conditions may include the presence of suicide ideation, intention, or past suicide attempts. It is important to note that an estimated 15% to 20% of patients who suffer from bipolar disorder and who do not receive medical attention commit suicide.

In one study, more than 50% of patients with bipolar I disorder attempted suicide; the risk was highest during depressive episodes. Other studies suggest that this figure is even higher in patients with bipolar II disorder or with major depression. Patients with mixed mania, possibly when it is marked by irritability and paranoia, are also at particular risk.

Other conditions that increase the risk of suicide attempts include:
- Personality disorder, especially borderline personality
- Alcohol and substance abuse
- Recent psychosocial stressors related to interpersonal conflicts, legal problems, or financial difficulties.

Personality Disorders. Several personality disorders—most commonly narcissistic, borderline, antisocial, obsessive-compulsive, and avoidant—may be present in the patient with bipolar disorder. In such patients, the symptoms of bipolar disorder may be more intense and more resistant to treatment, and the risk of suicide is higher.

Alcohol and Substance Abuse or Dependence. Patients may present with alcohol- or substance-induced depression or manic-like clinical symptoms; on closer investigation, they may not actually have bipolar disorder. In patients with diagnosed bipolar disorder, the alcohol or substance abuse can occur during a mood disturbance or in between such episodes. In patients with bipolar I disorder and alcohol and/or substance abuse, the risk of committing suicide is estimated to be as high as 61%.

Anxiety Disorders. Anxiety disorders, which affect mostly patients with bipolar I disorder, have been reported to decrease the response to anticonvulsant drugs but not to lithium.

Differential Diagnosis

Bipolar Disorder vs. Schizophrenia
Clinicians may attribute the presence of psychotic symptoms, especially hallucinations and delusions, to schizophrenia. However, not every psychosis is schizophrenia. When other causes of psychotic symptoms have been excluded, a mood disorder should be ruled out before a diagnosis of schizophrenia is considered. A longitudinal course that includes depressive, manic, or mixed episodes concurrent with psychotic symptoms is not consistent with a diagnosis of schizophrenia. Although atypical antipsychotics are used for both conditions, the prog-

noses of schizophrenia and bipolar disorder differ, in that schizophrenia is generally less likely to involve a robust response to treatment and a return to the previous level of functioning.

An accurate diagnosis is required to help anticipate the future course of the illness and better plan for long-term management. Patients with bipolar disorder may be well maintained on anticonvulsant or lithium monotherapy, whereas this treatment is inadequate for patients with schizophrenia.

Bipolar Disorder vs. Schizoaffective Disorder

Schizoaffective disorder is primarily a psychotic disorder with two subtypes: depressive and bipolar. Bipolar-type schizoaffective disorder is manifested by an uninterrupted period of illness during which symptoms of schizophrenia are concurrent with symptoms of major depression, mania, or mixed episodes of both; also, during the same period psychotic symptoms were present for at least 2 weeks in the absence of prominent mood symptoms. Treatment is similar to the treatment of bipolar disorder.

Unipolar Depression vs. Bipolar Depression

People with bipolar disorder are more likely to first seek help because of a depressive episode. Indeed, about 16% of persons with bipolar disorder do not have a manic episode until they have experienced three or more depressive episodes. In such cases, the condition is often diagnosed as depression (unipolar). An accurate diagnosis is important because patients with bipolar disorder who are inappropriately medicated with antidepressants have a higher incidence of rehospitalization than other patients with this disorder. A diagnosis of bipolar disorder cannot be established until a manic or hypomanic episode has occurred.

Bipolar disorder should be suspected in patients who have previously been treated for depression and who had an initial fast and good response that was followed by failure. Furthermore, they were then treatment-resistant to other antidepressants.

Bipolar Disorder vs. Substance-Induced Mood Disorder

Up to 60% of patients with bipolar disorder abuse alcohol and drugs at some point in the course of their illness. Both diagnosis and treatment are difficult in such cases because substance abuse is often a method of self-treatment, and withdrawal can produce symptoms of mania or severe depression.

The effects of cocaine in a heavy user can produce abnormal mood swings that closely resemble those of bipolar disorder. In such cases, maintenance of abstinence for 2 to 8 weeks may be required in order to differentiate the symptoms of the substance-induced mood disorder from those of the bipolar disorder.

Considerations in Children and Adolescents

Bipolar disorder in children and adolescents may be inappropriately diagnosed as attention deficit hyperactivity disorder (ADHD). In some cases, ADHD in children or adolescents can be a marker for an emerging bipolar disorder. Both ADHD and bipolar disorder often cause inattention and distractibility, and the two disorders may be difficult to distinguish, particularly in children. It is important to remember that manic or hypomanic episodes occur in bipolar disorder but not in ADHD. (For a detailed review of psychiatric emergencies in children and adolescents, see Chapter 18.)

Management

Immediate management of patients with acute mania often requires hospitalization. It is inadvisable for family members to transport the patient from the ED to the hospital, because they may not appreciate the irrationality of manic thinking and the unpredictability of manic behavior. Often, the police or ambulance transportation with trained personnel must be involved.

The clinician has the responsibility to inform family members about the possible need for the family to petition the court for the patient's admission to a psychiatric unit. It is important to recognize, and to try to allay, the guilt and regret family members often feel in these circumstances.

Special Considerations

Bipolar Disorder during Pregnancy

Management of the pregnant patient with bipolar disorder requires sustained collaboration between the patient's physician and the ED clinician. Patients with bipolar disorder should be encouraged to plan pregnancy so that their psychiatric medications can be slowly tapered. The risk of relapse is increased with abrupt discontinuation of medications. Relapse during pregnancy must be treated aggressively with mood stabilizers. Patients may need to be admitted to the hospital. See also Chapter 25.

If lithium therapy is required, patients should be educated and advised regarding the increased risk of cardiovascular malformations in fetuses exposed to lithium. Breast-feeding during lithium therapy is discouraged because lithium is excreted in breast milk.

During the postpartum period, worsening of mood symptoms may occur, including rapid cycling, which is sometimes refractory to pharmacological therapy. Patients who experience worsening of symptoms during the postpartum period have an increased risk of bipolar disorder recurrence.

Bipolar Disorder in Geriatric Patients
See Chapter 17 for a detailed discussion of geriatric patients.

Pharmacological Management

Contemporary treatment of bipolar disorder focuses almost exclusively on psychopharmacological therapy; most often, combination medications may be needed.

If necessary, and if patients have been in good general health, administration of mood stabilizers, as well as other medication used in the treatment of bipolar disorder, can be initiated, especially if the need to begin treatment is urgent. Medications can be given even before laboratory test results are obtained.

The treatment of depression associated with bipolar disorder differs somewhat from that of unipolar disorder (for detailed discussion of depression, see Chapter 7). Mild cases of bipolar depression can be treated with a mood stabilizer such as lithium. When an antidepressant is required, adequate mood stabilization is recommended before initiation of treatment. Alternatively, lamotrigine may be used.

 Psychotic symptoms during a manic episode should be treated with antipsychotic agents. Atypical antipsychotic agents are first-line choices; these agents may also be effective for treatment of acute mania itself. Short-term use of a benzodiazepine may also be required for anxiety or agitation.

With the exception of clozapine (Clozaril)—an atypical antipsychotic that is approved for treatment-resistant schizophrenia and for preventing suicide attempts in patients with schizo-phrenia and schizoaffective disorder—little is known about the ability of atypical antipsychotics to reduce the risk of suicidal ideation and behavior.

Pharmacological agents used for the treatment of bipolar disorder are summarized in Table 8-2.

Combinations of Atypical Antipsychotics with Lithium or Anticonvulsants

The use of lithium or divalproex in conjunction with an atypical antipsychotic can be implemented primarily in treatment of acute mania. The advantages of this augmentation become evident when the first medication has been given at doses that are therapeutic but not necessarily high enough to achieve optimal therapeutic effects, due to adverse effects associated with a higher dose. Drug combinations also may prevent the recurrence of manic relapse associated with maintenance treatment with lithium or divalproex alone.

Role of Antidepressants

Combinations of antipsychotic agents and antidepressants are used for treatment of depression in bipolar I disorder, and the combination drug of olanzapine and fluoxetine hydrochloride (Symbyax) has received the approval of the Food and Drug Administration (FDA) for that indication.

 Use of antidepressant monotherapy for bipolar disorder remains controversial due to the possibility of precipitating mania or a rapid-cycling pattern. In February 2004, an FDA advisory panel identified apparent risks associated with sev-eral antidepressants for increasing suicide-related behaviors in children and adolescents with depression. Although no specific risks of these behaviors were observed in adult patients with depression, the FDA extended a warning label advisory about the potential association between antidepressant use and suicidality in adults as well.

Some Other Pharmacological Interventions
(see also Chapters 3, 4, and 7)
Neuroleptics
Conventional high-potency antipsychotics such as haloperidol (Haldol) and thiothixene (Navane) can be used to treat mania while a mood stabilizer such as lithium or valproate takes effect. Side effects such as extrapyramidal syndromes (EPS),

Text continues on page 177.

Table 8–2

Pharmacological Agents Used in the Treatment of Bipolar Disorder

Medication	Class	FDA Indications	Dose and Titration	Side Effects and Precautions
Chlorpromazine HCl (Thorazine); available as tablets, syrup, suppositories, IM injection; now considered obsolete due to the advance of the newer atypical antipsychotics	Conventional (typical antipsychotic, major tranquilizer, neuroleptic)	Approved in 1970 for the treatment of manic type of manic-depressive illness	Dosage unclear; can start at 25 mg tid; product label states that 500 mg a day is generally sufficient, but gradual increases up to 2000 mg/day may be necessary; however, there is usually little therapeutic gain by exceeding 1000 mg/day for extended periods	EPS, TD, hypotension, weight gain, hepatitis with jaundice
Lithium; available as capsules, controlled-release and extended-release tablets, syrup	Mood stabilizer (antimanic agent)	Approved in 1970 for the treatment and maintenance of bipolar mania	Generally started at 900 mg/day, divided dose titrated to achieve serum trough level of 0.8–1.2 mEq/L acutely and 0.8–1.0 mEq/L long-term; serum levels	Cognitive slowing, nausea, diarrhea, polyuria, polydipsia, weight gain, tremor, metallic taste in the mouth, worsening of skin conditions (especially psoriasis), diabetes insipidus;

Continued

Table 8–2

Pharmacological Agents Used in the Treatment of Bipolar Disorder—cont'd

Medication	Class	FDA Indications	Dose and Titration	Side Effects and Precautions
Lithium—cont'd (Cibalith-S, Eskalith, Lithane, Lithobid, Lithonate, Lithotabs)			should be measured 10-12 hours after the last oral dose, and levels should not be drawn sooner than 4-5 days after latest change in dosage	because of narrow therapeutic-toxic range, lithium levels should be monitored periodically; renal function indicators (BUN and serum creatinine) and TSH should be measured every 6 months; different oral formulations are not interchangeable in dosing
Divalproex sodium (Depakote); available as delayed-release and extended-release tablets, sprinkles; also available as	Anticonvulsant (antiepileptic, mood stabilizer, antimigraine)	Only Divalproex sodium was approved in 1995 for bipolar mania	May be orally loaded at 20-30 mg/kg in acute mania to achieve serum trough level of 50-100 µg/mL	Weight gain; rarely associated with fatal hepatotoxicity and hemorrhagic pancreatitis; monitor hepatic function and platelet levels; controversy about reproductive safety

Medication	Class	FDA Indications	Dose and Titration	Side Effects and Precautions
Divalproex—cont'd Valproate (valproic acid), and Depakene				
Olanzapine (Zyprexa); available as tablets, orally disintegrating tablets (Zydis), IM injection	Atypical antipsychotic second-generation antipsychotic	Approved in 2000 for bipolar mania (monotherapy or add-on therapy) maintenance and for agitation associated with bipolar I mania (IM formulation)	Start at 10-15 mg/day; may increase to 20 mg/day in increments of 5 mg/day; IM dose is 10 mg per injection	Weight gain; monitor metabolic parameters associated with bipolar mania; risk for hyperlipidemia and diabetes type II, orthostatic hypotension
Olanzapine plus fluoxetine HCl (Symbyax); available as capsules	Atypical antipsychotic second-generation antipsychotic	Approved in 2003 for acute bipolar depression	Start with 6 mg olanzapine/25 mg fluoxetine capsule in evening; also available in 6 mg/50 mg, 12 mg/25 mg, and 12 mg/50 mg capsules	Weight gain, clinical worsening and suicide risk (now included in labeling for all antidepressants); monitor metabolic parameters; risk for hyperlipidemia and diabetes type II, orthostatic hypotension

Continued

Table 8-2

Pharmacological Agents Used in the Treatment of Bipolar Disorder—cont'd

Medication	Class	FDA Indications	Dose and Titration	Side Effects and Precautions
Risperidone (Risperdal); available as tablets, orally disintegrating tablets, oral solution, long acting IM injection (approved for schizophrenia)	Atypical antipsychotic second-generation antipsychotic	Approved in 2004 for bipolar mania (monotherapy or add-on therapy)	Initial dose, 2-3 mg/day; increase by 1 mg/day to maximum of 6 mg/day	EPS symptoms at higher doses, hyperprolactinemia, weight gain; monitor metabolic parameters; risk for hyperlipidemia and diabetes type II, orthostatic hypotension
Quetiapine fumarate (Seroquel); available as tablets	Atypical antipsychotic second-generation antipsychotic	Approved in 2004 for bipolar mania (monotherapy or add-on therapy)	Initial dose, 100 mg/day in two divided doses; increase by 100 mg/day up to 400 mg/day by day 4; target range, 400-800 mg/day	Weight gain; monitor metabolic parameters; risk for hyperlipidemia and diabetes type II, orthostatic hypotension

Medication	Class	FDA Indications	Dose and Titration	Side Effects and Precautions
Ziprasidone (Geodon); available as capsules); IM form available for the treatment of agitation in schizophrenia	Atypical antipsychotic second-generation antipsychotic	Approved in 2004 for bipolar mania (monotherapy)	Start at 40 mg bid with food; increase to 60-80 mg bid on day 2	Anorexia, weight loss, prolongation of QTc interval (probably not clinically relevant in patients without predisposing cardiac risk factors)
Aripiprazole (Abilify); available as tablets, oral solution	Atypical antipsychotic second-generation antipsychotic	Approved in 2004 for bipolar mania (monotherapy)	Start at target dose of 30 mg/day 15% of patients (in clinical trials had dose decreased to 15 mg on basis of tolerability)	Essentially well tolerated, but akathisia and nausea may occur; seems to be weight-neutral
Carbamazepine extended-release tablets (Equetro); carbamazepine (Tegretol, Atretol)	Anticonvulsant, mood stabilizer	Only the extended release form was approved in 2004 for bipolar I disorder, acute manic and mixed episodes	Start at 400 mg/day in two divided doses; adjust in 200-mg daily increments to achieve optimal clinical response; doses >1600 mg/day have not been studied	Sedation; small risk of liver toxicity, aplastic anemia, and agranulocytosis; induction of cytochrome P450 isoenzymes may occur, which initially decreases its own level, which may require dose adjustments of further carbamazepine and other drugs taken concurrently

Continued

Table 8–2

Pharmacological Agents Used in the Treatment of Bipolar Disorder—cont'd

Medication	Class	FDA Indications	Dose and Titration	Side Effects and Precautions
Lamotrigine (Lamictal); available as tablets, chewable dispersible tablets	Anticonvulsant, mood stabilizer	Approved in 2003 for bipolar I disorder maintenance (monotherapy)	25 mg/day for 2 wk, then 50 mg/day for 2 wk, then 100 mg/day for 1 wk, then 200 mg/day (target); for patients also taking divalproex, the titration is in smaller increments to a target dose of 100 mg/day by wk 6; for those taking carbamazepine, the titration is in larger increments to a target dose of 400 mg/day by wk 7	Skin rashes in about 10% of patients, serious skin rashes in about 0.03% (highest risk if dosing rate exceeds recommendations); Stevens-Johnson syndrome (blistering/burnlike lesions on soft mucocutaneous tissues and systemic illness, warranting drug cessation and rapid medical attention)

Adapted from: Goldberg JF, Citrome L: Latest therapies for bipolar disorder. Looking beyond lithium. Postgrad Med 2005;117:25-26, 29-32, 35-36. BUN, blood urea nitrogen; EPS, extrapyramidal symptoms; TD, tardive dyskinesia; FDA, Food and Drug Administration; IM, intramuscular; TSH, thyroid-stimulating hormone.

akathisia, and tardive dyskinesia (TD) can be severe. Symptoms of TD include difficulty in speaking or swallowing, loss of balance control, muscle spasms, severe restlessness, stiffness of arms and legs, tremors in fingers and hands, twisting body movements, and weakness in the limbs.

Bupropion (Wellbutrin, Zyban)
Bupropion is a heterocyclic antidepressant that is effective in regulating bipolar depression in some patients. Side effects include agitation, anxiety, confusion, tremor, dry mouth, fast or irregular heartbeat, headache, and insomnia. Other adverse effects include seizures and anorexia. Although it has been reported not to trigger mania, the possibility of its occurrence should not be overlooked.

Benzodiazepines
Benzodiazepines such as clonazepam (Klonopin) and alprazolam (Xanax) are used to calm and sedate patients until mania or hypomania has waned and mood-stabilizing agents can take effect. Sedation is a common effect. Other side effects include clumsiness, lightheadedness, and slurred speech.

Clozapine (Clozaril)
This atypical antipsychotic medication is FDA-approved for treatment of resistant schizophrenia. It can be used to stabilize manic episodes in treatment-resistant patients; it is useful as a prophylactic, or preventative, in some bipolar patients. Common side effects of clozapine include tachycardia, hypotension, constipation, and weight gain. Agranulocytosis, a potentially serious but reversible condition, is a possible adverse effect. Patients being treated with clozapine should undergo weekly blood tests to monitor white blood cell counts.

Calcium Channel Blockers (Nimodipine, Nimotop)
These agents, typically used to treat angina and hypertension, can be effective in treating rapid-cycling bipolar disorder. Calcium channel blockers are usually given in conjunction with other mood stabilizers. Side effects include hypotension and worsening of preexisting cardiac conditions.

Alpha Adrenergic Agonists
Drugs such as clonidine (Catapres), typically used to treat hypertension, can be used as adjunctive treatment in certain

treatment-resistant cases of bipolar disorder. Side effects include hypotension and bradycardia in addition to fatigue and feelings of weakness.

Nonpharmacological Treatment

Electroconvulsive Therapy (ECT)

Commonly called "shock treatment," ECT has received bad press since it was introduced in the 1930s. Over the years, however, the technology has been improved, and it may now be safer than pharmacological intervention. ECT may be particularly beneficial for the following patients:

- Patients who need immediate stabilization of their condition and who cannot wait for medications to become effective
- Most patients with mania (it may be particularly useful for elderly patients with severe mania). Patients with suicidal thoughts and guilt during the depressive phase of bipolar disorder
- Patients with coexisting Parkinson's disease
- Patients who simply prefer ECT
- Pregnant patients
- Patients who cannot tolerate medications
- Patients with certain cardiac conditions

Repeated Transcranial Magnetic Stimulation (TMS)

TMS is a new and still experimental treatment for the depressive phase of bipolar disorder. In TMS, a large magnet is placed on the patient's head and magnetic fields of different frequency are generated to stimulate the left front cortex of the brain. Unlike ECT, TMS requires no anesthesia and does not induce seizures.

Psychotherapy

Psychotherapy is indicated for improving social and interpersonal relationships, supporting medication compliance, teaching techniques of stress management, and providing psychoeducation. In addition to supportive psychotherapy, cognitive behavioral therapy (CBT) in conjunction with psychopharmacological treatment may be beneficial in preventing relapses, alleviating symptoms, and promoting social functioning.

Typical goals of CBT for bipolar disorder include:

- Recognition of the prodromal phase of manic episodes before they become full-blown

- Modification or change of behaviors that could precipitate a manic episode
- Learning techniques for coping with depressive episodes by developing behaviors and thoughts that can modify or prevent the depression.

Other Nonpharmacological Treatment Strategies

The clinician also may recommend (and supply referrals when applicable) the following nonpharmacological treatment strategies.

Bipolar Support Groups. These self-help groups provide ongoing support to patients and their families. They also can provide sources of community and social support networks.

Optimizing Sleep Patterns. Educational activities related to techniques of sleep hygiene and relaxation training.

Substance Abuse Treatment. Initiate referral to treatment and rehabilitation programs for patients with alcohol and illicit drug abuse.

Monitoring and Grading Mood. This technique for helping patients to predict or recognize an impending episode uses a graph and diary to record and grade the effect of the patient's mental state on energy level and physical activity.

Interpersonal and Social Rhythm Therapy (IPSRT). Interpersonal conflicts and disruptions in daily routines or social rhythms may trigger a relapse in patients with bipolar disorder into mania or depression. IPSRT is a form of psychosocial treatment that focuses on minimizing these potential triggers.

Role of the Family

It is important to encourage family members to get involved in support groups in order to acquire coping and problem-solving skills. An important issue to address with the family is the need to initiate protective financial measures for both the family and the patient during manic episodes. The teaching of family coping techniques improves the patient's chances of treatment compliance.

Summary

In many patients with bipolar disorder, early episodes occur years apart. Episodes tend to occur more frequently with the passage of time, with associated worsening of functioning. Although some patients may experience only a single manic episode, most experience recurrent episodes. Between episodes, patients may be symptom-free, although many patients have some residual symptoms.

 Women with bipolar disorder tend to have more episodes of depression, whereas men tend to have more episodes of mania. Rapid-cycling bipolar disorder may develop over time and tends to be associated with poorer outcome.

Effective treatments of bipolar disorder now extend to several options that include various anticonvulsants and antipsychotics. Although lithium still has an important role, particularly in the classic treatment of bipolar disorder and relapse prevention, other FDA-approved agents are better tolerated and more efficacious for mixed states and rapid cycling. It is not uncommon to use combination therapy for the latter. The FDA has approved olanzapine, risperidone, quetiapine, ziprasidone, and aripiprazole in combination with lithium or divalproex for acute mania, and the combination medication of olanzapine and fluoxetine for acute bipolar depression. Maintenance treatments that have received FDA approval include olanzapine and lamotrigine. Off-label use of adjunctive medications may be required to target residual symptoms.

Bipolar disorder causes substantial psychosocial impairment, affecting multiple aspects of the patient's life, including interpersonal relationships and causing occupational and financial difficulties. These complications require adjunctive psychosocial and spiritual interventions, which will also involve family and significant others. By accurately identifying and diagnosing bipolar disorder, the ED clinician plays a pivotal and essential role in initiating urgent treatment and assuring maintenance and long term follow-up care. The various ED interventions and referrals will surely result in improving the long-term prognosis of this chronic and debilitating illness.

Further Reading

American Psychiatric Association. Diagnostic and Statistical Manual of Mental Disorders, 4th ed. Text Revision. Washington, DC. American Psychiatric Association, 2000, pp 181-190 and 345-428.

Bauer MS, Mitchner L: What is a "mood stabilizer"? An evidence-based response. Am J Psychiatry 2004;161:13-18.

Berrettini W: Bipolar disorder and schizophrenia: Convergent molecular data. Neuromolecular Med 2004;5:109-117.

Bowden C, Maier W: Bipolar disorder and personality disorder. Eur Psychiatry 2003;18:S9-S12.

Brieger P, Ehrt U, Marneros A: Frequency of comorbid personality disorders in bipolar and unipolar affective disorders. Compr Psychiatry 2003;44:28-34.

Citrome L, Goldberg JF: The many faces of bipolar disorder. How to tell them apart. Postgrad Med 2005;117:15-16, 19-23.

Ernst CL, Goldberg JF: Antisuicide properties of psychotropic drugs: A critical review. Harv Rev Psychiatry 2004;12:14-41.

Geddes JR, Burgess S, Hawton K, et al: Long-term lithium therapy for bipolar disorder: Systematic review and meta-analysis of randomized controlled trials. Am J Psychiatry 2004;161:217-222.

Geller B, Tillman R, Craney JL, et al: Four-year prospective outcome and natural history of mania in children with a prepubertal and early adolescent bipolar disorder phenotype. Arch Gen Psychiatry 2004;61:459-467.

Ghaemi SN, Boiman EE, Goodwin FK: Diagnosing bipolar disorder and the effect of antidepressants: A naturalistic study. J Clin Psychiatry 2000;61:804-808.

Gijsman HJ, Geddes JR, Rendell JM, et al: Antidepressants for bipolar depression: A systematic review of randomized, controlled trials. Am J Psychiatry 2004;161:1537-1547.

Goldberg JF, Citrome L: Latest therapies for bipolar disorder. Looking beyond lithium. Postgrad Med 2005;117:25-26, 29-32, 35-36.

Goldberg JF, Harrow M, Sands JR: Lithium therapy in the longitudinal course of bipolar disorder. Psychiatr Ann 1996;26:651-658.

Hirschfeld RM, Calabrese JR, Weissman MM, et al: Screening for bipolar disorder in the community. J Clin Psychiatry 2003;64:53-59.

Judd LL, Akiskal HS, Schettler PJ, et al: A prospective investigation of the natural history of the long-term weekly symptomatic status of bipolar II disorder. Arch Gen Psychiatry 2003;60:261-269.

Kafantaris V, Coletti DJ, Dicker R, et al: Lithium treatment of acute mania in adolescents: A placebo-controlled discontinuation study. J Am Acad Child Adolesc Psychiatry 2004;43:984-993.

Keck PE Jr, McElroy SL, Havens JR, et al: Psychosis in bipolar disorder: Phenomenology and impact on morbidity and course of illness. Compr Psychiatry 2003;44:263-269.

Khouzam HR, Emery PE, Reaves B: Secondary mania in late life. J Am Geriatr Soc 1994;42:85-87.

Regier DA, Farmer ME, Rae DS, et al: Comorbidity of mental disorders with alcohol and other drug abuse: Results from the Epidemiologic Catchment Area (ECA) Study. JAMA 1990;264:2511-2518.

Sachs GS, Printz DJ, Kahn DA, et al: The Expert Consensus Guideline Series: Medication Treatment of Bipolar Disorder 2000. Minneapolis: McGraw-Hill Healthcare Information Group, 2000:1-104 (Postgrad Med: A Special Report, Apr 2000).

Tohen M, Vieta E, Calabrese J, et al: Efficacy of olanzapine and olanzapine-fluoxetine combination in the treatment of bipolar I depression. Arch Gen Psychiatry 2003;60:1079-1088.

Other Resources

Lithium Information Center, 7617 Mineral Point Rd, Suite 300, Madison, WI 53717. Tel: 608-827-2470. General information is provided over the phone; literature searches on specific topics cost a nominal fee. The center also publishes many patient guides and reference books.

National Alliance for the Mentally Ill (NAMI), 200 N. Glebe Rd., Arlington, VA 22203-3754. Tel: 800-950-6264 (http://www.nami.org/). NAMI is a national grass roots organization providing ways for self-help and support organizations to help individuals and families of people with psychological disorders.

National Depressive and Manic-Depressive Association, 730 N. Franklin St., Suite 501, Chicago, Ill. 60610. Tel: 800-826-3632; 312-642-0049 (http://www.ndmda.org/). Makes referrals to local support services and offers a free information package.

National Foundation for Depressive Illness, PO Box 2257, New York, NY 10116. Tel: 800-239-1265; 212-268-4260 (http://www.depression.org/).

National Institute of Mental Health, D/ART (Depression Awareness, Recognition, and Treatment) Program, Room 15-C-05, 5600 Fishers Lane, Rockville, MD 20857. Tel: 800-421-4211 (http://www.nimh.nih.gov/).

National Mental Health Association, 1021 Prince St., Alexandria, VA 22314-2971. Tel: 703/684-7722 or the Mental Health Information Line (800-969-6642) (http://www.nmha.org/). This organization can supply the names and numbers of regional chapters and provides information on two hundred mental health topics.

POSTSCRIPT

When you have eliminated the impossible, whatever remains, however improbable, must be the truth.
Sir Arthur Conan Doyle—1859-1930

CHAPTER 9

The Violent Patient

Tirath S. Gill, MD

KEY POINTS

- Examine the chart for history of assault, incarceration, psychiatric illness, ongoing medical problems, substance abuse, and allergies.
- Look for abnormal vital signs and try to determine the cause.
- Treat patients with respect and let them know that you are there to help resolve the cause of their anger.
- Have an exit available, keep a safe distance from the patient, and have security personnel present to thwart and prevent aggressive behavior toward yourself or others.
- Do not try to verbally de-escalate a patient with signs of increasing hostility or paranoia.

Overview (Fig. 9-1)

The violent patient can be a diagnostic and management challenge for the emergency department (ED) clinician. Violent behavior can have many causes. These include medication, alcohol, and substance abuse and primary psychiatric disorders.

To arrive at a suitable plan of intervention, it is useful, when feasible, to observe the patient, perform a physical examination, and review any laboratory data. Following the initial assessment and acute stabilization of the patient, decisions must be made regarding hospitalization and the duty to warn any potential victims of threats.

Epidemiology

Several studies report a higher prevalence of violence among patients with mental illness and substance abuse. This risk may

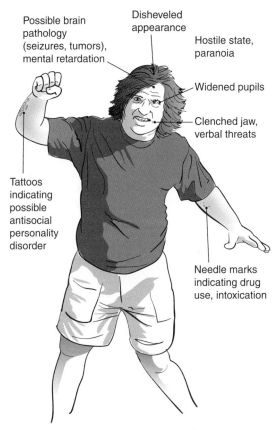

Possible brain pathology (seizures, tumors), mental retardation

Disheveled appearance

Hostile state, paranoia

Widened pupils

Clenched jaw, verbal threats

Tattoos indicating possible antisocial personality disorder

Needle marks indicating drug use, intoxication

The Violent Patient
Aggressive posture
Pacing
Clenched fists

FIGURE 9–1

The violent patient.

be two to four times that in the normal population. Violent behavior in itself, however, does not automatically imply the presence of mental illness or substance abuse.

The Neurochemistry of Aggression

The underlying neurochemistry of aggression is not totally clear, but studies indicate a possible role for low serotonin levels in the central nervous system. Patients that exhibit violence have been noted to have low levels of 5-HIAA (a serotonin metabolite) in their cerebrospinal fluid. Subtle aberrations in the levels of acetylcholine, gamma-aminobutyric acid (GABA), norepinephrine, and dopamine may have a role in aggression as well.

Some women may have a tendency for aggressive behaviors during certain periods of the menstrual cycle. Anabolic steroids and androgens used in competitive sports and body-building regimens may also lead to violent and aggressive behaviors.

Assessment

Interviewing the Violent Patient

Before the ED clinician proceeds with the interview, the patient should be screened by security personnel for any weapons or articles that could be used as weapons. The presence of another staff member is recommended. The clinician should convey a sense of control and self-assurance while speaking respectfully to the patient.

When beginning the interview, the following sequence is recommended:
- Introduce yourself and reassure the patient that you will try to identify and resolve the cause of his or her distress.
- Restate the problem as you understand it and ask any clarifying questions in an empathetic and nonjudgmental tone.
- Ask about physical distress, hunger, and thirst; supply pain relief, food, and liquids as needed. This helps to build trust and an alliance with the patient.

It is important to ascertain the level of risk of violence during the first few minutes of the interview, as evidenced by the level of psychomotor activity and signs of escalation such as clenching of the jaw or hands, straightening of the spine, pacing, cursing, and verbal threats. This may progress to knocking over furniture, slamming doors, invasion of personal space, punching, kicking, or assault in other ways such as biting, pulling, and choking.

Prudence and good sense are advisable; it is dangerous to carry on a lengthy interview with a potentially violent patient. The salient and necessary details should be obtained, and a more detailed assessment can be made when the patient is calmer and poses less of a risk.

If the patient expresses thoughts of harming a specific person, that person should be informed so that protective measures can be instituted.

When possible, it is useful to obtain collateral information from the family, friends, and other personnel who may know the patient.

Handling an Attack by the Violent Patient

If you are attacked, it is important to deflect kicks and punches away from vital body areas, call for help, and flee if necessary to save yourself from injury. If you are caught in a chokehold, consciousness may be lost in as little as 20 seconds, and urgent action is mandatory. To free yourself, tuck in your chin to protect the airway, shout loudly to startle the patient, stomp on the arch of the patient's foot, apply other aversive physical stimuli to break the hold, and strike the panic button, if one is available. In short, you may do whatever is needed short of mortal injury if the attack is life-threatening and no escape is possible.

 To a large degree, the presence of security personnel and other staff and interviewing the patient in an open area and behind a barrier will prevent such mishaps. Most fatal attacks on clinicians have occurred when the previous recommendations were ignored, and the clinician was alone with the patient in the room and failed to take some basic precautions.

Laboratory Studies

The laboratory workup should include a urine drug screen, a chemistry panel, complete blood count (CBC), and urinalysis. The decision to do other laboratory tests should be dictated by the history and physical examination.

Assessment and Differential Diagnosis

The clinician must be sensitive when making the diagnosis to the fact that aggressive and impulsive behaviors have varied and complex causes and manifestations. For example, the manic patient tends to be talkative, loud, and labile and often sarcastic and demanding, whereas the schizophrenic patient may show disorganization in thought and speech and reveal a paranoid and bizarre delusional belief system. The intoxicated patient may reveal an odor of alcohol or signs of drug abuse such as needle marks, nystagmus, and tremor.

The medical workup is an important part of the diagnostic assessment and should include a physical examination, if possible, and review of vital signs and the medical history. The medically compromised patient may show signs of a specific medical illness such as cyanosis or jaundice or nonspecific signs such as wandering focus, fluctuating levels of alertness, and abnormal vital signs.

Psychiatric illnesses also should be considered in the differential diagnosis. Violent behaviors are associated most frequently with bipolar disorder, psychotic states with prominent paranoia, active hallucinations, posttraumatic stress disorder (PTSD), and certain personality disorders in the Cluster B spectrum, which are characterized by antisocial, narcissistic, borderline, and histrionic patterns of relating to others (Table 9-1). More than one of these traits may be present in a patient.

Depression may be associated with violence towards others, and this risk is increased if psychotic features are present, as may be the case with postpartum depression and severe major depression with nihilistic delusions.

A prior history of violent episodes is a strong predictor of future violence and should be given due weight when determining disposition of the patient. The combination of a personality disorder, substance and alcohol abuse, and major mental illness increases the risk of violence in a cumulative manner.

In addition to the above-mentioned psychiatric conditions, violent behaviors also are associated with developmental disabilities and dementia of any cause, but especially that related to orbitofrontal pathology or right-sided strokes. Substance withdrawal, delirium, delusional disorder, acute emotional trauma, and adjustment disorders may be implicated at times.

Table 9–1

Some Psychiatric Disorders and Drug Intoxications Associated with Violent Behaviors

Diagnosis	Clinical Features	Physical Signs and Symptoms	Intervention
Cocaine intoxication	Rapid speech, paranoia, agitation, impulsive acting out, formication, and ritualized behaviors.	Lesions in the nose such as ulceration, bleeding, burn marks on lips from crack pipes, skin infection at injection sites	Rest; monitor for suicidal acting out and assault; may need emergency medication
Amphetamine intoxication	Similar to cocaine; agitation may be of longer duration; paranoid delusions and tics; obsessive ritualized behaviors such as picking up specks of dirt and lint from the ground or furniture.	Patches of reddened skin caused by skin picking related to formication	Low-potency antipsychotic such as Thorazine or one of the atypical antipsychotics such as quetiapine or olanzapine; long-term treatment with antipsychotics usually not necessary if the patient abstains
Alcohol withdrawal	History of alcoholism, odor of alcohol on breath	Elevated vital signs, tremors; severe withdrawal may lead to disorientation, ophthalmoplegia, ataxia, symptoms of Wernicke's syndrome and delirium tremens	Thiamine, 100 mg IV or IM, if patient is being fed parenterally, to avoid acute thiamine deficiency; benzodiazepine is a safe detoxification strategy

Continued

Table 9-1

Some Psychiatric Disorders and Drug Intoxications Associated with Violent Behaviors—cont'd

Diagnosis	Clinical Features	Physical Signs and Symptoms	Intervention
Alcohol intoxication	Excessively talkative, grandiose, irritable, over-friendly or boorish	Elevated blood alcohol level, ataxia; with increasing level of intoxication, stupor, coma, and death may ensue	Verbal de-escalation; thiamine and folic acid; monitor vital signs along with supportive measures as indicated
Anticholinergic toxicity	Disoriented, visual hallucinations, loud and rambling speech	Classic signs of elevated temperature ("hot as a hare"), elevated pulse due to vagal blockade, flushed appearance ("red as a beet") and apparent responses to internal stimuli ("mad as a wet hen")	Physostigmine, 1-2 mg IM; cholinergic toxicity possible; also, risk of arrhythmia; otherwise conservative supportive measures are indicated
Schizophrenia	Catatonic features; active auditory hallucinations and paranoia; disheveled, guarded appearance	Malnutrition, comorbid substance abuse and intoxication or withdrawal	Antipsychotic agent such as Risperdal, 1-2 mg, along with lorazepam, 1-2 mg, may help to calm acutely psychotic patient
Manic disorder	Overdressed, flamboyant; excessively talkative, with flight of ideas	Signs of exhaustion; sometimes calluses and sores on feet from excessive walking; signs of venereal disease	Olanzapine, 20-30 mg acutely, with anticonvulsant or lithium; lorazepam may be added for sedation

Diagnosis	Clinical Features	Physical Signs and Symptoms	Intervention
Antisocial personality	May have ulterior motives for seeking admission; may present with features of malingered illness	A higher likelihood of prison tattoos; features of substance intoxication	Security personnel may need to be called in; legal prosecution of violent acts or threats may be a suitable option
Narcissistic personality disorder	Sense of entitlement; demand for special treatment	May wear colorful clothing, expensive jewelry	Low-dose benzodiazepines; respectful interactions in attempt to problem-solve
Histrionic personality disorder	Exaggerated style of expression; attention-catching clothing	No specific signs; may act out on threats of impulse and should not be ignored	Low-dose benzodiazepines; supportive and respectful interactions
Borderline personality disorder	Acutely dysphoric and angry or psychotic when anger or stress is extreme	Scars on arms or legs related to prior attempts at cutting or burning self	Antipsychotic such as Risperdal, 1-2 mg, along with a benzodiazepine for acute agitation
Delirium due to medical causes	Disoriented; may be responding to internal stimuli	Elevated or suppressed vital signs, abnormal neurologic findings	Discontinue any offending medications; treat underlying medical cause; haloperidol, 2-5 mg PO, with lorazepam, 1-2 mg PO or IV, to control agitation

IM, intramuscularly; IV, intravenously; PO, by mouth.

Acute Management

After the clinician has determined what medications have helped in the past, the patient can be offered a choice of oral medications. If oral medication is refused and there is persistent danger from agitation, the patient can be treated with a combination of an antipsychotic and lorazepam given intramuscularly (IM). A list of these agents is included in Table 9-2. Any benzodiazepine can be given orally, but only lorazepam is reliably absorbed by the intramuscular route. Lorazepam can be given IM in a dose of 1 to 3 mg, depending on the patient's size and body habitus and the level of agitation. It is important to note that intramuscular lorazepam is contraindicated if the patient is taking clozapine, as there have been some cases of respiratory arrest and death with this combination. Its use should also be avoided if alcohol levels are increased or if other sedative hypnotic intoxication is suspected.

Used in conjunction with lorazepam, oral and intramuscular antipsychotics may be particularly useful in the violent psychotic or manic patient. These agents include haloperidol (Haldol), 5 to 10 mg by mouth (PO) or IM, and fluphenazine (Prolixin), 2.5 to 5 mg PO or IM. The dose may be repeated every half hour to 45 minutes if needed, and may be combined with benztropine (Cogentin), 1 to 2 mg PO, or diphenhydramine (Benadryl), 50 mg PO, to prevent stiffness, tremor, and other extrapyramidal syndrome (EPS) side effects. Diphenhydramine is preferable because it is less expensive and may provide greater sedation. Anticholinergics, should be avoided if the agitation is suspected to be related to anticholinergic toxicity. A common strategy is to use a combination of haloperidol or Prolixin, 5 mg, combined with diphenhydramine, 50 mg, and lorazepam, 1 to 2 mg, given PO or IM.

Atypical antipsychotics have become available for intramuscular use and have proved their efficacy. However, they tend to be expensive and may not be readily available in the ED.

One example is ziprasidone (Geodon), 20 mg IM. Clinical experience indicates that it is an effective agent for short-term control of agitation. Another atypical agent available for parenteral use is olanzapine. It is available for injection in 10-mg vials. The peak blood levels in the first hour with intramuscular olanzapine are four to five times higher than with oral olanzapine and provide strong level of sedation and some genuine antipsychotic and antimanic effects. Other agents that are equally

Table 9-2

Medications for Violent Behaviors

Medication	Usual Dose	Comments
Ziprasidone (Geodon)	20 mg IM	Very helpful in sedating agitated patients
Olanzapine (Zyprexa)	10 mg IM Rapid-dissolving Zydis tablets, 5 mg, 10 mg, 15 mg, and 20 mg	Olanzapine, 5 mg IM, may be equivalent to Zydis, 20 mg PO
Haloperidol (Haldol)	5 mg IM or 10 mg PO, given with lorazepam, 2 mg PO or IM, and diphenhydramine (Benadryl), 50 mg PO or IM	May be repeated at 45-minute intervals if significant agitation persists
Fluphenazine (Prolixin)	2.5-5 mg IM combined with lorazepam, 2 mg PO or IM, and diphenhydramine, 50 mg PO or IM	May be repeated at 45-minute intervals if significant agitation persists
Lorazepam (Ativan)	1-2 mg PO or IM for mild agitation	May be combined with an antipsychotic for greater efficacy in treating psychotic, manic, and borderline personality disorders
Chlorpromazine (Librium)	50-100 mg IM or PO as tablet or concentrate	Injection site may be painful; risk of fall in blood pressure, dizziness (orthostatic), and anticholinergic side effects
Quetiapine (Seroquel)	50- and 100-mg tablets; parenteral form not available	May help to calm some patients; risk of orthostasis as with chlorpromazine; minimal extrapyramidal and anticholinergic effects

IM, intramuscularly; PO, by mouth.

effective include oral risperidone liquid or its rapid-dissolving M-tabs, and Zyprexa Zydis, a rapidly dissolving formulation of olanzapine.

If the patient is somewhat cooperative, intravenous or intramuscular droperidol may be used for acute agitation. However, its use in psychiatry has fallen out of favor and it is now mostly used in anesthesiology. Droperidol does carry some risk of QTc prolongation and it should be avoided if patient has cardiac conduction delay or is taking other agents that may have similar effects on cardiac conduction. Its calming effects tend to wear off within the hour.

Acute management of the violent patient may also involve seclusion, restraints, and other medications to calm the patient (see Chapter 3 for guidelines in this regard).

Long-Term Management

Long-term management of the violent patient is predicated on accurate diagnosis and specific treatment of the manifested symptom complex.

For the depressed patient, antidepressants including tricyclic agents and serotonin reuptake inhibitors (SSRIs) may be useful. There is evidence that SSRIs may increase thoughts of violence toward oneself and others in the first few weeks of therapy, and close monitoring during this period is warranted. Some role for decreasing aggressive and impulsive behaviors may be present in these agents independent of their antidepressant effects.

Lithium has been used to reduce aggression, and classic trials among prison inmates indicate an efficacy for impulsive aggression independent of the drug's antimanic effects. Anticonvulsants have been used with some success in reducing impulsivity and aggression.

Gabapentin (Neurontin) has had mixed reviews but has been noted to be of benefit in some cases for mood stabilization. Double-blinded trials, however, have not shown a significant effect of treatment of the bipolar spectrum disorders for which it was initially used. Gabapentin has been reported to be of some benefit to lessen anxiety and impulsivity associated with borderline personality disorder.

The nonbenzodiazepine anxiolytic buspirone (BuSpar) has been used as an agent at times for depression, anxiety, agitation, and aggression.

Beta-blockers have been used to treat aggression. Propranolol (Inderal) has been used for aggressive behaviors related to akathisia in low doses of 10 to 20 mg PO three to four times a day. The dose requires upward titration to avoid side effects such as slowing of the heart rate and dizziness related to decrease in blood pressure. It has been used at gradually titrated higher doses in cases of impulsivity related to brain injury and in patients with intermittent explosive disorder. Doses up to 1000 mg in divided doses have been used. Tapering of dosage is necessary before discontinuing administration of beta-blockers such as propranolol to avoid rebound symptoms such as tachycardia and anxiety.

Beta- and alpha-blockers appear to be useful in some cases of nightmares associated with PTSD and for impulsivity in dementia. Beta-blockers that have been used for the chronically violent patient include oral nadolol, 40 to 120 mg/day, and metoprolol, 200 to 300 mg/day. Clonidine and guanfacine may also be useful for some patients.

Benzodiazepines such as clonazepam may be helpful in some cases of impulsive aggression. Disinhibition has been reported as a side effect of benzodiazepine therapy; if this occurs, it should be noted in the patient history and in the future, use of benzodiazepines should be avoided.

Psychostimulants may be of some use for impulsive aggression in children with attention deficit disorder (ADD) and attention deficit hyperactivity disorder (ADHD). It may also be of some use for symptoms of residual ADHD in adults; bupropion and desipramine also have been used for this disorder with benefit for some patients.

Nonpharmacological Therapy

Referral to anger management programs using psychotherapeutic approaches is helpful. In these programs, patients learn nonviolent techniques for self-assertion, such as expressing their frustration and distress verbally instead of physically and examining their thoughts and dissociating them from automatic behavioral responses. Patients in anger management groups may have untreated psychiatric disorders that can be helped with appropriate medications.

Group therapy with others who are trying to deal with anger issues may also be useful. Such therapy, however, should not be used in isolation from psychiatric assessment of other possible causes of violent behavior, such as paranoia and bipolar disorder with manic impulsivity.

The legal consequences of threats and violent acts may be deterrents over the long term.

Summary

The combination of medication and psychotherapy may be more effective than either modality alone. Long-term management of the patient with a tendency toward violence hinges on a seamless continuity of care between different caregivers, use of long-acting depot medications, and case management. Follow-up of missed appointments and encouragement of treatment compliance can avoid much misery for the patient and those that may become the targets of their violence.

Further Reading

Albert JE, Spellman MK: Psychotherapeutic approaches to aggressive and violent patients. Psychiatr Clin North Am 1997;20:453-472.

Awalt RM, Reilly PM, Shopshire MS: The angry patient: An intervention for managing anger and substance abuse treatment. J Psychoactive Drugs 1997;29:353-358.

Balaban E, Alper JS, Kasamon YL: Mean genes and the biology of aggression: A critical review of recent animal and human research. J. Neurogenet 1996;11:1-43.

Blue HC, Griffith EE: Sociocultural and therapeutic perspectives on violence. Psychiatr Clin North Am 1995;18:571-587.

Gerberich SG, Church TR, McGovern PM, et al: Risk factors for work-related assaults on nurses. Epidemiology 2005;16:704-709.

Lee SS, Gerberich SG, Waller LA, et al: Work-related assault injuries among nurses. Epidemiology 1999;10:685-691.

Skeem J, Schubert C, Stowman S, et al: Gender and risk assessment accuracy: Underestimating women's violence potential. Law Hum Behav 2005;29:173-186.

Skeem JL, Mulvey EP, Odgers C, et al: What do clinicians expect? Comparing envisioned and reported violence for male and female patients. J Consult Clin Psychol 2005;73:599-609.

Zun LS, Downey L: The use of seclusion in emergency medicine. Gen Hosp Psychiatry 2005;27:365-371.

CHAPTER 10

The Acutely Psychotic Patient

Doris T. Tan, DO

KEY POINTS

- Psychosis presenting in the emergency department (ED) can have many etiologies, including substance-induced toxicity, medical conditions, and psychiatric disorders.
- Proper emergency interventions and treatment can assist the patient's own handling of the crisis.
- The ED clinician may require the help of family members, who can supply collateral information, and of the patient's outpatient provider in baseline assessment of the patient.
- It is essential that medications are on hand for emergent calming and immediate crisis intervention so that patients can participate in their own evaluation and treatment.
- Plans for disposition of the patient following intervention should be discussed and finalized.

Definitions

The term psychosis implies a marked impairment in reality testing. This can be due to a myriad of medical problems and psychiatric disorders. In general, the threshold for psychosis is reached due to mounting stressors that exceed the person's ability to cope and to the breakdown of emotional boundaries. Following are definitions of some common manifestations of impaired reality:

Hallucinations. Abnormal sensations perceived in the absence of external stimuli. Hallucinations are usually auditory, less often visual, and even less commonly tactile and olfactory.

Delusions. Firmly held false beliefs generally due to incorrect inference of reality; for example, a patient believes that several policemen, the mayor, and the governor are waiting in the driveway in order to catch her doing something illegal in order to remove her from the community.

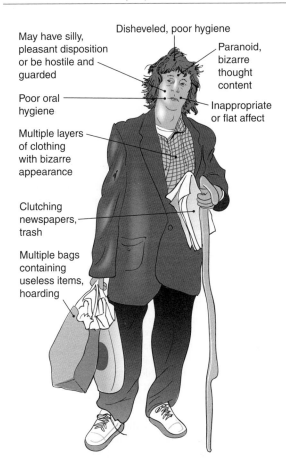

The Homeless Psychotic Patient
May be brought into the ED from the community due
to bizarre behaviors or agitation

FIGURE 10–1

The psychotic patient.

Thought disorder. A disturbance in the form or organization of thought. Types of thought disorder include flight of ideas (going from one subject to another, unrelated subject), thought blocking (completely blocking the topic at hand), perseveration (repetition of a thought pattern or of a subject even after the conversation is over), incoherence or "word salad" (stringing words together in phrases that do not make any sense ("some sky create tomorrow headphone"), and paranoia (believes others are out to harm them).

Evaluation of the Psychotic Patient

In order to properly triage psychotic patients in the ED, the clinician should determine whether the psychotic episode is an acute presentation or a manifestation of a chronic disorder. The patient's primary outpatient provider, if one is available, should be contacted to determine the patient's baseline presentation and whether there have been any recent changes in treatment that might have caused or precipitated the episode.

Collateral information from family members can be useful. If possible, the clinician should obtain the patient's written consent to gather information from the patient's family. In a life-threatening situation, this consent could be waived.

 A medical evaluation may be necessary before decisions are made about treatment, especially in patients presenting with acute-onset psychosis. Such patients may have a reversible medical condition such as delirium and its many causes. Often, symptomatic treatment must precede evaluation and diagnosis (see Chapter 3 for discussion of medications used in psychiatric emergencies).

The clinician should decide whether the patient will require a temporary hold for further psychiatric evaluation. Most states allow a 72-hour civil commitment for such evaluations (see Chapter 23 for details).

Hospitalization may be necessary, based on one or more of the following criteria:
- The patient is dangerous to self or others.
- The patient is unable to care for self (e.g., regarding adequate food, clothing, and shelter) due to impaired judgment or to extreme crisis or distress.
- Past treatment failures or resistance to treatment leading to the patient experiencing exacerbation of a chronic psychosis.
- The patient is severely intoxicated.

- Hospitalization is necessary to determine a particularly difficult diagnosis.

Disorders Causing Psychosis Commonly Seen in the ED

Psychosis can be due to medical reasons, such as seizure disorders (see Chapter 16); delirium (see Chapter 5); infections, neoplasms, endocrinopathies, and CNS lesions (see Chapter 4); alcohol abuse (see Chapter 14); and drug abuse (see Chapter 15). Psychoses induced by over-the-counter (OTC) medications and some "street drugs" are described here, as well as psychotic disorders commonly seen in the ED.

Drug-Induced Psychosis

Phencyclidine (PCP)
PCP is a hallucinogen often sprinkled in smoking materials such as tobacco or marijuana. At lower doses, it may produce euphoria and illusions. At higher doses, it may produce symptoms of psychosis such as delusions, paranoia, catatonia, hallucinations, a sense of being distant from one's environment, and disordered thought. At even higher doses, muscular hypertonicity, myoclonus, and ataxia may occur. Seizure is an unusual presentation; hypertension, hyperthermia, and coma may result. The excessive salivation (sialorrhea) seen in PCP users may distinguish its use from that of other hallucinogens. Hallucinations, as if in a flashback, have been reported to recur periodically up to a year later, when PCP ingestion is repeated.

Initial intervention includes reduction of anxiety with benzodiazepines and treatment of seizures, if they occur. Drug-related psychosis resulting from a small amount of PCP generally resolves without medication, but haloperidol may be administered if necessary. In cases of overdose, gastric lavage should be used to reduce drug levels as PCP may have gastroenteric circulation (excreted into the stomach and when re-alkalinized in the duodenum is reabsorbed). Support life-functioning with glucose, hydration, and respiratory aid as needed.

Ketamine
Ketamine use is on the rise. It is one of the choice drugs used at rave clubs and often is sold as Ecstasy. It is a dissociative anesthetic used in both humans and animals.

Its effects are similar to those of PCP but with a shorter duration. It can produce hallucinations, dissociation from sensory perceptions, mood changes, and outright psychosis. It is tasteless and odorless and has been used in drinks to cause sedation and amnesia in sexual assaults.

MDMA (3,4-methylene dioxymethamphetamine)

MDMA, commonly known as Ecstasy, is one of the most popular club drugs, especially at rave clubs. It has properties that produce the autonomic hyperactivity of both amphetamines and hallucinogens. MDMA intoxication can quickly progress to become a medical emergency. This drug has a rapid release of serotonin and probably also inhibits serotonin reuptake. Due to autonomic hyperactivity, cardiac arrhythmias and hypertension are common. Hyperthermia due to catecholamine surges may occur.

The intense heat generated by dancing and crowding increases body temperature, enhancing the effects of MDMA and resulting in increased dehydration and possibly severe hyperthermia. Strokes, renal failure, rhabdomyolysis, and heart failure are other adverse effects associated with MDMA intoxication. The most severe psychiatric manifestation is paranoia, followed by anxiety, depression, confusion, and sleep problems. Long-term use of MDMA may cause memory loss and depression.

LSD (Lysergic Acid Diethylamide)

The effects of LSD include mood shifts, time and space distortions, synesthesia ("seeing" sounds and "hearing" colors), and impulsive behavior that may progress to pyschosis. Although LSD users rarely land in the ED, when psychosis is severe, such individuals may present with symptoms of paranoia and aggression.

Treatment may consist of measures to decrease patients' anxiety and perhaps placing them in a safe environment until the effects of LSD have diminished. There have been reports of patients dying because of distorted thought patterns caused by LSD (e.g., trying to stop a train with one's bare hands).

Dextromethorphan (DXM)

DXM, an ingredient in numerous OTC cough and cold medications, is a cough suppressant and antitussive; it has no significant analgesic or sedative properties. Its mechanism of action is unknown, but it has been shown to increase serotonin surges and is thought to have activities as a glutamate and NMDA antagonist; also it may increase dopamine levels by blocking its reuptake.

Medications containing DXM are popular among adolescents and young adults seeking a "high." A 4-oz bottle of generic cough syrup contains about 240 mg of DXM. DXM is safe in the 20-mg doses recommended for treating coughs or colds; however, in large doses, it can cause hallucinations and feelings of unreality.

Lower, "recreational" doses (up to 90 mg) result in euphoria and feelings of dissociation. Doses of 200 mg may have stimulant effects and signs and symptoms such as confusion, dilated pupils, and altered perception of time. Higher doses of up to 500 mg can cause feelings of drunkenness or of being "stoned," similar to the effects of ketamine. Higher doses of up to 1000 mg can cause central nervous system (CNS) perceptual abnormalities such as hallucinations, dissociative feelings, and thought disturbance. Doses higher than 1000 mg can cause outright dissociation.

Chronic use does not seem to cause physiologic dependence; hence there are no withdrawal symptoms. However, craving does occur, creating a subjective desire for the drug and psychological dependence. Please refer to Chapter 15 for other illicit substances (e.g., cocaine) that may also cause psychosis.

Mood Disorders

Bipolar Disorder

Psychosis is a common symptom in both the manic phase and the depressed phase of bipolar disorder (see Chapter 8). Patients often present with grandiose delusions. Psychosis may also be a manifestation of a severe depressive episode. The patient may have paranoid ideation and command or persecutory hallucinations and may pose a danger to self and others. In addition, the depressive episode may fit the criteria for major depression with psychotic features.

Schizoaffective Disorder

Schizoaffective disorder is defined as an uninterrupted period of illness during which there is a major depressive, manic, or mixed episode concurrent with symptoms that meet the first criteria for schizophrenia in the *Diagnostic and Statistical Manual of Mental Disorders, 4th Edition, Text Revision* (DSM-IV-TR). See Box 10-1, criteria A.

During their illness, when patients are euthymic (not manic or depressed), they experience psychotic symptoms for a period of at least 2 weeks. These psychotic symptoms include two or more of the following: delusions, hallucinations, disorganized speech, grossly disorganized behavior, catatonia, and negative symptoms such as alogia, avolition, and affective flattening.

Treatment depends on the predominant presentation. It is recommended that patients receive both mood stabilizers and treatment for psychotic symptoms.

Noncompliance with medication occurs often in this patient population, and hospitalization may be necessary.

Major Depressive Disorder with Psychotic Features

Hallucinations or delusions are present in the context of this depressive disorder. Generally, psychosis will recur when the patient experiences another episode of depression. Hallucinations typically are auditory, and delusions and hallucinations are mostly mood-congruent in theme. When the delusions and hallucinations are not mood-congruent, they may consist of thought broadcasting or other ideas of reference. Mood-incongruent psychosis in the setting of a major depression carries a poor prognosis.

Treatment consists of antidepressants and antipsychotics combined. When the psychosis has subsided, a trial of discontinuation of antipsychotics may begin, but antidepressant therapy should be continued for at least 6 to 12 months.

Electroconvulsive therapy (ECT) has been found to be useful, especially in cases resistant to psychopharmacologic treatment. Transcranial magnetic stimulation (TMS) is another method that is currently being studied as a possible treatment option, and at the time of this writing is not yet approved by the U.S. Food and Drug Administration.

Delusional Disorders

A *bizarre* delusion is a belief that is clearly implausible. For example, a patient believes that the entire room is charged with lethal electrical current and only an alien implanted by the patient prevents this electricity from electrocuting every living thing in the room.

Delusional disorders, in contrast, accompany *non-bizarre* delusions—they are possible but highly improbable beliefs. For example, a patient believes that he has been implicated in sexual molestation of a child in the neighborhood but does not know who this child is. He may present to the ED fearing for his life due to the belief that the neighborhood has collected a reward fund and has asked the Mafia to kill him and that the police are after him to collect this reward.

Delusional disorders are notoriously difficult to treat even with antipsychotics. Long-term psychotherapy is usually recommended.

Schizotypal Personality Disorder

Patients with schizotypal personality disorder usually present to the ED with symptoms of depression, anxiety, and obsessive-compulsive behavior. At times, they may suffer from a brief psychotic episode (see the following section).

Their appearance may be odd, with eccentric behaviors, and they may have perceptual distortions, odd thinking, and beliefs such as magical thinking (the belief that events are not objectively determined but mediated by their own thoughts, wishes, and actions). They have discomfort with, and reduced capacity for, close relationships. Occasionally, their symptoms fit the criteria for brief psychotic disorder.

Temporary antipsychotics may be required for acute symptoms, but hospitalization is rarely needed. Outpatient psychotherapy is usually recommended.

Brief Psychotic Disorder

Brief psychotic disorder is a short-term (1 day to 1 month) time-limited disorder in which the psychosis completely remits and the patient returns to a premorbid level of functioning. Treatment may include hospitalization if the symptoms fit the DSM-IV-TR criteria, which may include delusions, hallucinations, disorganized speech, grossly disorganized behavior, and catatonic behavior. A short course of benzodiazepines may be useful to reduce anxiety. Antipsychotics for symptomatic treatment may be justified, but if long-term use is necessary, then reevaluation of the diagnosis is warranted.

Schizophreniform Disorder

Schizophreniform disorder is characterized by a first-break onset of psychotic episode for at least 1 month but less than 6 months in duration; its symptoms fit the DSM-IV-TR criteria (see Box 10-1, criteria A) under Schizophrenia. As in the case of brief psychotic disorder, patients return to baseline functioning after the initial episode.

Treatment usually requires hospitalization to ensure a safe environment, especially for patients with catatonia. Antipsychotics may be necessary, and occasionally ECT may be required. Patients generally respond well to antipsychotic therapy.

The risk for depression and suicide rate is high in patients following resolution of the psychosis. Thus psychotherapy is recommended to help patients deal with their illness.

A first-break psychotic episode is a very frightening experience. Family support and understanding is important in this period and may help in attaining the best possible outcome. The family is the clinician's best resource for ensuring compliance and effective treatment.

Schizophrenia

No single pathognomonic symptom leads clinicians to conclude that the patient sitting in front of them is suffering from this devastating illness. Generally a myriad of symptoms hinders the patient's social, interpersonal, and occupational functioning. These symptoms are broadly categorized into two types: positive (meaning "in excess of," "in addition to," or "plus") symptoms and negative (meaning "deficit in" or "lacking") symptoms.

Positive Symptoms
- Hallucinations—auditory (hearing voices or noises), visual (seeing people, animals or objects), olfactory, (smell), tactile (touch).
- Delusions—persecutory, religious or grandiose, somatic or guilt-ridden, thought broadcasting, thought insertion (the belief that one's thoughts are not really one's own but have been placed in one's mind by an external force).
- Positive thought disorder, disorganized speech— derailment (loosening of association, deviation of the train

of thought without totally blocking it), circumstantiality (disturbance in the thought process by details that are often tangential and irrelevant), tangentiality (switching rapidly from one topic under discussion to other topics that arise through association), clanging (thinking driven by word sounds; e.g., rhyming or punning may give the appearance of logical connections, when in fact none exist), illogia (illogical conclusions), incoherence.

- Bizarre behaviors—repetitive, stereotyped, aggressive, agitated; odd clothing, wearing multiple layers of clothing not appropriate for the temperature, odd social or sexual behaviors. Behaviors may be catatonic as well as disorganized (see Fig. 10-1).

Negative Symptoms

- Affective flattening—nearly absent or markedly diminished emotionality with hypoprosody (absence of stress, pitch, and rhythm in speech).
- Avolition—a general lack of desire, motivation.
- Anhedonia—inability to gain pleasure from normally pleasurable activities; often associated with depression.
- Apathy and social withdrawal, poverty of thought or speech.

In order to fit the DSM-IV-TR criteria for schizophrenia, the patient must have at least two of the characteristic symptoms shown in Box 10-1. Also, the duration of the illness must be more than 6 months. Subtypes of schizophrenia are listed in Box 10-2.

Psychosis Not Otherwise Specified (NOS)

Psychosis with symptoms that do not meet the full criteria for a particular diagnosis are categorized as psychosis NOS. This category is useful as a working diagnosis in the ED, where often it is not possible to make a complete psychiatric evaluation because of a poor history and inadequate collateral information.

For example, a patient is brought in by the police because she was found huddled in the local interstate bus station, screaming that there were snakes in the room. You are unable to obtain laboratory data such as urine drug screening, the patient has a history of treatment noncompliance, and you have no one to call for collateral information.

Box 10–1. DSM-IV-TR Diagnostic Criteria for Schizophrenia*

A. Two or more of the following characteristic symptoms are present in a significant portion of 1 month's time (less if treated successfully):
   1. Delusions (diagnosis can be confirmed if bizarre delusions are present even without the symptoms in criteria 2-5)
   2. Hallucinations (diagnosis can be confirmed with only auditory hallucinations if they include a running commentary on patient's behavior, or more than one voice conversing with each other)
   3. Disorganized speech
   4. Disorganized or catatonic behavior
   5. Negative symptoms
B. Social, interpersonal, occupational, or self-care functioning is below the level achieved before the onset of the illness.
C. Symptoms are present for at least 1 month (less if treated successfully) during the active phase, and signs of the disturbance (which can be in an attenuated form) are continuously present for at least 6 months.
D. Mood disorder with psychotic features or schizoaffective disorder has been ruled out.
E. Substance-induced mood disorder or psychosis due to a medical condition has been ruled out.
F. If there is overlap of symptoms of schizophrenia with pervasive developmental disorder, schizophrenia may be added as a separate diagnosis only if prominent delusions or hallucinations are present for at least 1 month (less if successfully treated).

*Adapted from the *Diagnostic and Statistical Manual of Mental Disorders, 4th ed, Text Revision* [DSM-IV-TR]. Washington, DC, American Psychiatric Association, 2000.

Treatment Options

The best approach is to identify and treat the root cause of the psychosis while initiating therapy for the psychotic symptoms.

Specific emergent psychotropics (see Chapter 3) may be necessary in the acute setting to achieve control of agitation as soon as possible. Assessment for acute intervention should

Box 10–2. Subtypes of Schizophrenia

Paranoid Type
In the context of relatively preserved cognitive functioning, symptoms include delusions that are predominantly persecutory or grandiose and are organized in a coherent theme. Auditory hallucinations that are related to the delusions may be seen, but disorganized thoughts, speech, and behavior and flat affects are not.

Disorganized Type
Features include disorganized speech and behavior, with flat affect.

Catatonic Type
The clinical picture is dominated by at least two or more of the following:
- Motor immobility as in cataplexy (waxy flexibility—staying in a placed position no matter how uncomfortable) and stupor
- Excessive, purposeless motor activity
- Mutism (no speech) or extreme negativism (motionless resistance to being moved or if instructed to move)
- Peculiar posturing and movements, prominent grimacing, stereotyped mannerisms
- Echolalia (repeating or parroting another's words) or echopraxia (pathologic imitation of another's movement)

Undifferentiated Type
The patient does not fit the criteria for the previously described types but has two or more of the following symptoms: delusions, hallucinations, disorganized speech, grossly disorganized or catatonic behavior, negative symptoms.

Residual Type
The patient has had at least one episode of schizophrenia, but the current presentation has no prominent positive symptoms. Two or more attenuated positive symptoms may be present. Negative symptoms continue to be present.

include evaluation of current stressors, including "why now" questions. This may require collateral information.

If the patient is uncooperative, volatile, angry, and irritable and possibly dangerous to self and others, then seclusion, restraints, or involuntary hospitalization may be necessary (see Chapter 23 for detailed discussion of medicolegal concerns and procedures for involuntary hospitalization).

An alliance for care with the patient and family members should be established. The outpatient treating clinician should be contacted for information about treatment history, including any treatment changes that may have precipitated the current episode.

Interventions based on the biopsychosocial and cultural model should be considered. Social aspects and living situations can be evaluated with the help of the social services department, if available.

Medications

Psychotropic medications include the newer atypical antipsychotics now available (Table 10-1). As a class, they are noted to have a lower incidence of dystonia, parkinsonism, and tardive dyskinesia (TD) than conventional antipsychotics. They are reported to be effective in the treatment of positive symptoms of schizophrenia and to have greater efficacy than conventional antipsychotics in the treatment of negative symptoms.

Management of compliance issues is improved with intramuscular administration of long-acting atypical antipsychotics such as risperidone (Risperdal Consta) every 2 weeks. The use of rapidly dissolving and disintegrating medications can lessen the cheeking of medications prescribed.

Conventional antipsychotics (Table 10-2) are recommended for patients whose condition had stabilized in the past as a result of therapy with these medications. Conventional antipsychotics also are useful as an adjunct to atypical antipsychotics when positive symptoms are still prominent even with maximized doses—for example, in a patient already taking 800 mg of Quetiapine who still has command hallucinations.

An advantage of conventional antipsychotics is their cost-effectiveness, which usually is less than that of atypical antipsychotics. A disadvantage is the side effects profile of conventional antipsychotics, which may include dystonias and TD.

Table 10–1

Some Atypical Antipsychotics and Some Common Adverse Effects

Generic (Brand) Name	Common Daily Dose Range	Effects			
		Sedation	Weight Gain	Orthostasis	Long QTc
Aripiprazole*[a] (Abilify)	15-45 mg	++	+	+	+
Clozapine (Clozaril)[†]	50-900 mg	+++	+++	+++	++
Olanzapine[‡][a] (Zyprexa)	2.5-30 mg	++	+++	+	+
Quetiapine[§] (Seroquel)	25-800 mg	++	++	+	+
Risperidone[‖][a] (Risperdal)	0.5-8 mg	++	+	+	+
Ziprasidone[¶] (Geodon)	40-160 mg	++	+	+/−	++

*The only partial agonist on the market; not known to increase prolactin levels.

[†]Requires close monitoring with weekly complete blood count because of risk of agranulocytosis; reserve for treatment-resistant cases after at least two other antipsychotics have been tried.

[‡]Available as short- and rapid-acting intramuscular preparations; can affect insulin tissue resistance; monitor for metabolic syndrome.

[§]Not known to increase prolactin levels.

[‖]Available as long-acting intramuscular preparation to be given every 2 weeks.

[¶]Available as short- and rapid-acting intramuscular preparations.

[a] Rapidly disintegrating tablets.

+/−, possible incidence, least likely; +, low incidence; ++, medium incidence; +++, high incidence.

Table 10–2

Some Conventional Antipsychotics

| | | Effects | |
Generic (Brand) Name	Possible Daily Oral Dose	*Anticholinergic*	*Sedation*
Chlorpromazine (Thorazine)	50-400 mg	high	high
Fluphenazine (Prolixin)*	2-20 mg	low	low
Haloperidol (Haldol)*	2.5-40 mg	low	low
Mesoridazine (Serentil)	100-400 mg	medium	high
Perphenazine (Trilafon)*	16-64 mg	low	low
Thioridazine (Mellaril)	50-800 mg	high	high
Thiothixene (Navane)	15-60 mg	low	low
Trifluoperazine (Stelazine)	4-20 mg	low	low

*Available in decanoate form that has an effective time range of 2 to 4 weeks.

Disposition Decisions

Hospitalization may be warranted if further stabilization is necessary (see Chapter 2). However, the least restrictive environment that will affect the patient's treatment positively should be the goal of the ED clinician.

Briefly, criteria for hospital admission include:

- Danger to self (high risk of suicide in psychotic patients) or danger to others
- Grave disability due to mental illness; unable to care for self or the failure of support system to care for the patient, in terms of food, clothing, shelter, and continuation of medical management
- Crisis or severe distress despite ED intervention
- Intoxication; no support system available following detoxification
- Diagnostic clarification needed for further treatment
- Exacerbation of illness due to noncompliance

- Treatment failure due to lack of support system
- Need for special services such as ECT and EMS

For disposition to home, the patient should meet the following qualifications:

- Is not suicidal, homicidal, or gravely disabled.
- Is capable of following up on outpatient treatment.
- Has enough medications to last until next outpatient appointment.
- Has adequate support system to continue with current level of functioning (which does not necessitate hospitalization).
- Will return to the ED if there should be other medical or psychiatric emergencies.

Further Reading

American Psychiatric Association: Diagnostic and Statistical Manual of Mental Disorders, 4th ed, Text Revision. Washington, DC, American Psychiatric Association, 2000.

Grunhaus L, Dannon PN, Schreiber S, et al: Repetitive transcranial magnetic stimulation is as effective as electroconvulsive therapy in the treatment of nondelusional major depressive disorder: An open study. Biol Psychiatry 2000;47:314-324.

Kaplan HI, Sadock BJ: Synopsis of Psychiatry. Behavioral Sciences/Clinical Psychiatry, 8th ed. Baltimore, Lippincott Williams & Wilkins, 1998.

Makram M, Dribben B: Toxicity: Hallucinogens, LSD. 2004. Available at http://www.emedicine.com/ped/topic2809.htm

National Highway Traffic Safety Administration: Dextromethorphan. http://www.nhtsa.dot.gov/people/injury/research/job185drugs/dextromethorphan.htm

Physicians' Desk Reference 2005, 59th ed. Montvale, NJ, Thompson PDR, 2005.

Kaplan H, Sadock B: Pocket Handbook of Psychiatric Drug Treatment, 3rd ed. Philadelphia, Lippincott Williams & Wilkins, 2001.

Torrey EF: Surviving Schizophrenia, 4th ed. New York, Quill (HarperCollins), 2001.

CHAPTER 11

The Acutely Anxious Patient

Doris T. Tan, DO

KEY POINTS

- Persons presenting with anxiety or panic in the emergency department (ED) may believe that they have a devastating life-threatening illness.
- Alleviation of anxiety in the ED begins with calming and reassurance by the ED clinician.
- There are many different causes of anxiety, and medical causes must first be ruled out.
- Referral for continuation of care is emphasized.

Definitions

Anxiety. *Common definition*—distress or a state of mind caused by fear of danger or misfortune; *in psychiatry*—a state of apprehension and psychic tension, occurring in some form of mental distress; *when pathologic*—reaction to an internal stimulus that is autonomous, intense, and exaggerated.

Anxious. Mentally distressed about possible danger or misfortune; apprehensive, uneasy, troubled.

Fear. An alerting signal in response to an external threat.

Anxiety can be distinguished from fear in that fear is a clear response to a threat that is definitely from an external source, whereas anxiety is the expression of an alerting signal arising from an internal conflict.

Overview

It is postulated that anxiety is a survival cue and an adaptation mechanism. During times of heightened arousal, such as in homing in on possibly dangerous prey, it is an expected, although a transient, response to stressful situations, characterized by an increased sympathetic discharge. When sympathetic discharges are inappropriate, miscued, or no longer transient, they can raise havoc with the functioning and adaptation of an individual. Anxiety disorder then may result.

Patients generally do not present to the ED until after they have experienced anxiety numerous times, or they may have experienced outright panic attacks. The disability and suffering that result from anxiety disorders should not be ignored, as they can be devastating to the social, occupational, and general well-being of the patient. The ED clinician who encounters the anxious patient is urged to be vigilant in making the appropriate referral for the continuation of care after the initial crisis is over.

Epidemiology

Approximately 25% of the U.S. population will suffer from pathologic anxiety over the course of a lifetime. The incidence may, in fact, be higher, because many patients who suffer from subclinical features of anxiety disorders do not seek treatment. Thus, anxiety is one of the most prevalent psychiatric disorders (Table 11-1).

Table 11–1

Estimated Lifetime Prevalence of Anxiety Disorders

Diagnosis	Prevalence
Anxiety due to a general medical condition	Varies
Substance-induced anxiety disorder	Varies
Acute stress disorder	Varies
Anxiety disorder NOS	1% to 10%
Panic disorder	3.8%
Panic attacks	5.6%
Specific anxiety disorders	11% to 13%
Social phobia	3% to 13%
Obsessive-compulsive disorder	2% to 3%
PTSD in the general population	7.8% to 13%
PTSD in Vietnam veterans	30%
Generalized anxiety disorder	24.1% to 45%

NOS, not otherwise specified; PTSD, posttraumatic stress disorder.

Gender differences are apparent in the incidence of anxiety disorders; the female-to-male ratio is estimated to be 2:1.

Studies of family histories suggest that genetic predisposition increases the likelihood of anxiety disorders. The risk for having this illness is increased four- to eightfold in patients who have a history of first-degree relatives with the disorder.

Environmental factors, such as divorce or changing jobs or schools, may play a role in the risk for anxiety disorders. Trauma and other stressful events, such as abuse or death of a loved one, may lead to posttraumatic stress disorder (PTSD) (see Chapter 20).

Assessment

 The ED clinician should speak in a reassuring and a calming tone during the interview (avoid giving the impression that you also are anxious about the patient's anxiety), because patients with panic disorder often believe that they have a devastating medical condition that may lead to death.

A full medical history should be obtained if possible. Collateral information (obtained with the patient's permission) from the primary physician, family members, and friends can be helpful.

The medical examination should include a thorough work-up of somatic symptoms or complaints. It is important to remember that many medical conditions (Table 11-2) and psychiatric disorders (Box 11-1) may have anxiety as a component or symptom.

The definitive treatment of patients experiencing anxiety due to a medical condition should be the treatment of any underlying medical condition.

If needed, referral to the appropriate specialty should be made.

Diagnosis

Diagnoses to consider in patients presenting with anxiety in the ED include:
- Generalized anxiety disorder
- Panic disorder
- Social phobia (social anxiety disorder)
- Acute stress disorder
- PTSD (see Chapter 20)
- Obsessive compulsive disorder

Text continues on page 224.

Table 11–2

Medical Conditions That May Cause Anxiety Symptoms

Condition	Associated Features
Endocrine Disorders	
Hyperthyroidism	Hypermetabolism, increased T_3 and T_4, low TSH, ocular signs (stare, lid lag), goiter, tachycardia, moist skin
Hypothyroidism	Slowed metabolism, elevated TSH, dry coarse skin, cold intolerance, sparse hair, facial puffiness, psychosis with myxedema
Hyperadrenocorticism	Na^+ and water retention, hypervolemia, hypertension, personality disturbance
Pheochromocytoma	Hypersecretion of catecholamines causing hypertension, headaches, diaphoresis, palpitations, pallor, tremors
Hypoglycemia	CNS dysfunction, stupor
Pituitary dysfunction	Hyperthyroidism, low gonadotropin levels
Parathyroid dysfunction	Hypercalcemia—constipation, ileus, confusion when severe, shortened QTc interval, bone lesions; hypocalcemia with hyperphosphatemia—tetany; hypercalciuria—renal damage
Virilization disorders in females	Hirsutism, short stature, clitoral enlargement, ambiguous sex determination, amenorrhea
Premenstrual syndrome	Mild mood swings dependent on phase of menstrual cycle

Continued

Table 11–2

Medical Conditions That May Cause Anxiety Symptoms—cont'd

Condition	Associated Features
Cardiovascular Disease	
Arrhythmias	Irregular heart beat, palpitations, SOB
Anemias	Fatigue, weakness, SOB on exertion, pale appearance, low Hgb, low Hct
Hypovolemia	Low blood pressure, orthostasis, fatigue
Hypotension	Dizziness, weakness, fainting spells
Hypertension	Headaches, chronic retinal changes, end organ damage (e.g., renal failure, microproteinuria, heart failure)
Congestive heart failures	SOB on exertion, heart enlargement, poor perfusion
Acute chest pain	SOB, feelings of heaviness and being smothered
Acute myocardial infarction	Heavy feeling in chest, SOB; pain radiating to left arm, abdomen, and/or back
Angina	Fatigue, weakness, ECG changes, elevated levels of troponin and other cardiac enzymes
Respiratory Disease	
COPD	Dyspnea, expiratory wheezing, cough, hyperinflation of the lung
Pneumonia	SOB, purulent sputum, fever, fatigue, leukocytosis with shift, chest pain (pleurisy)
Hyperventilation	Feeling of tingling around the mouth and fingertips, SOB with subjective feeling of inability to exchange air; may lead to dizziness and syncope

Condition	Associated Features
Sleep apnea	Snoring, daytime drowsiness, morning headache, slowed mentation, oxygen desaturation during sleep
Asthma	Intermittent dyspnea, bronchospasm mediated by inflammation of airway; occasionally lethal when not treated
Acute and chronic bronchitis	Productive cough with edematous mucosa
Neurologic Disorders	
Cerebrovascular disease	Sudden change in mentation, hemiparesis, aphasia
Cerebral neoplasms	Vary, depending on size, site, and type
Encephalitis	Fever, malaise, neck stiffness, headache, vomiting
Seizure disorders	May be partial or tonic-clonic, may have loss of consciousness
Migraines	With or without aura; intermittent severe headache, sensitivity to light
Subarachnoid hemorrhage	Generally due to trauma; sudden headache, varying degrees of neurologic deficits
Closed head injuries	Mild deficit with concussion headache, dizziness; severe injuries can cause coma and death
Multiple sclerosis	Various neurologic symptoms, apathy, euphoria, pseudobulbar palsy
Wilson's disease	Unexplained hepatic, neurologic, or psychiatric symptoms, persistent transaminasemia
Vestibular dysfunctions	Positional vertigo, nausea
Dementias	Progressive memory impairment, aphasia, agnosia
Delirium	Waxing and waning of consciousness, altered mental status with memory impairment

Continued

Table 11–2

Medical Conditions That May Cause Anxiety Symptoms—cont'd

Condition	Associated Features
Huntington's disease	Depression, choreoathetotic movements, anhedonia, dementia-like
Psychomotor epilepsy	Aura, seizures (may be focal, tonic-clonic or partial). See Chapter 16.
Temporal lobe diseases	Hallucinations, aphasia, anomia, prosody changes
Metabolic Disorders	
Vitamin deficiencies	Vary, depending on deficiency
Porphyria	Abdominal pain with neurovisceral symptoms, muscle weakness, painful skin eruptions in reaction to sunlight
Pellagra	Cutaneous lesions, tongue and mucosal redness; abdominal discomfort from nausea, vomiting, diarrhea; psychosis, confusion
Uremia	Weight loss, fatigue, nausea and vomiting, itching, peripheral neuropathy, encephalopathy
Hypocalcemia	Generally without symptoms; with severely low calcium levels, symptoms range from neuromuscular irritability to tetany
Hypokalemia	Generally without symptoms; with severely low K⁺ levels, muscle weakness, cramping, fasciculation, tetany, rhabdomyolysis, ECG changes
Inflammatory Disorders	
Systemic lupus erythematosus	Fever, malaise, arthralgia, cutaneous lesions, pleurisy, adenopathy, pericarditis, vasculitis, headaches, personality changes, renal involvement
Rheumatoid arthritis	Nodules, hand erosions, positive rheumatoid factor, joint pain

Condition	Associated Features
Temporal arteritis	Elevated sedimentation rate, severe headache at temporal region, amaurosis fugax, blurred vision
Costochondritis	Reproducible pain in affected rib segment(s) on palpation or movement
Autoimmune disease	Vary
Fibromyalgia	Myofascial pain, achiness, muscle and tendon tenderness, presence of trigger points
Allergic reactions	Vary; range from mild skin eruptions to anaphylaxis
Toxicity	
Caffeine intoxication	Heart palpitations, wakefulness, restlessness, anorexia, dehydration; seizures possible
Amphetamines	Insomnia, irritability, anorexia, arrhythmia, chest pain, hyperactivity, heart block, psychosis
Heavy metals	Headaches, abdominal pain, diarrhea, insomnia, vomiting, ataxia, restlessness, mania, confusion; convulsions if severe
Vasopressors and sympathomimetic agents	High blood pressure, arrhythmia, strokes
Organophosphates	Nausea, vomiting, abdominal cramps, sialorrhea, rhinorrhea, blurred vision, miosis, respiratory distress, altered mental status; if severe, possible coma and death
Alcohol	Incoordination, labile mood, nausea, vomiting, stupor; may lead to coma
Opiates	Miosis, sedation, respiratory depression or failure
Phencyclidines (PCPs)	Hypertension; visual, tactile, and auditory hallucinations; severe psychosis, paranoia

Continued

Table 11-2

Medical Conditions That May Cause Anxiety Symptoms—cont'd

Condition	Associated Features
Cocaine	Autonomic hyperstimulation, hypertension, dilated pupils, increased pain threshold, chest pain, tremors, nausea, vomiting, delirium, myocardial infarction; respiratory or circulatory failure possibly leading to death
Ecstasy	Autonomic overstimulation, dehydration, panic attacks, rarely visual hallucinations/illusions, psychosis
Infectious and Other Processes	
Septicemia	Temperature spikes, fatigue, malaise, shaking chills; when in septic shock, altered mental status, tachypnea
Carcinoid syndrome	Abdominal cramps, diarrhea, flushed skin, striking skin color changes
Infectious mononucleosis	Pharyngitis, fever, fatigue, lymphadenopathy, malaise; splenomegaly in 50% of cases
AIDS	Initial flu-like symptoms, seroconversion; may be latent, with lowered immune system, low CD4 count, opportunistic infections, candidiasis, *Pneumocystis carinii* pneumonia, Kaposi's sarcoma
Systemic malignancies	Weight loss, fatigue, pain, wasting, obstruction by neoplasm.
Subacute bacterial endocarditis	Low-grade fever, night sweats, weight loss, fatigue, valvular insufficiency, heart murmur, Roth's spot, possible embolism
Gastrointestinal hemorrhage	Hematemesis, hematochezia, melena, pallor, fatigability, orthostatic hypotension; may precipitate hepatic encephalopathy with altered mental status

Condition	Associated Features
Miscellaneous Disorders	
Irritable bowel syndrome	Abdominal pain relieved by defecation; bloating; colicky pain varies, depending on whether syndrome is constipation- or diarrhea-dominant
Dyspepsia	Abdominal gaseous fullness, indigestion, early satiety, epigastric burning
GERD	Heartburn, regurgitation of gastric contents, esophageal burning (may lead to Barrett's esophagus)
Shingles (herpes zoster)	Painful, fluid-filled vesicles; chills, fever, malaise may precede appearance of skin vesicles; neuralgia, may persist for years after vesicular eruptions have resolved (postherpetic neuralgia)
Akathisias	Restlessness, inability to sit or stand still; generally due to medication

AIDS, acquired immunodeficiency syndrome; COPD, chronic obstructive pulmonary disease; ECG, electrocardiogram; GERD, gastroesophageal reflux disease; Hct, hematocrit; Hgb, hemoglobin; HIV, human immunodeficiency virus; SOB, shortness of breath; T_3, triiodothyronine; T_4, thyroxine; TSH, thyroid-stimulating hormone.

> **Box 11–1. Psychiatric Disorders That May Be Associated with Anxiety or Panic Attacks**
>
> Bipolar disorder
> Comorbid depression
> Eating disorders
> Obsessive compulsive disorder
> Personality disorders
> Schizoaffective disorders
> Schizophrenia
> Schizophreniform disorder

Generalized Anxiety Disorder

Criteria for the diagnosis of generalized anxiety disorder include:
- Excessive anxiety or worry more days than not for the past 6 months
- Difficulty controlling such worry or anxiety
- Worry or anxiety are associated with three or more of the following:
  - Restlessness, feeling on edge or keyed up
  - Easily fatigued
  - Difficulty concentrating
  - Irritability
  - Muscle tension
  - Sleep disturbance
  - Focus of the anxiety and worry not confined to the features of a primary psychiatric or an axis I disorder.

Panic Disorder

The essential feature of panic disorder is the presence of recurrent unexpected panic attacks followed by persistent worry (for at least 1 month) about having another attack.

Panic Attack
Panic attack is defined as a discrete and abrupt period of intense discomfort or intense fear that peaks within 10 minutes or less and includes four or more of the following symptoms:
- Palpitations, accelerated heart rate, pounding heart beat
- Sweating

- Trembling or shaking
- Feeling of choking
- Feeling of smothering; shortness of breath
- Chest pain or chest discomfort
- Nausea or abdominal distress
- Numbness or tingling sensations around the mouth and extremities
- Autonomic instability such as chills or hot flashes
- Lightheadedness or fainting spell; feeling unsteady or dizzy
- Feeling detached from one's mind or body (depersonalization)
- Feeling that things are not real (derealization)
- Fear that one may be losing one's mind
- Fear of losing self-control
- Fear of dying

Panic attacks can occur with no precipitating factors and for no discernible reason. They may happen while the patient is asleep, although they are not necessarily associated with dreams or nightmares. Certain situations, especially if they are associated with a previous attack, seem to precipitate a recurrence—for example, entering an elevator or a tunnel or driving a car.

Complications of panic disorder may include physiologic changes associated with enhanced autonomic responses. Some studies indicate that there is a higher incidence of suicide attempts by suicidal patients with anxiety disorder.

Panic Disorder with Agoraphobia

The central feature of agoraphobia is anxiety about being in places or situations from which escape might be difficult or embarrassing or where help may not be available in the event of having a panic attack or panic-like symptoms. Although agoraphobia can exist both with and without panic disorder, in the majority of individuals the restrictions in behavior occur as part of their fear of having a panic attack in an "unsafe" or public place. Such persons can become more anxious about the anticipation of an attack than about the attack itself, which may or may not arise.

This type of anticipatory unease can lead to poor socialization; individuals essentially imprison themselves due to their attempts to avoid any possibility of inducing anxiety or panic. They are unable to leave the perceived "safe place" or are able to leave only if accompanied by a trusted companion or a "safe person."

See Boxes 11-2 and 11-3, respectively, for criteria for panic disorder with agoraphobia and without agoraphobia. Note that the only difference in the criteria is the presence of agoraphobia.

Social Phobia (Social Anxiety Disorder)

Social phobia is characterized by persistent fear of social or performance situations in which embarrassment or humiliation may occur. Persons with social phobia know that their fear is unreasonably excessive but nonetheless experience anxiety or panic. The feared situations are either avoided or are endured with intense anxiety or distress, which interferes significantly with their normal routine, occupational and social functioning, and social relationships.

Treatment with the beta blocker propranolol, 125 mg to 25 mg PO, before exposure to anxiety-provoking situations has been shown to be helpful in some cases.

Acute Stress Disorder

The important feature of acute stress disorder is the development of anxiety, increased arousal, dissociation (characterized by a subjective sense of detachment, derealization, or depersonalization), occurring within 1 month after exposure to a traumatic event.

The person's response includes intense fear, a sense of helplessness, and/or horror. The event is persistently re-experienced in recurrent thoughts, images, illusions, flashbacks, or dreams.

According to the *Diagnostic and Statistical Manual of Mental Disorders, Fourth Edition, Text Revision* (DSM-IV-TR) criteria for acute stress disorder, the above-mentioned symptoms should persist for a minimum of 2 days and a maximum of 4 weeks and should occur within 4 weeks of the traumatic event. If the duration is more than 1 month, the diagnosis of PTSD should be considered.

Associated symptoms include increased arousal that was not present before the traumatic event, difficulty falling asleep or staying asleep, increased irritability and anger outbursts, hypervigilance, exaggerated startle responses, and increased risk-taking behaviors and impulsiveness. The person may avoid any stimuli associated with the trauma.

Box 11–2. Criteria for Panic Disorder without Agoraphobia*

A. Both (1) and (2):
   (1) Recurrent unexpected panic attacks
   (2) At least one of the attacks has been followed by (a) 1 month (or more) of persistent concerns about having additional attacks, (b) worry about the consequences of the attack, or (c) a significant change in behavior related to the attacks
B. Absence of agoraphobia
C. The panic attacks are not due to a general medical condition or the direct effects of a substance (e.g., illicit drugs or medications)
D. The panic attacks are not better accounted for by another mental disorder (see DSM-IV criteria for other anxiety disorders)

Adapted from the *Diagnostic and Statistical Manual of Mental Disorders, 4th Edition, Text Revision* (DSM-IV-TR).

Box 11–3. Criteria for Panic Disorder with Agoraphobia*

A. Both (1) and (2):
   (1) Recurrent unexpected panic attacks
   (2) At least one of the attacks has been followed by (a) 1 month (or more) of persistent concerns about having additional attacks, (b) worry about the consequences of the attack, or (c) a significant change in behavior related to the attacks
B. **Presence** of agoraphobia
C. The panic attacks are not due to a general medical condition or the direct effects of a substance (e.g., illicit drugs or medications)
D. The panic attacks are not better accounted for by another mental disorder (see DSM-IV criteria for other anxiety disorders)

*Note that this box is included here to emphasize the presence of agoraphobia.
Adapted from the *Diagnostic and Statistical Manual of Mental Disorders, 4th Edition, Text Revision* (DSM-IV-TR).

Obsessive Compulsive Disorder

The most significant feature of obsessive compulsive disorder is marked distress or impairment resulting from recurrent obsessions or compulsions. The terms *obsession* and *compulsion* can be defined in the context of this illness as follows:

Obsession—persistent impulses, thoughts, or images that are experienced as intrusive and inappropriate that cause marked anxiety or distress

Compulsion—behaviors or mental acts that the person feels driven to perform in response to an obsession or according to rigidly applied rules

Following are DSM-IV-TR criteria for obsessive compulsive disorder:

- At some point during the course of the illness, the person recognizes that the obsessions or compulsions are excessive or unreasonable.
- The obsessions or compulsions are time-consuming (take up more than 1 hour a day) and significantly interfere with the person's normal routine, occupational functioning, and usual social activities and relationships.
- The disorder is not due to the direct physiologic effects of a substance (e.g., drug of abuse or medication) or a general medical condition.

Obsessions and compulsions may displace useful behaviors, and thus the person may not be able to perform formerly satisfying tasks, such as reading or going to work.

Situations or objects that may provoke a compulsion or obsession are avoided at all costs—for example, a person who is obsessed about dirt will not touch a prized book because there is a speck of dust on it.

Management

Anxiety is a common manifestation of psychiatric disorders such as schizophrenia and bipolar disorder (see Box 11-1). In these cases, akathisia (bodily restlessness) should be ruled out as the cause of the anxiety if psychotropic medications are prescribed. The focus of treatment should be on the suspected psychiatric disorder rather than merely relieving the symptoms of anxiety.

Pharmacologic Therapy

A short course of a benzodiazepine for anxiolytic effects, such as lorazepam, 0.5 mg to 2 mg given orally (PO) or intramuscularly (IM), can be effective for symptomatic relief, making further evaluation and treatment possible. A short course (less than 2 weeks) is less likely to become habitual or addictive, given at the lowest dose that controls the symptoms, and is advisable, especially in the elderly. Elderly persons are at particular risk for respiratory depression and delirium as a complication of benzodiazepine therapy and should be monitored closely. Table 11-3 lists commonly used benzodiazepines.

Once the medical workup is completed and it has been determined that the anxiety symptoms are caused by chronic generalized anxiety or panic disorder rather than by another psychiatric condition, treatment with buspirone (BuSpar), 10 mg

Table 11–3
Recommended Dosages for Benzodiazepines

Generic (Brand) Name	Initial Dose (mg)	Daily Dose Range* (mg)	Frequency
Alprazolam (Xanax)	0.25-0.5	1-6	qid
Xanax XR	0.5	0.5-6	daily
Chlordiazepoxide (Librium)	5-10	5-100	tid
Clonazepam (Klonopin)	0.25	0.5-4	bid
Diazepam (Valium)	2.5	5-40	tid
Lorazepam (Ativan)	0.5	1-10	tid-qid
Oxazepam (Serax)	15	30-120	tid
Temazepam (Restoril)	15	30-120	tid

*Dose ranges are approximations only. Tolerance to benzodiazepines when used over a long period of time may require higher dosages; monitoring for respiratory depression is essential when taking greater than the approved recommended dose.

tid, or with one of the antidepressants discussed here should be initiated.

Selective Serotonin Reuptake Inhibitors (SSRIs)

Table 11-4 lists recommended dosages for some SSRIs.

Fluoxetine (Prozac) therapy should be started at a low dose of 10 mg or 20 mg daily for a few days to a week because it may cause akathisia, irritation, agitation, and even increased anxiety. Hence the "go low and slow" rule of thumb is a good guide to therapy with this drug.

Citalopram (Celexa) therapy (initial dose of 10-20 mg/day) can be increased to 60 mg if necessary, but its efficacy at greater doses is questionable. It is generally accepted that it may take 6 to 8 weeks or more before a substantial reduction in anxiety is noted. However, some studies report positive responses of anxiety reduction after 2 to 3 weeks of therapy.

Obsessive compulsive disorders are thought to be responsive to higher doses of SSRIs.

Serotonin/Norepinephrine Reuptake Inhibitors (SNRIs)

SNRIs are useful in the treatment of anxiety, especially anxiety associated with depression. Recommended dosages for the SNRIs discussed here are listed in Table 11-5.

Table 11–4

Recommended Dosages for Selective Serotonin Reuptake Inhibitors

Generic (Brand) Name	Initial Dose (mg)	Daily Dose Range* (mg)	Frequency
Citalopram (Celexa)	10	10-60	daily
Escitalopram (Lexapro)	5-10	10-20	daily
Fluoxetine (Prozac)	10-20	10-80	daily
Fluvoxamine (Luvox)	25-50	50-300	daily to bid
Paroxetine (Paxil)	10	10-60	daily
Sertraline (Zoloft)	25-50	50-200	daily

*Dose ranges are approximations.

Table 11–5

Recommended Dosages for Serotonin/Norepinephrine Reuptake Inhibitors

Generic (Brand) Name	Initial Dose (mg)	Daily Dose range* (mg)	Frequency
Duloxetine (Cymbalta)	20	20-60	bid
Mirtazapine† (Remeron)	15	15-45	at bedtime
Venlafaxine (Effexor)	37.5	37.5-375	bid-tid
Venlafaxine Extended Release (Effexor XL)	37.5	37.5-225	daily

*Dose ranges are approximations.
† Although mirtazapine is a tetracyclic in its chemical structure, its clinical effects are similar to those of SNRIs and hence are included in this section.

Duloxetine (Cymbalta) is useful in treating anxiety symptoms in the context of depression.

Mirtazapine (Remeron) has a side effect profile that includes increased drowsiness (which at times is a welcome feature for those with difficulty sleeping) and weight gain due to increased appetite.

Venlafaxine (Effexor) (initial dose of 37.5 mg/day) is an immediate-release drug. For patients who are sensitive to this medication, dosage can be started at 37.5 mg and increased in increments of up to 75 mg/day to a maximum of 375 mg/day in three divided doses. Venlafaxine Extended Release (Effexor XR) (same dosage as Effexor, but maximum of 275 mg/day) is indicated for general anxiety disorder and social anxiety disorder.

Tricyclic Antidepressants

Tricyclic antidepressants are known to be helpful in treatment of panic disorders, generalized anxiety disorders, phobia, and obsessive compulsive disorders. Table 11-6 lists recommended dosages for some tricyclic antidepressants.

Because persons with panic disorder can be particularly sensitive to side effects of tricyclics, a very low initial dose and slow titration to the lowest effective daily dose are advised. In

Table 11-6

Recommended Dosages for Tricyclic Antidepressants

Generic (Brand) Name	Initial Dose (mg)	Daily Dose Range* (mg)	Frequency
Imipramine (Tofranil)	10-25	150-300	daily to tid
Desipramine (Norpramin)	10-25	100-300	daily to bid
Amitriptyline (Elavil)	10-25	50-300	daily to tid
Nortriptyline (Pamelor)	10-25	25-150	daily to tid
Amoxapine (Ascendin)	25-50	50-600	daily to tid
Doxepin (Sinequan)	10-50	50-300	daily to tid
Trazodone (Desyrel)	25-50	50-600	at bedtime
Clomipramine (Anafranil)	25	50-250	tid

*Dose ranges are approximations.

some cases, benzodiazepines may be co-administered with tricyclic antidepressants early in treatment and discontinued when symptoms are controlled.

Benzodiazepines

Benzodiazepines are very effective anxiolytics, but they should be used for only a short time, less than 2 weeks if possible, and should be given at the lowest dose that alleviates anxiety. Continued administration carries with it a high propensity for tolerance and both physiologic and psychological dependence and it also comes with a risk for respiratory depression. Benzodiazepine therapy is contraindicated in cases of alcohol abuse.

Nonpharmacologic Therapy

Cognitive behavioral therapy (CBT) involves recognizing automatic negative patterns of thinking and behavior and replacing them with more realistic and helpful ones. CBT is particularly useful in the treatment of anxiety disorder, panic disorder, and (especially in conjunction with psychopharma-cologic therapy) of obsessive compulsive disorder.

Desensitization therapy has been effective in persons with panic disorder. In a controlled environment, the person is taken to a point where anxiety or panic is felt and is then counseled about its harmlessness; with repeated sessions, the patient gradually gains control of the panic attacks.

Biofeedback, now used to treat a wide variety of conditions and diseases ranging from epilepsy to hypertension, has been effective in the treatment of anxiety when administered by a trained and experienced therapist.

The family and significant others of a patient who is under-going psychotherapy should be educated about the patient's condition and the type of therapy. Referral to an outpatient psychologist or psychiatrist may be necessary. Associations such as the National Alliance on Mental Illness offer support, education, and advice about further management.

Further Reading

American Psychiatric Association: Diagnostic and Statistical Manual of Mental Disorders, 4th ed, Text Revision. Washington, DC, American Psychiatric Association, 2000.

Dunner DL, Goldstein DJ, Mallinckrodt C, et al: Duloxetine in treatment of anxiety symptoms associated with depression. Depress Anxiety 2003;18:53-61.

Hall RC, Platt DE, Hall RC: Suicide risk assessment: A review of risk factors for suicide in 100 patients who made severe suicide attempts. Psychosomatics 1999;40:18-27.

Hermida T, Malone D: Anxiety Disorders. The Cleveland Clinic Medicine Index, 2003, 2004. http://www.clevelandclinicmeded.com/diseasemanagement/psychiatry/anxiety/anxiety.htm

Kaplan HI, Sadock BJ: Synopsis of Psychiatry: Behavioral Sciences/Clinical Psychiatry, 8th ed. Philadelphia, Lippincott, 1998, pp 581-623.

Physicians' Desk Reference, 59th ed. Montvale, NJ, Thompson PDR, 2005.

CHAPTER 12

The Personality-Disordered Patient

Doris T. Tan, DO

KEY POINTS

- Personality disorder is a constellation of inflexible and maladaptive behaviors that begins in adolescence and early adulthood and results in an enduring pattern of behaviors that impact negatively on a person's social, interpersonal, and occupational functioning.
- Emergency department (ED) clinicians should keep in mind that personality disorders often co-exist with Axis I (primary psychiatric) disorders such as mood disorders and psychiatric disorders due to medical conditions or to alcohol or substance abuse. Medical causes of anxiety, depression, and agitation must always be ruled out.
- ED clinicians should examine their own emotions for clues that may be helpful in the evaluation of patients with personality disorder.
- Acute presentations may necessitate hospitalization if suicidality or homicidality is present. Because of the chronic presentation of personality disorder, outpatient psychotherapy is usually recommended.

Overview

Patients with personality disorders often exhibit symptoms mimicking those of primary psychiatric disorders such as anxiety, depression, and psychosis.

Although personality disorder by definition consists of a pervasive, chronic, and enduring pattern of behaving, thinking, and relating to others, the emergent psychiatric presentation often is so intense that it merits psychiatric evaluation focused on imminent lethality and on the treatment of the acute current presentation; other psychological issues should be reserved for long-term outpatient psychotherapy when the patient is not in a state of acute crisis. Treatment should be focused on alleviating symptoms that could lead to dangerous actions and on supporting the patient's ego structure.

The ED clinician and supporting staff should be aware of the possible negative impact of the personality-disordered patient's actions on treatment; transference and countertransference issues should not be allowed to interfere with the patient's evaluation and disposition. When a patient arouses feelings of frustration, anger, or irritation in the clinician, the diagnosis of personality disorder should be considered.

Treatment of medical and other primary psychiatric disorders is often hindered by the inflexibility of the co-morbid personality disorder; hence successful treatment is less likely in this population than in those without personality disorder.

General Diagnostic Criteria for Personality Disorder

General diagnostic criteria for personality disorder are listed in Box 12-1. According to the DSM-IV-TR, to be considered a personality disorder, these patterns of behavior must have been evident in or be traceable back to adolescence or early adulthood. Normal people may have personality traits with the same symptomatology as in personality disorder. Only when the inflexibility of an individual affects important aspects of life, such as social and occupational functioning, are these behaviors categorized as personality disorder. Often a person may have symptoms of, or fit the criteria for, more than one type of personality disorder.

Epidemiology

A landmark study by the 2001-2002 National Epidemiologic Survey on Alcohol and Related Conditions (NESARC) reported that personality disorders affect 14.8% of the U.S. population (Table 12-1).

Patients with personality disorder are at higher risk than the general population for many primary psychiatric disorders. Mood disorders are a particular risk across all personality disorder diagnoses.

> ### Box 12–1. General Diagnostic Criteria for Personality Disorder
>
> A. An enduring pattern of inner experience and behavior that deviates markedly from that person's cultural expectations. This pattern is shown in two or more of the following areas:
>   1. Cognition—their ways of perceiving and interpreting self, other people, and events
>   2. Affectivity—the range, intensity, lability, and appropriateness of emotional response
>   3. Interpersonal functioning
>   4. Impulse control
> B. The enduring pattern of behavior is inflexible and pervasive, leading to clinically significant distress or impairment in social, occupational, and other important areas of functioning.
> C. The pattern is stable and of long duration, and its onset can be traced back at least to adolescence or early adulthood.
> D. The enduring pattern is not better accounted for as a manifestation or consequence of another mental disorder.
> E. The enduring pattern is not due to the direct physiologic effects of a substance (e.g., drug of abuse, medication) or a general medical condition (e.g., head trauma).

Adapted from the DSM-IV-TR (*Diagnostic and Statistical Manual of Mental Disorders, Fourth Edition, Text Revision*).

Possible Causes of Personality Disorder

Psychological Causes

Theories abound as to the causes of personality disorder, such as childhood or adolescent developmental trauma, chronic abuse, and an overindulgent or overbearing relationship with caregivers, leading to maladjustment and/or incomplete development of underlying personal characteristics. Often, trust is broken, and without trust the continuation of healthy character development is difficult. In-depth coverage of these theories is beyond the scope of this chapter; see Kaplan and Sadok (2003) for a detailed discussion.

Medical Causes

Numerous medical conditions can cause personality changes, including neurodegenerative diseases, such as the dementias,

Table 12–1

The NESARC Report on Patients Affected by Personality Disorders*

Disorder	Affected (%)	Number Affected (millions)
Dependent personality	0.5	1.0
Histrionic personality	1.6	3.8
Avoidant personality	2.4	4.9
Schizoid personality	3.1	6.5
Antisocial personality	3.6	7.6
Paranoid personality	4.4	9.2M
Obsessive compulsive personality	7.9	16.4

*According to the *Diagnostic and Statistical Manual of Mental Disorders, Fourth Edition, Text Revision* (DSM IV-TR), the prevalence of narcissistic personality disorder is less than 1% and that of borderline personality is 2%. NESARC, National Epidemiologic Survey on Alcohol and Related Conditions.

and traumatic brain injuries, especially those that involve the frontal lobes. Post-stroke personality changes often are associated with a right-sided hemispheric lesion. Other conditions include Huntington's disease, human immunodeficiency virus (HIV), neurosyphilis, and systemic lupus erythematosus (SLE).

It is imperative that the medical workup be the first priority in the ED assessment so that any medical conditions can be identified and reversible conditions can be treated. When distinguishing between personality changes due to a medical condition and personality disorder, it is helpful to remember that the former occur after the onset of the medical condition, whereas personality disorder by definition has its origin before or in early adulthood.

Clinical Presentation and Management of Specific Personality Disorders

This chapter discusses the clinical manifestations and management of the personality disorders grouped by the DSM-IV-TR into three clusters:

- Cluster A—paranoid, schizoid, and schizotypal personality disorders
- Cluster B—antisocial, borderline, histrionic, and narcissistic personality disorders

- Cluster C—avoidant, dependent, and obsessive compulsive personality disorders

Cluster A Disorders

Paranoid Personality Disorder (Box 12-2)
Clinical Presentation
Patients with paranoid personality disorder often exhibit suspiciousness and distrust and may believe that other people have malevolent intentions to exploit them. Although often sharp in their thinking, their false premises lead to distorted and even bizarre conclusions.

These patients usually present to the ED not because of the disorder but because of a medical emergency. Often, the ED clinician is asked to see such patients because of their mistrust

---

Box 12–2. DSM-IV-TR Criteria for Paranoid Personality Disorder

A. A pervasive distrust and suspiciousness of others such that their motives are interpreted as malevolent, beginning by early adulthood and present in a variety of contexts, as indicated by four or more of the following:
1. Suspects, without sufficient basis, that others are exploiting, harming, or deceiving him/her
2. Is preoccupied with unjustified doubts about the loyalty or trustworthiness of friends or associates
3. Is reluctant to confide in others because of unwarranted fear that the information will be used maliciously against him/her
4. Reads hidden demeaning or threatening meanings into benign remarks or events
5. Persistently bears grudges (i.e., is unforgiving of insults, injuries, or slights)
6. Perceives attacks on his/her character or reputation that are not apparent to others and is quick to react angrily or to counterattack
7. Has recurrent suspicions, without justification, regarding fidelity of spouse or other partner

Adapted from the DSM-IV-TR (*Diagnostic and Statistical Manual of Mental Disorders, Fourth Edition, Text Revision*).

and refusal to be treated based on their belief that the recommended treatment may be harmful.

Management

Assess for medical conditions that may explain the presenting complaint and treat any underlying comorbid primary psychiatric condition.

It is imperative to remain nonconfrontational but firm regarding the reality of the situation. To foster trust, clearly explain all procedures and the reasons for performing them. Any wavering or inconsistency only confirms the patient's suspiciousness. Use continued reality testing during the evaluation and treatment, although with this, it may not be possible to get past the patient's distorted convictions.

Assess for dangerousness and whether hospitalization may be necessary.

Schizoid Personality Disorder (Box 12-3)
Clinical Presentation

Patients with schizoid personality disorder often have difficulty forming close and intimate relationships. The consequence is isolation, although they may still long for relationships. They prefer to work in a relatively socially isolated environment and usually live alone. They are cognitively intact.

They usually present to the ED because of a medical emergency or due to a comorbid primary psychiatric disorder.

Management

Assess for medical conditions that may explain the presenting complaint and treat any underlying comorbid primary psychiatric condition.

The focus of treatment is the underlying condition that brought the patient to the ED. The patient's treating physician should be informed about the need for privacy. Such patients may appear quite aloof and indifferent to praise or empathy, but they may be more responsive than they seem on the surface.

Schizotypal Personality Disorder (Box 12-4)
Clinical Presentation

Patients with schizotypal personality disorder are odd in behavior and strange in their eccentric ways and beliefs. Such patients are often oddly attired. Their behaviors do not fit the criteria for schizophrenia but may share some of this disorder's

---

Box 12–3. DSM-IV-TR Criteria for Schizoid Personality Disorder

A. A pervasive pattern of detachment from social relationships and a restricted range of expression of emotions in interpersonal settings, beginning by early adulthood and present in a variety of contexts, as indicated by four or more of the following:
   1. Neither desires nor enjoys close relationships, including being part of a family
   2. Almost always chooses solitary activities
   3. Has little, if any, interest in having sexual experiences with another person
   4. Takes pleasure in few, if any, activities
   5. Lacks close friends or confidants other than first-degree relatives
   6. Appears indifferent to the praise or criticism of others
   7. Shows emotional coldness, detachment, or flattened affectivity

Adapted from the DSM-IV-TR (*Diagnostic and Statistical Manual of Mental Disorders, Fourth Edition, Text Revision*).

---

perceptual illusions. At times, patients may experience brief psychotic episodes, anxiety, depression, or obsessive compulsive episodes, and these are usually the reason for their presentation to the ED.

Management

Assess for medical conditions that may explain the presenting complaint and treat any underlying primary psychiatric comorbid condition.

Brief psychotic episodes are usually self-limited and they respond well to low-dose antipsychotic therapy.

During the evaluation, do not seem "pushy" or abrupt, because the sense of reality of such patients is fragile, and they seem to need more reality-affirming explanations than other patients. Scaffolding for emotional support may be needed during times of crisis.

Assess for dangerousness and whether hospitalization may be necessary, although this is unusual in patients with schizotypal personality disorder.

Box 12–4. DSM-IV-TR Criteria for Schizotypal Personality Disorder

A. A pervasive pattern of social and interpersonal deficits marked by acute discomfort with, and reduced capacity for, close relationships as well as by cognitive or perceptual distortions and eccentricities of behavior, beginning by early adulthood and present in a variety of contexts, as indicated by five or more of the following:

1. Ideas of reference (excluding delusions of reference)
2. Odd beliefs or magical thinking that influences behavior and is inconsistent with subcultural norms (e.g., superstitions, belief in clairvoyance, telepathy, or "sixth sense"; in children and adolescents, bizarre fantasies or preoccupations)
3. Unusual perceptual experiences, including bodily illusions
4. Odd thinking and speech (e.g., vague, circumstantial, metaphorical, overelaborate, or stereotyped)
5. Suspiciousness or paranoid ideation
6. Inappropriate or constricted affect
7. Behavior or appearance that is odd, eccentric, or peculiar
8. Lack of close friends or confidants other than first-degree relatives
9. Excessive social anxiety that does not diminish with familiarity and tends to be associated with paranoid fears rather than negative judgments about self

Adapted from the DSM-IV-TR (*Diagnostic and Statistical Manual of Mental Disorders, Fourth Edition, Text Revision*).

Cluster B Disorders

Antisocial Personality Disorder (Box 12-5)
Clinical Presentation
As with other personality disorders, patients with antisocial personality disorder usually do not present to the ED because of the disorder. Often, comorbid conditions such as substance abuse or other medical illnesses bring them to the ED. They may, however, come to the ED to gain access to hospitalization in an attempt to avoid the consequences of their actions, such as after a fight or a criminal act.

> ## Box 12–5. DSM-IV-TR Criteria for Antisocial Personality Disorder
>
> A. There is a pervasive pattern of disregard for and violation of the rights of others occurring since age of 15 years, as indicated by three or more of the following:
>   1. Failure to conform to social norms with respect to lawful behaviors as indicated by repeatedly performing acts that are grounds for arrest
>   2. Deceitfulness, as indicated by repeated lying, use of aliases, or conning others for personal profit or pleasure
>   3. Impulsivity or failure to plan ahead
>   4. Irritability and aggressiveness, as indicated by repeated physical fights or assaults
>   5. Reckless disregard for safety of self or others
>   6. Consistent irresponsibility, as indicated by repeated failure to sustain work behavior or honor financial obligations
>   7. Lack of remorse, as indicated by being indifferent to or rationalizing having hurt, mistreated, or stolen from another
> B. The individual is at least 18 years of age.
> C. There is evidence of conduct disorder with onset before age 15.
> D. The antisocial behavior does not occur exclusively during the course of schizophrenia or a manic episode.

Adapted from the DSM-IV-TR (*Diagnostic and Statistical Manual of Mental Disorders, Fourth Edition, Text Revision*).

People with antisocial personality disorder often are manipulative, deceitful, and adept at hiding their intentions and using their considerable charm to gain whatever they are seeking. They feel no remorse or guilt about their actions and consider the feelings of others inconsequential.

They have little impulse control and may be abusive to spouses. They may show rage and anger if they are the recipient of others' criminal or manipulative acts.

They may express suicidal threats and have complaints of a somatic nature.

Clinicians of the same sex may experience countertransference of anger and irritation when they encounter such patients, whereas clinicians of the opposite sex may be completely won over by their charm.

Management

Assess for medical conditions that may explain the presenting complaint and treat any underlying comorbid primary psychiatric condition, such as substance abuse.

Once the personality disorder is established, it runs an unrelenting course and treatment is difficult and often unsuccessful. However, you should continue to set limits, affirm the reality of the situation, and not allow patients to manipulate or con you.

Assess for dangerousness and whether hospitalization may be necessary. Suicidal threats must always be treated as serious until proven otherwise.

Psychopharmacologic therapy with a selective serotonin reuptake inhibitor (SSRI) such as fluoxetine may have a beneficial effect on temperament, and studies have shown that anti-androgens may be beneficial. Administration of the latter should be discussed with the patient's treating psychiatrist, if available, or perhaps in consultation with forensic psychiatry. Treatment with lithium and other anticonvulsants may decrease impulsiveness and acting out.

Psychosocial therapy by a qualified psychotherapist in a highly structured setting (e.g., in a forensic psychiatry setting) may be beneficial. Anger management therapy may also be beneficial.

Some studies indicate that people with antisocial personality disorder mellow over time and that their symptomatology decreases by the time they reach their 50's.

Borderline Personality Disorder (Box 12-6)
Clinical Presentation

Often dreaded in the ED setting, patients with borderline personality disorder present with one form of crisis after another. They are heavy users of medical and psychiatric resources and often present with suicidal ideations with or without plans and may have perceptual symptoms such as auditory and visual hallucinations. They may also present with dissociative identity disorder and may even assume another persona and associated behaviors.

 Such patients may present to the ED after an ambulance was called due to a suicide attempt, a suicidal gesture, or a para-suicidal act, such as cutting themselves. They generally do not wish to die but may accidentally kill themselves while seeking attention after a perceived rejection or a rift in a volatile relationship.

Box 12–6. DSM-IV-TR Criteria for Borderline Personality Disorder

A. A pervasive pattern of instability of interpersonal relationships, self-image, and affects, and marked impulsivity beginning by early adulthood and present in a variety of contexts, as indicated by five or more of the following:

1. Frantic efforts to avoid real or imagined abandonment (NOTE: Do not include suicidal or self-mutilating behavior covered in criterion 5)
2. A pattern of unstable and intense interpersonal relationships characterized by alternating between extremes of idealization and devaluation
3. Identity disturbance: markedly and persistently unstable self-image or sense of self
4. Impulsivity in at least two areas that are potentially self-damaging (e.g., spending, sex, substance abuse, reckless driving, binge eating) (NOTE: Do not include suicidal or self-mutilating behavior in criterion 5)
5. Recurrent suicidal behavior, gestures, or threats, or self-mutilating behavior
6. Affective instability due to a marked reactivity of mood (e.g., intense episodic dysphoria, irritability, or anxiety usually lasting a few hours and only rarely more than a few days)
7. Chronic feelings of emptiness
8. Inappropriate, intense anger or difficulty controlling anger (e.g., frequent displays of temper, constant anger, recurrent physical fights)
9. Transient, stress-related paranoid ideation or severe dissociative symptoms

Adapted from the DSM-IV-TR (*Diagnostic and Statistical Manual of Mental Disorders, Fourth Edition, Text Revision*).

They see the world in black or white and are unable to modulate their affective range. They see others as either good or bad; hence they either idealize or devalue others.

Patients with borderline personality disorder have a very poor sense of personal identity and may attach themselves emotionally to others in an attempt to establish some stability.

They are usually very lonely because relationships are bound to be imperfect, and their emotional status is dependent on how the "other" is keeping them fulfilled. The "other" most likely will not be able to satisfy their emotional needs. Due to this, they often feel "empty" and may go to drastic extremes to feel "human" again, such as cutting or otherwise mutilating themselves. The feeling of pain may supply temporary relief of this emptiness.

The chaotic life of people with borderline personality disorder often leads to sexual promiscuity or sexual abuse, sexual orientation difficulty, and drug and/or alcohol abuse, if not dependence. The basis of their wide range of emotional needs probably can be found in their environment when growing up. Their history often includes some form of emotional, sexual, or physical abuse during childhood. Many report dissociation, the feeling that their body is in one place but their person is in another.

Borderline personality disorder must be distinguished from bipolar disorder and attention deficit hyperactivity disorder (ADHD).

Management
Assess for medical conditions that may explain the presenting complaint and treat any underlying comorbid primary psychiatric condition.

Attend to the medical issues at hand, such as a suicidal gesture or a suicide attempt. Keep in mind that the presence of the "other" may be necessary to obtain collateral information. Consultation with a physician or surgeon may be necessary, especially for overdose (a common suicidal gesture) and self-mutilation.

Avoid countertransference when evaluating the patient. This is easier said than done. ED clinicians must be prepared emotionally for whatever issue the borderline personality patient may throw at them, including anger, spitting, and manipulativeness.

Recruit case managers and outpatient providers to identify the source of the current crisis and to help with management.

Assess for dangerousness (see Chapters 6 and 10) while considering disposition decisions. If the patient is admitted to the medical floor, evaluate the need for one-to-one (one staff member with the patient at all times) close observation. A temporary civil confinement (legal hold) may be required (see Chapter 23).

Supportive therapy is a must. Such patients often have very low self-esteem, and they need to feel that you are on their side. If they do not feel this, at this point they may easily "split" you out as "bad" and devalue you. If this occurs, it will be difficult to be effective with the patient. Be aware that with projection, patients at times are able to "lob" this projection and manipulativeness to the ED administration. Also be aware of projective identification. This is a primitive defense by which the patient projects anger toward the clinician.

Consider the following vignette:

ED physician: "I understand you're here because of feelings of suicidality. How long have you been feeling this way?"

Patient: "I'm not here for suicide, I'm here because I want you to tell my lover that I'm going to kill myself if I don't get to go to the office Christmas party."

ED physician: "I'm sure you have already tried to tell him that, but why did you have to scratch your wrists today?"

Patient: "Don't you understand? Nobody understands me—what kind of a dumb question is that? Where's your boss? I want another doctor."

The ED physician does not have a chance. The patient projected anger toward the physician within the first two sentences of the conversation. Now the physician, if unguarded or unaware that this is happening, may react in anger, justifying the continued anger of the patient.

As with most personality disorders, outpatient psychotherapy (e.g., group, cognitive, dialectal therapy or psychoanalysis) is usually indicated. Medication to alleviate any comorbid primary psychiatric disorder may be needed.

 Opinions differ about the use of medications for symptoms of the disorder itself. On the one hand, medication may help manage anger, anxiety, sleeplessness, and depression so that patients can be more responsive to outpatient psychotherapy. On the other hand, patients may use medications to hurt themselves, perhaps overdosing on them.

Histrionic Personality Disorder (Box 12-7)
Clinical Presentation

There is little evidence that the incidence of histrionic personality disorder is higher in women than in men (Grant, 2004; Golomb, 1995) as is commonly believed, perhaps due to innate bias (missing the male histrionic personality, but not the seductive, flamboyant female).

Box 12–7. DSM-IV-TR Criteria for Histrionic Personality Disorder

A. A pervasive pattern of excessive emotionality and attention-seeking, beginning by early adulthood and present in a variety of contexts, as indicated by five or more of the following:

1. Is uncomfortable in situations in which he/she is not the center of attention
2. Interaction with others often characterized by inappropriate, sexually seductive, or provocative behavior
3. Displays rapidly shifting and shallow expression of emotions
4. Consistently uses physical appearance to draw attention to self
5. Has a style of speech that is excessively impressionistic and lacking in detail
6. Shows self-dramatization, theatricality, and exaggerated expression of emotion
7. Is suggestible—i.e., easily influenced by others or by circumstances
8. Considers relationships to be more intimate than they actually are

Adapted from the DSM-IV-TR (*Diagnostic and Statistical Manual of Mental Disorders, Fourth Edition, Text Revision*).

Patients with histrionic personality disorder usually present to the ED for reasons other than their disorder. They may come in to attract attention, acting in a grandiose manner. They have a very strong need for admiration and strive to be the center of attention, creating a scene or resorting to somaticizing behaviors if necessary. They tend to spend an excessive amount of money, time, and energy to keep their appearance attractive.

If they happen to have a medical condition, they will surely drag this out to their advantage to keep attention focused on themselves. By the same token, medical illness may adversely affect the attractiveness, strength, and flamboyant behaviors that make them the center of attention.

Their emotional expression shifts rapidly and is exaggerated, dramatic, and theatrical, often embarrassing their friends and relatives. Their speech often has a dramatic flair, with exaggerated and flamboyant intonation, but lacks substance.

They are influenced easily by fashion and fads. They crave novelty and become bored with the same routine quite easily.

They may be overly trusting and credulous, and their opinions and convictions may be easily swayed by others. Often they regard relationships with others as deeper and more intimate than they really are.

They are easily frustrated if they are not able to achieve "instant gratification." They tend to alienate friends because of their excessive demand for attention. They also foster deep dependency in their relationships because of their inexhaustible craving for attention.

It is the author's opinion that this type of craving is at some level akin to dependency on alcohol or other substances (the need for more and more attention, the use of excessive amounts of energy, planning, thinking, and resources in order to obtain attention, with a concurrent decline in social, occupational, and interpersonal functioning).

Management
Assess for medical conditions that may explain the presenting complaint and treat any underlying comorbid primary psychiatric condition.

Assess for dangerousness and suicidality, keeping in mind that such patients are overly expressive and flamboyant, and that their actions may only be a means to attract attention or to gain control over a relationship.

Determine whether the patient has had any recent loss that is integral to the patient's self-esteem, such as loss of function or beauty (e.g., had to go to surgery, will leave a scar, will lose a leg due to diabetes).

Due to such patients' vulnerability and sensitivity to rejection, depression can ensue. Antidepressants may be beneficial in these cases.

Outpatient psychotherapy is usually the treatment of choice.

Narcissistic Personality Disorder (Box 12-8)
Clinical Presentation
Narcissistic personality disorder is more common in men than in women. The criteria for this disorder have some similarity to those for antisocial, histrionic, dependent, and borderline personality disorders.

Patients may present to the ED because of a comorbid primary psychiatric disorder or dysphoria (from sensitivity to

Box 12–8. DSM-IV-TR Criteria for Narcissistic Personality Disorder

A. A pervasive pattern of grandiosity (in fantasy or behavior), need for admiration, and lack of empathy, beginning by early adulthood and present in a variety of contexts, as indicated by five or more of the following:

1. Has a grandiose sense of self-importance (e.g., exaggerates achievements and talents, expects to be recognized as superior without commensurate achievements)
2. Is preoccupied with fantasies of unlimited success, power, brilliance, beauty, or ideal love
3. Believes that he/she is "special" and unique and can only be understood by, or should associate with, other special or high-status people (or institutions)
4. Requires excessive admiration
5. Has a sense of entitlement—i.e., unreasonable expectations of especially favorable treatment or automatic compliance with his/her expectations
6. Is interpersonally exploitative—i.e., takes advantage of others to achieve his/her own ends
7. Lacks empathy; is unwilling to recognize or identify with the feelings and needs of others
8. Is often envious of others or believes that others are envious of him/her
9. Has arrogant, haughty behaviors or attitudes

Adapted from the DSM-IV-TR (*Diagnostic and Statistical Manual of Mental Disorders, Fourth Edition, Text Revision*).

criticism). Occasionally, patients may present in a narcissistic rage (deep-seated anger in reaction to an imagined slight that is usually directed at the person believed responsible for the slight).

At the core of narcissistic personality disorder are feelings of self-importance, egocentricity, and entitlement, a lack of empathy for others, and a craving for admiration (often a person with this disorder may form relationships solely to satisfy this need).

Narcissists are surprised and/or furious when they do not receive the entitlement and admiration that they consider their right. They expect others to regard them as unique, superior beings. They tend to be exploitative and shallow and are preoccupied with wealth, power, achievement, and glory.

Management
Assess for medical conditions that may explain the presenting complaint and treat any underlying comorbid primary psychiatric condition, which in these patients is most likely to be depression, substance use, or anorexia nervosa.

Assess for dangerousness, including homicidality if the patient presents in a narcissistic rage, and whether hospitalization may be necessary. Suicidal threats must always be treated as serious until proven otherwise. Consider hospitalization if crisis intervention is unsuccessful.

Outpatient psychotherapy is the treatment of choice, although its efficacy is not known.

Cluster C Disorders

Avoidant Personality Disorder (Box 12-9)
Clinical Presentation
Avoidant personality disorder is characterized by social inhibition, feelings of inadequacy, and hypersensitivity to negative evaluation. People with this disorder avoid social, work, and school activities due to their fear of criticism or rejection. They avoid making new friends unless they are sure they will be liked and accepted without criticism.

They are capable of having intimate relationships (in contrast with persons with schizoid personality, who are indifferent to others), although they withhold their feelings because of their fear of criticism and ridicule. They tend to be shy, quiet and "invisible." Some marry and have children but greatly limit their social interaction.

Management
Because of their sensitivity to negative evaluation, patients with avoidant personality disorder are unlikely to present to the ED due to psychological problems. They may, however, present for medical reasons.

Assess for medical conditions that may explain the presenting complaint and treat any underlying comorbid primary psychiatric condition. Assess for co-existing anxiety and depressive disorders.

Box 12–9. DSM-IV-TR Criteria for Avoidant Personality Disorder

A. A pervasive pattern of social inhibition, feelings of inadequacy, and hypersensitivity to negative evaluation, beginning by early adulthood and present in a variety of contexts, as indicated by four or more of the following:
1. Avoids occupational activities that involve significant interpersonal contact, because of fears of criticism, disapproval, or rejection
2. Is unwilling to get involved with people unless certain of being liked
3. Is restrained in intimate relationships because of the fear of being shamed or ridiculed
4. Is preoccupied with being criticized or rejected in social situations
5. Is inhibited in new interpersonal situations because of feelings of inadequacy
6. Views self as socially inept, personally unappealing, or inferior to others
7. Is unusually reluctant to take personal risks or to engage in any new activities because they may prove embarrassing

*Adapted from the DSM-IV-TR (*Diagnostic and Statistical Manual of Mental Disorders, Fourth Edition, Text Revision*).*

Be aware of the patient's extreme insecurity and sensitivity and avoid any hint of criticism while establishing rapport.

Psychiatric hospitalization is rarely necessary. Outpatient psychotherapy is the recommended treatment.

Dependent Personality Disorder (Box 12-10)
Clinical Presentation
Persons with dependent personality disorder have an excessive need to be taken care of that results in submissive and clinging behaviors and morbid fear of separation from those on whom they are dependent. They have a self-perception of being incapable of caring for themselves without the help of others and need others to assume responsibility and make decisions for them.

Because of fear of loss of approval, they may do things that are unpleasant or wrong. They may repress appropriate reactions (such as justifiable anger) and tolerate abuse in a relationship.

Box 12–10. DSM-IV-TR Criteria for Dependent Personality Disorder

A. A pervasive and excessive need to be taken care of that leads to submissive and clinging behavior and fears of separation, beginning by early adulthood and present in a variety of contexts, as indicated by five or more of the following:
   1. Has difficulty making everyday decisions without an excessive amount of advice and reassurance from others
   2. Needs others to assume responsibility for most major areas of his/her life
   3. Has difficulty expressing disagreement with others because of fear of loss of support or approval (NOTE: Do not include realistic fears of retribution)
   4. Has difficulty initiating projects or doing things on his/her own because of lack of self-confidence in judgment or abilities rather than a lack of motivation or energy
   5. Goes to excessive lengths to obtain nurturance and support from others, to the point of volunteering to do things that are unpleasant
   6. Feels uncomfortable or helpless when alone because of exaggerated fears of being unable to care for himself/herself
   7. Urgently seeks another relationship as a source of care and support when a close relationship ends
   8. Is unrealistically preoccupied with fears of being forced to take care of himself/herself

Adapted from the DSM-IV-TR (*Diagnostic and Statistical Manual of Mental Disorders, Fourth Edition, Text Revision*).

They may avoid appearing or becoming competent, fearing that competence may lead to abandonment.

They usually present to the ED accompanied by "important others" (the person or persons on whom they depend) and will not make decisions without consulting them.

Management
Assess for medical conditions that may explain the presenting complaint and treat any underlying Axis I comorbid condition, including anxiety and excessive fear.

Crisis intervention is highly dependent on the availability of a support system. The important others may be controlling, domineering, and overprotective.

If the patient's occupational functioning is severely diminished, referral to social services may be advisable.

 Patients with dependent personality disorder, known as "frequent flyers," use hospitalization as a temporary substitute for a broken relationship until a new relationship is formed. To avoid this, do not consider hospitalization if the patient does not pose a danger to self or others and is not gravely disabled due to mental illness.

Outpatient therapy is the recommended treatment. Assertiveness and social skills training may be helpful.

 Note: It is difficult for the individual with dependent personality disorder to make decisions, but many patients, when ill—even egosyntonic individuals—tend to have some behavioral regression to dependency. The clinician should keep this in mind when evaluating ED patients.

Obsessive Compulsive Personality Disorder
(Box 12-11)
Clinical Presentation
The core features of obsessive compulsive personality disorder* (OCPD) are perfectionism, constrictedness, and excessive mental and interpersonal discipline at the expense of efficiency, openness, and flexibility.

Persons with this disorder are restricted in their behavior by rigid rules, including moral rules, to the detriment of friendship and other relationships, because others are expected to follow these rules.

They are often indecisive and tormented when faced with making decisions about trivial matters. Their perfectionism may interfere with completion of their work in a timely manner.

The patient with OCPD usually presents to the ED because of a medical condition. The presenting symptom may be anxiety due to failure to exert control or make decisions. Some studies suggest an association between OCPD and mood disorder and eating disorder.

Management
Assess for medical conditions that may explain the presenting complaint and treat any underlying primary psychiatric comorbid condition.

---

*Note that this is not the same as obsessive compulsive disorder.

Box 12–11. DSM-IV-TR Criteria for Obsessive Compulsive Personality Disorder

A. A pervasive pattern of preoccupation with orderliness, perfectionism, and mental interpersonal control, at the expense of flexibility, openness, and efficiency, beginning by early adulthood and present in a variety of contexts, as indicated by four or more of the following:

1. Is preoccupied with details, rules, lists, order, organization, or schedules to the extent that the major point of the activity is lost
2. Shows perfectionism that interferes with task completion (e.g., is unable to complete a project because his/her own overtly strict standards are not met)
3. Is excessively devoted to work and productivity to the exclusion of leisure activities and friendships (not accounted for by obvious economic necessity)
4. Is overly conscientious, scrupulous, and inflexible about matters of morality, ethics, or other values (not accounted for by cultural or religious identification)
5. Is unable to discard worn-out or worthless objects even when they have no sentimental value
6. Is reluctant to delegate tasks or to work with others unless they submit to exactly his/her way of doing things
7. Adopts a miserly spending style toward both self and others; money is viewed as something to be hoarded by future catastrophes
8. Shows rigidity and stubbornness

Adapted from the DSM-IV-TR (*Diagnostic and Statistical Manual of Mental Disorders, Fourth Edition, Text Revision*).

Assess for dangerousness and whether hospitalization may be necessary. Although suicide by patients with OCPD is rare, suicidal threats must always be treated as serious unless proved otherwise.

Outpatient psychotherapy is the treatment of choice. Carefully outline the proposed therapy and give the patient ample time to make decisions about treatment; such patients will ask more questions than usual.

Psychosis Not Otherwise Specified

People with psychosis not otherwise specified have features of more than one personality disorder but do not fit the full criteria of any of the aforementioned DSM-IV-TR criteria of a specific personality disorder. However, they do continue to suffer the constellation of inflexible and maladaptive behaviors cited in Box 12-1.

 People with one personality disorder often fit the criteria for another personality disorder, usually within the same cluster (e.g., borderline and histrionic personality disorders).

Further Reading

Ahles SR: Our Inner World: A Guide to Psychodynamics and Psychotherapy. Baltimore, The Johns Hopkins University Press, 2004.

American Psychiatric Association: Diagnostic and Statistical Manual of Mental Disorders, 4th ed, Text Revision. Washington, DC, American Psychiatric Association, 2000.

Golomb M, Fara M, Abraham M, Rosenbaum JF: Gender differences in personality disorders. Am J Psychiatry 1995;152:579-582.

Grant BF, Hasin DS, Stinson FS, et al: Prevalence, correlates, and disability of personality disorders in the United States: Results from the National Epidemiologic Survey on Alcohol and Related Conditions. J Clin Psychiatry 2004;65:948-958.

Hall RW, Platt DE, Hall RW: Suicide risk assessment: A review of risk factors for suicide in 100 patients who made severe suicide attempts. Evaluation of suicide risk in a time of managed care. Psychosomatics 1999;40:18-27.

Kaplan HI, Sadock BJ: Synopsis of Psychiatry, 9th ed. Philadelphia, Lippincott Williams & Wilkins, 2003, pp 275-286, 775-796.

Torgersen S, Kringlen E, Cramer V: The prevalence of personality disorders in a community sample. Arch Gen Psychiatry 2001;58:590-596.

CHAPTER 13

The Chronically Somatizing Patient

Doris T. Tan, DO

KEY POINTS

- Treatment of chronically somatizing patients accounts for a disproportionate expenditure of medical services.
- Iatrogenic injuries due to unnecessary procedures and pursuit of false negative testing are a major component of these services.
- Presentation of patients suspected of having a somatization disorder places a burden on the emergency department (ED) clinician, because correct diagnosis and decisions about treatment are extremely difficult, especially ruling out potentially dangerous conditions.
- It may be best to obtain collateral information from an old chart and the primary care physician(s) for a more rounded history that may affect the ED clinician's decisions.
- The emphasis of management should be on treatment of comorbid psychiatric disorders such as anxiety and depressive disorders.
- Somatization disorders must be distinguished from factitious disorder and malingering.

 - Remain alert for true illness presentation.

Definitions

Somatization. Symptom or a syndrome manifested by somatic complaints in the absence of a physiologically explainable medical etiology. Physical complaints generally are experienced over several years, involving clinically significant distress, causing significant impairment in functioning, and resulting in unnecessary medical treatment. The somatic symptoms are neither intentionally produced nor feigned and appear to be unconscious.

Factitious Disorder. A psychopathology characterized by physical or psychological symptoms that are intentionally feigned, exaggerated, or self-induced to assume the sick role, thus gaining attention and nurturance.

Malingering. The intentional production of physical or psychological symptoms in order to obtain some external gain, such as disability payments or narcotic drugs.

Somatoform Disorders

Patients with somatoform disorders may have physical or psychological symptoms that suggest a medical condition. The physical symptoms are not intentionally produced and are not voluntarily controlled as in factitious disorders or malingering. They cause considerable distress and may impair social and occupational functioning.

The Diagnostic and Statistical Manual of Mental Disorders, Fourth Edition, Text Revision (DSM-IV-TR) classifies somatoform disorders in the following categories:
- Somatization disorder
- Conversion disorder
- Pain disorder
- Hypochondriasis
- Body dysmorphic disorder
- Undifferentiated somatoform disorder
- Somatoform disorder not otherwise specified (NOS)

Somatization Disorder (Box 13-1)

The main feature of somatization disorder (also known as *Briquet's syndrome*) is recurrent, chronic, and multiple somatic complaints not accounted for by a medical diagnosis. If there are related medical findings, the physical symptoms are in excess of what would be expected.

Epidemiology
Somatization disorder occurs more often in women (0.2% to 2%) than in men (0.2%). A study by Fink et al (1999) reported that the prevalence in a general practice setting could be as high as 30.3%; a study by DeWaal et al (2004) indicated that the prevalence could be as high as 21.9%. Age of onset usually is less than 30 years of age.

Box 13–1. DSM-IV-TR Diagnostic Criteria for Somatization Disorder

A. A history of many physical complaints beginning before age 30 that occur over a period of several years and result in treatment being sought or significant impairment in social, occupational, or other important areas of functioning.

B. Each of the following criteria must have been met, with individual symptoms occurring at any time during the course of the disturbance:

1. A history of pain symptoms related to at least four different sites or functions
2. A history of at least two gastrointestinal symptoms other than pain
3. A history of at least one sexual or reproductive symptom other than pain
4. A history of at least one symptom or deficit suggesting a neurologic condition not limited to pain

C. Either (1) or (2):

1. After appropriate investigation, each of the symptoms in criterion B cannot be fully explained by a known general medical condition or the direct effects of a substance (drug of abuse or medication).
2. When there is a related general medical condition, the physical complaints or resulting social or occupational impairment are in excess of what would be expected from the history, physical examination, or laboratory findings.

D. The symptoms are not intentionally produced or feigned (as in factitious disorder or malingering).

Adapted from the *Diagnostic and Statistical Manual of Mental Disorders, Fourth Edition, Text Revision* (DSM-IV-TR).

Clinical Presentation

Patients may have a chaotic lifestyle, are "physician shoppers" (consult a number of physicians), give inconsistent histories, make conflicting requests, and may receive multiple work-ups for their multitude of symptomatic presentations.

They may have a family history of somatization disorder, antisocial personality disorder, or substance abuse disorder.

Medical history may include comorbid psychiatric illnesses, including personality disorders, major depression, anxiety or panic disorder, and substance abuse.

Management

Assess for medical conditions that may explain the presenting complaint and treat any underlying comorbid disorder.

The goal of treatment is to help patients learn to control their symptoms. Often there is an underlying mood disorder, such as depression, that may respond to conventional treatment.

A supportive relationship with a sympathetic therapist is the most important aspect of treatment. Regularly scheduled follow-up appointments with their primary care provider should be maintained to review patients' symptoms and coping mechanisms.

 It is not helpful to tell patients that their symptoms are imaginary.

Conversion Disorder (Box 13-2)

Conversion disorder involves unexplained symptoms affecting voluntary motor or sensory function that suggest a neurologic or other general medical condition. Its onset often is preceded by a stressful event.

Symptoms generally do not follow a known anatomic pathway, but rather run in a pattern based on the patient's conceptualization of the condition. Common symptoms are blindness, paralysis, and mutism.

The course of the disorder usually is self-limited, but symptoms may recur or become more chronic.

In some cases, conversion disorder may precede a medical condition.

Epidemiology

Conversion disorder is the most common of all somatoform disorders; its prevalence is estimated as 11 to 300 per 100,000 in the general population. It occurs more often in women than in men.

Onset is rare before age 10 and after age 35. When the disorder does occur at a later age, the probability of an occult neurologic or medical condition increases.

A family history of conversion disorder has been reported in people with the disorder.

Clinical Presentation

The patient may present with any of four different types of symptoms: (1) motor, (2) sensory, (3) seizures, or (4) mixed presentation. Symptoms are not intentionally produced or feigned.

> ### Box 13–2. DSM-IV-TR Diagnostic Criteria for Conversion Disorder
>
> A. One or more symptoms or deficits affecting voluntary motor or sensory function that suggest a neurologic or other general medical condition.
> B. Psychological factors are judged to be associated with the symptom or deficit because the initiation or exacerbation of the symptom or deficit is preceded by conflicts or other stressors.
> C. The symptom or deficit is not intentionally produced or feigned (as in factitious disorder or malingering).
> D. The symptom or deficit cannot, after appropriate investigation, be fully explained by a general medical condition or by the direct effects of a substance, or as a culturally sanctioned behavior or experience.
> E. The symptom or deficit causes clinically significant distress or impairment in social, occupational, or other important areas of functioning or warrants medical evaluation.
> F. The symptom or deficit is not limited to pain or sexual dysfunction, does not occur exclusively during the course of Somatization Disorder, and is not better accounted for by another mental disorder.

Adapted from the *Diagnostic and Statistical Manual of Mental Disorders, Fourth Edition, Text Revision* (DSM-IV-TR).

Management

It is imperative to perform a complete medical and neurologic examination, because 25% to 50% of these patients go on to develop a neurologic or a medical condition.

The patient may be susceptible to suggestion, and such ploys as giving benign normal saline eye drops for the patient's "blindness" may be effective. There is no need to confront the patient about the reality of the symptoms as this only worsens the situation.

Psychotherapy is usually the recommended treatment.

Pain Disorder (Box 13-3)

The key feature of pain disorder is the presentation of pain with sufficient severity to warrant a medical evaluation. The pain may become a major focus of the patient's life, often causing discord within the family due to changes in lifestyle.

Box 13–3. DSM IV-TR Diagnostic Criteria for Pain Disorder

A. Pain in one or more anatomic sites is the predominant focus of the clinical presentation and is of sufficient severity to warrant clinical attention.

B. The pain causes clinically significant distress or impairment in social, occupational, or other important areas of functioning.

C. Psychological factors are judged to have an important role in the onset, severity, exacerbation, or maintenance of the pain.

D. The symptom or deficit is not intentionally produced or feigned (as in factitious disorder or malingering).

E. The pain is not better accounted for by a mood, anxiety, or psychotic disorder and does not meet criteria for dyspareunia.

Adapted from the *Diagnostic and Statistical Manual of Mental Disorders, Fourth Edition, Text Revision* (DSM-IV-TR).

Functional impairment includes inability to work or attend school. Iatrogenic narcotic dependence may ensue from chronic use of pain-killers.

The onset, severity, exacerbation, recurrence, and duration of the pain are believed to have psychological undertones.

The DSM-IV-TR divides pain disorder into three subtypes:

1. Pain associated with psychological factors
2. Pain associated with both psychological and medical factors
3. Pain as a symptom of a general medical condition (not considered a mental disorder and therefore coded as an Axis III disorder [general medical conditions])

Epidemiology

Prevalence is unknown, but it is estimated that 10% to 15% of adults suffer from chronic back pain, a common manifestation of pain disorder. The peak age of onset is the fourth or fifth decade. The disorder is thought to be more frequent in women, and is more likely to occur in those with first-degree relatives affected with pain disorder.

Clinical Presentation

Chronic pain may cause inactivity and decreased physical endurance, leading to social isolation, which in turn can lead to additional psychological problems such as anxiety and depression.

Patients who have associated depression are at high risk for suicide. Therefore, depression and suicidality should be assessed in every patient with pain disorder.

Management

In the ED setting, treat psychiatric illnesses as they arise and refer to the patient's primary caregiver for continued support.

The emphasis of treatment should be teaching the patient to live with the pain and avoid iatrogenic complications that can result from excess diagnostic procedures or overmedication (e.g., side effects of nonsteroidal anti-inflammatory drugs, such as gastrointestinal symptoms or bleeding, or hepatic injury resulting from acetaminophen therapy).

Hypochondriasis (Box 13-4)

Even when appropriate medical assessment shows negative results, patients with hypochondriasis continue to fear or believe that they have a serious illness and cannot be reassured of the contrary, resulting in significant distress and impairment.

Onset usually occurs in early childhood. Episodes may be precipitated by stress, such as the death of a loved one. The disorder is chronic but severity waxes and wanes.

Epidemiology

Incidence varies in different cultures. In the United States, hypochondriasis is estimated to affect up to 5% of the population, whereas only 1% of the population is affected in African nations.

The affliction does not seem to be gender-specific.

Clinical Presentation

Patients generally present to the ED with a detailed history of their symptoms. They may have come to the ED because they were alarmed by information regarding their presumed illness or because they recently learned that an acquaintance had succumbed to the illness.

They may misinterpret normal bodily functions (such as peristalsis) or minor, vague, physical sensations (such as loose stool) as symptoms of their feared illness (such as colon cancer). Definitive test results such as negative colonoscopy, guaiac stool, and CT scan will not reassure these patients.

Box 13–4. DSM IV-TR Diagnostic Criteria for Hypochondriasis

A. Preoccupation with fears of having, or the idea that one has, a serious disease based on the person's misinterpretation of bodily symptoms.

B. The preoccupation persists despite appropriate medical evaluation and reassurance.

C. The belief in A above is not of delusional intensity and is not restricted to a circumscribed concern about appearance (as in body dysmorphic disorder).

D. The preoccupation causes clinically significant distress or impairment in social, occupational, or other important areas of functioning.

E. The duration of the disturbance is at least 6 months.

F. The preoccupation is not better accounted for by generalized anxiety disorder, obsessive compulsive disorder, panic disorder, a major depressive disorder, separation anxiety disorder, or another somatoform disorder.

G. The person does not recognize that the concern about having a serious illness is excessive or unreasonable.

Adapted from the *Diagnostic and Statistical Manual of Mental Disorders, Fourth Edition, Text Revision* (DSM-IV-TR).

 Their relationship with their primary physician is often strained and frustrating. They may demand excessive diagnostic workups, which may result in iatrogenic injuries, or the exasperated, sorely tried physician may perform only a cursory evaluation, missing the presence of a medical condition.

Social and work relationships may be strained due to patients' preoccupation with their supposed illness.

Patients with very severe hypochondriasis may become total invalids.

Management

Assess for medical conditions that may explain the presenting complaint, and treat any underlying comorbid disorder, such as anxiety and depression.

If available, obtain collateral information from the primary care physician, family, and friends.

The focus of treatment should be reassurance rather than excessive procedures and tests.

Body Dysmorphic Disorder (Box 13-5)

Body dysmorphic disorder (BDD) is characterized by an obsessive preoccupation with an imagined defect in appearance or excessive concern about a minor physical anomaly.

Epidemiology

Prevalence is unknown. Rates of 6% to 15% have been reported in cosmetic surgery and dermatology settings.

Onset occurs during adolescence or childhood, but diagnosis may not be made until patients are in their 30s. There is no strong evidence of gender differences.

Clinical Presentation

Because people with BDD feel ashamed of their perceived deformity, they usually do not present to the ED for treatment of the defect. When they do present for treatment, it may be because they have subjected themselves to multiple procedures to compensate for the perceived imperfection but are not satisfied with the results.

ED presentation also may be due to suicidality. Isolation and avoidance of social encounters are common and may lead to depression and anxiety. There may be a history of multiple

---

Box 13–5. DSM IV-TR Diagnostic Criteria for Body Dysmorphic Disorder

A. Preoccupation with an imagined defect in appearance. If a slight physical anomaly is present, the person's concern is markedly excessive.

B. The preoccupation causes clinically significant distress or impairment in social, occupational, or other important areas of functioning.

C. The preoccupation is not better accounted for by another mental disorder (e.g., dissatisfaction with body shape and size in anorexia nervosa).

Adapted from the *Diagnostic and Statistical Manual of Mental Disorders, Fourth Edition, Text Revision* (DSM-IV-TR).

hospitalizations due to comorbid psychiatric illnesses and suicidal ideation; therefore, a psychiatric evaluation is mandatory for suicidal intent and comorbid pathology, such as major depressive disorder.

Management

Psychotherapy is the recommended treatment. The therapist should be a specialist in the treatment of BDD or the closely related obsessive compulsive disorder. Educate the patient and family about the features of BDD and about measures to alleviate symptoms. Prevention of iatrogenic injuries should be a priority.

Antidepressants (e.g., fluvoxamine [Luvox], fluoxetine [Prozac], imipramine) have been known to help in about 50% of cases.

Undifferentiated Somatoform Disorder

(Box 13-6)

Undifferentiated somatoform disorder, considered a subthreshold somatization disorder, is characterized by one or more physical complaints that persist for greater than 6 months, including poorly defined discomfort with fatigue and weakness. Symptoms may overlap with those of medical illnesses such as fibromyalgia, chronic fatigue syndrome, and ecological allergies.

Patients with this diagnosis seldom present to the ED. Management includes assessment for medical conditions that may explain the presenting complaint and treatment of any underlying comorbid disorder. Referral to the patient's primary care physician may be advisable.

Somatoform Disorder Not Otherwise Specified (NOS)

This category includes disorders with symptoms that do not meet the criteria for specific somatoform disorders.

Examples include:

- Pseudocyesis (false pregnancy)
- Disorders involving hypochondria lasting less than 6 months
- Disorders that are not due to a medical disorder but involve unexplained physical symptoms (e.g., fatigue and weakness) of less than 6 months' duration

Box 13–6. DSM IV-TR Diagnostic Criteria for Undifferentiated Somatoform Disorder

A. One or more physical complaints (e.g., fatigue, loss of appetite, gastrointestinal or urinary complaints.
B. Either (1) or (2):
   1. After appropriate investigation, the symptoms cannot be fully explained by a known general medical condition or the direct effects of a substance (e.g., drug of abuse or medications).
   2. When there is a related general medical condition, the physical complaints or resulting social or occupational impairment is in excess of what would be expected from the history, physical examination, or laboratory findings.
C. The symptoms cause clinically significant distress or impairment in social, occupational, or other important areas of functioning.
D. The duration of the disturbance is at least 6 months.
E. The disturbance is not better accounted for by another mental disorder (e.g., another somatoform disorder, sexual dysfunction, mood disorder, anxiety disorder, sleep disorder, or psychotic disorder).
F. The symptoms are not intentionally produced or feigned (as in factitious disorder or malingering).

Adapted from the *Diagnostic and Statistical Manual of Mental Disorders, Fourth Edition, Text Revision* (DSM-IV-TR).

Factitious Disorder and Malingering

Factitious Disorder (Box 13-7)

Factitious disorder is a psychopathology characterized by physical or psychological symptoms that are intentionally produced, including the following:
- Fabrication of subjective complaints and falsification of objective signs; self-inflicted wounds or self-administration of noxious agents or exaggeration of previous ailments in order to assume the sick role or to extend the stay in the hospital.
- Absence of any external incentive for the behavior except for the specific reason of assuming the sick role.

Box 13–7. DSM IV-TR Diagnostic Criteria for Factitious Disorder

A. Intentional production or feigning of physical or psychological signs or symptoms.
B. The motivation for the behavior is to assume the sick role.
C. External incentives for the behavior (e.g., economic gain, avoiding legal responsibility, or improving physical well-being, as in malingering) are absent.

Adapted from the *Diagnostic and Statistical Manual of Mental Disorders, Fourth Edition, Text Revision* (DSM-IV-TR).

- Pseudologia fantastica—a fantastic explanation to intrigue the listener about an extraordinary history or physical symptom (e.g., describing a body scar that was obtained in childhood as a war injury).
  A severe form of this illness is called Munchausen syndrome.

Epidemiology

Factitious disorder is more frequent in men and in hospital and health care workers, but the incidence is unknown.

Clinical Presentation

Patients with factitious disorder usually have an average or above-average IQ. Their simulated somatic complaints are made consciously but for unconscious reasons (e.g., to assume a sick role to obtain the care that comes with medical treatment).

Their history may reveal visits to many physicians and stays in various hospitals; they may have changed names in order to continue to receive medical treatment and maintain the sick role.

While they are in the hospital, they often subject themselves to numerous procedures and tests. They may insist on surgical procedures and analgesic and narcotic therapy. They may accuse physicians of incompetence and threaten litigation. They may demand to leave against medical advice when they suspect that the medical staff is about to confront them, and repeat the cycle in other hospitals.

Management

Management of these cases is a daunting challenge for ED clinicians. It may be years before factitious disorder is finally diagnosed.

Keep in mind that these patients may present with a true medical condition that needs to be addressed. They often have a comorbid psychiatric illness such as borderline personality disorder.

If there is a registry in your ED for these patients, it may be worthwhile checking it.

Munchausen Syndrome by Proxy

Munchausen syndrome by proxy is thought to be a subtype of factitious disorder in which an individual (usually a mother or other caregiver) makes another person (usually an unwitting victim such as a child) ill in order to maintain a sick role by proxy. Such individuals are overly protective and concerned about the victim; more often than not their concern is admired by others rather than recognized as a symptom of this disorder. Some authors challenge this diagnosis and the debate is a reminder of the difficulty in practicing with uncertainty when diagnosing conditions for which evidence is not easy to obtain.

Malingering

Malingering is the intentional production of physical or psychological symptoms in order to obtain some form of secondary gain (e.g., to avoid responsibilities, punishment, or unpleasant situations or consequences or to receive compensation).

Epidemiology
The incidence is unknown, but malingering occurs more often in situations where men congregate, such as in the military and in prisons.

Clinical Presentation
Malingerers generally are vague about their symptoms but exaggerate their severity. There is generally a marked discrepancy between the objective findings and the claims of stress and disability.

Drug abusers may come to the ED for a warm bed and food or for drugs. Malingering is often seen in patients with antisocial personality disorder.

The feigned illness dissipates once the desired objective is attained.

Management

The ED clinician should, as always, perform a thorough examination and assess for medical conditions that may explain the presenting complaint.

Continue to be a good listener and control the anger that is often felt when assessing malingering patients. Give a clear explanation of the evaluation results without confrontation.

Ganser Syndrome

Ganser syndrome (also known as *prison psychosis* because it was first observed in prisoners) is a type of malingering characterized by short-term episodes of odd behavior similar to those seen in serious mental disorders. A classic symptom of Ganser syndrome is "approximate answers" in which the person gives nonsense answers to simple questions (e.g., 2 + 2 = 5). There is some evidence that Ganser syndrome may be a variant of malingering.

Further Reading

American Psychiatric Association: Diagnostic and Statistical Manual of Mental Disorders, 4th ed, Text Revision. Washington, DC, American Psychiatric Association, 2000.

De Waal M, Arnold IA, Eekhof JA, van Hemert AM: Somatoform disorders in general practice: Prevalence, functional impairment and comorbidity and anxiety and depressive disorders. Br J Psychiatry 2004;184:470-476.

Dickinson WP, Dickinson LM, deGruy FV, et al: A randomized clinical trial of a care recommendation letter intervention for somatization in primary care. Ann Fam Med 2003;1:228-235.

Fink P, Sorensen L, Engberg M, et al: Somatization disorder in primary care: Prevalence, health care utilization, and general practitioner recognition. Psychosomatics 1999;40:330-338.

Kaplan HI, Sadock BJ: Synopsis of Psychiatry, 8th ed. Philadelphia, Lippincott Williams & Wilkins, 1998, pp 629-659.

CHAPTER 14

The Alcohol-Dependent Patient and Related Emergencies

Tirath S. Gill, MD

KEY POINTS

- One should maintain a high index of suspicion for alcohol-related withdrawal syndromes in the hospitalized medically ill. Their medical illness in the context of unknown alcohol dependence may make them more prone to delirium tremens.
- Cocaine and stimulant intoxication can cause serious problems during the intoxication phase of alcohol dependence.
- Treatment of alcohol abuse is effective in a surprisingly high number of people. The emergency department (ED) may provide an opportunity for intervention at a time of crisis when patients may be receptive to offers of help.
- The incidence of alcohol and substance abuse is high in the mentally ill. Alcohol and substance abuse can cause a unique psychiatric pathology that usually remits when the abuse and dependence patterns are overcome with treatment.
- Negative attitudes toward this subset of the population hinder the provision of effective care and should be examined if they arise in the clinician.
- Urine drug screen testing on a routine basis in patients with unusual behaviors is recommended. It almost doubles the detection rate of substance abuse compared with relying on the history alone.

Overview (Fig. 14-1)

Alcohol is the most dangerous of the drugs of abuse. The fact that it is readily accessible and legal makes it even more of a

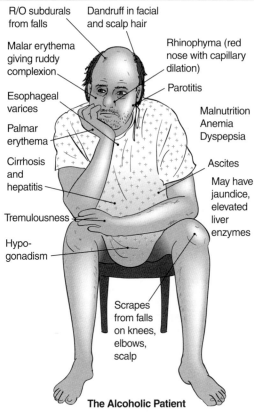

The Alcoholic Patient

Risk factors are
- Family history
- Other psychiatric illness
- Unemployed
- Divorced or single
- Male
- White and Native American race
- Homeless or displaced

FIGURE 14–1

The alcoholic patient.

problem. National surveys indicate that alcohol abuse and dependence are responsible for an inordinately large number of visits to the ED. The specter of alcoholism haunts EDs worldwide, not only as the ambulance brings in an innocent slaughtered by a drunk driver but also with regard to its corrosive effects on the physical, mental, and social well-being of the individual. Shootings, stabbings, sexual assault, and other trauma are often preceded by the use of alcohol.

Systemic alcohol toxicity affects many organs and causes a plethora of medical conditions, including gastritis, anemia, dementia, amnestic syndromes, Wernicke's syndrome, pancreatitis, cancer of the gastrointestinal tract, hepatitis, cirrhosis, and cardiomyopathy. The alert clinician recognizes the underlying alcohol-related issues and may consult a mental health professional for assistance in providing an intervention. ED evaluation provides a unique opportunity to break through the denial that is so prominent in these individuals.

Alcohol-Related Emergencies

Epidemiology

In the United States, 30% to 45% of adults have had at least one episode of complications due to alcohol use. It is estimated that 10% of women and 20% of men in this population meet the criteria for alcohol abuse during their lifetime and that 3% to 5% of the women and 10% of the men meet the criteria for alcohol dependence.

Clinical Assessment

It is important to gather information from collateral sources when available about the extent of alcohol use by the patient and the circumstances that led to the ED presentation. It is also useful to note whether there were recent expressions about suicide. There is a high risk for suicide in alcoholic patients who show signs of depression and a sense of hopelessness.

Alcoholic patients usually have a deep sense of guilt about their problem and may naturally be defensive. Approach such patients with respect and try to put them at ease, conveying a non-judgmental attitude by your verbal and nonverbal expressions.

Ask patients if they are in physical distress or pain and if they have any specific worries that they want cleared up (e.g., the safety of other passengers in a vehicle that may have crashed; illegal and/or violent acts they might have committed during a black-out period that they are unable to recall).

It is important when evaluating patients to let them tell their story without interruption, if possible. One may gain much data by such an open-ended approach.

If patients are obtunded or appear to be in a state of delirium, it is vital to ascertain stat alcohol levels and finger-stick glucose measurements. To avoid the emergence of Wernicke's syndrome (i.e., ataxia, ophthalmoplegia, disorientation, and paresis of the lateral rectus muscle), thiamine, 100 mg, should be administered by the intramuscular (IM) or intravenous (IV) route before giving any fluids or food with caloric value.

During the first few minutes of the interview, check for the presence of a medical bracelet around the wrist, ankle, or neck.

If the patient is alert and oriented but shows clear signs of withdrawal such as tremulousness and elevated heart rate, give IM, IV, or PO (per os; by mouth) benzodiazepine before proceeding further with the interview, which may take some time.

Determine when the last drink was taken and check if recent laboratory tests have been done. If indicated, order a blood alcohol level measurement, urine drug screen, chemistry panel, complete blood count (CBC), liver function tests, and prothrombin time (PT) and partial thromboplastin time (PTT) measurements.

This is also a good time to review the medical history and determine whether patients have been taking street drugs and/or prescribed medications that may have had an effect on their medical conditions. For example, an elevated blood pressure and tachycardia can be due to alcohol withdrawal but it also may be rebound hypertension and tachycardia due to missed doses of clonidine or beta blockers. A history of delirium tremens is a risk factor in the recurrence of this dangerous condition.

When performing the mental status examination, look for issues with depression, hallucinosis, delusions, memory problems, and cognitive problems in particular. The tests for cognition and memory, however, may be affected by the anxiety related to withdrawal and to the circumstances necessitating the visit to the ED.

If the patient is depressed, ask about suicidal or homicidal ideations and any specific plans for such acts.

Physical Examination

It is an axiom that complications such as delirium tremens almost always develop in the malnourished alcoholic who is also suffering from infections such as pneumonia, urinary tract infection, dehydration, or uncontrolled medical issues due to the dysfunction caused by the addiction.

As described previously, perform a thorough physical examination. Check for bruising, occult head injuries (bumps and bruises in various stages over the forearms, lower legs, knees, and head are common in alcohol-dependent patients), and cracked ribs. Look for evidence of malnutrition, subdural and extradural hemorrhages, tuberculosis, human immuno-deficiency virus (HIV) infection, and sexually transmitted disease (STD). Electrolyte abnormalities such as hypokalemia, hyponatremia, hypomagnesemia, elevated liver enzyme levels, cirrhosis, and ascites may be noted. Cardiomyopathy, hypogonadism, and gynecomastia may be noted in the later stages of alcoholism as well.

Spider nevi (dilated peripheral veins and capillaries) may be present over the nose (rhinophyma), cheeks, and abdomen (caput medusae). The palms may have a red, splotchy appearance (palmar erythema), and recalcitrant dandruff may be seen on the scalp, as well as on the eyebrows and beard areas at times.

Laboratory Test Parameters (Table 14-1)

The following laboratory parameters may give clues to the presence of alcohol abuse: increased mean corpuscular volume (MCV), anemia, deficiencies in vitamin B_{12} and folic acid, elevated liver enzyme, gamma-glutamyltransferase (GGT), aspartate transaminase (AST), and alanine aminotransferase (ALT) levels, prolonged PT and PTT, decreased albumin levels, and hypokalemia, hyponatremia, and hypomagnesemia.

Signs and Symptoms of Alcohol Withdrawal

Tremulousness is one of the most common signs of withdrawal and tends to develop within 6 to 8 hours of significant reduction in alcohol intake.

Symptoms can progress to visual hallucinations and seizures after 12 to 24 hours following alcohol withdrawal. Other symptoms include nausea and vomiting, increased irritability, insomnia, easy startle reflex, and sensitivity to light and noise.

Table 14–1

Laboratory Test Parameters Suggesting Alcohol Abuse

Parameters	Associated Complications
Elevated GGT, ALT, and AST levels; increased MCV, low platelet count; hyponatremia, hypokalemia, hypomagnesemia; megaloblastic anemia	Cirrhosis (ascites, pedal edema); gastritis (hematemesis, epigastric pain), esophageal varices, increased incidence of cancer of mouth and GI tract; malnutrition (low body weight); dementia (disorientation); cardiomyopathy (CHF); hypogonadism (impotence); increased rate of seborrheic dermatitis

ALT, alanine aminotransferase; AST, aspartate transaminase; CHF, congestive heart failure; GGT, gamma-glutamyltransferase; GI, gastrointestinal; MCV, mean corpuscular volume.

There are also signs of autonomic arousal such as tachycardia, elevation of blood pressure, and diaphoresis.

Treatment of Alcohol Dependence

The Detoxification Phase

Perform a complete physical examination (as previously described) and identify and treat any active medical problems.

Monitor vital signs every 4 hours for the first 48 hours while the patient is awake; if the patient's condition is stable, the frequency can be decreased to three times/day for the next 2 or 3 days.

Benzodiazepines are preferred for managing the withdrawal. Any of various brands can be used, but keep in mind that generic formulations vary in their bioavailability. A reliable choice is temazepam (Restoril), 30 mg PO every 6 hours for 24 hours, then 30 mg PO every 8 hours for 24 hours, then 30 mg PO bid, and then 30 mg PO/day for the last day. The advantage of formulations such as lorazepam, temazepam, and oxazepam is that they impose less of a metabolic burden on the liver compared with other benzodiazepines as they require only conjugation prior to excretion from the body. They are hence preferred in those with significant liver disease. In the intensive care unit (ICU) setting, where oral intake is not possible, IV diazepam and lorazepam offer an advantage. Temazepam 30 mg every

4 hours on a prn (as needed) basis should also be ordered for any residual withdrawal symptoms for 5 days.

Dehydration can be treated with oral or intravenous fluids. Administer thiamine by the parenteral route, if possible. If magnesium levels are low, magnesium supplementation is recommended.

Clonidine and beta blockers should be avoided because they can mask the signs and symptoms of alcohol withdrawal. Anticonvulsants such as Tegretol and Depakote for detoxification are not generally recommended in view of the increased incidence of adverse side effects. Close monitoring of liver function is indicated if these agents are used.

The Long-term Recovery and Abstinence Phase

Success depends on the motivation of the individual to quit drinking. It is important to link the individual while an inpatient and motivated with a sponsor of a rehab program (Box 14-1) such as an Alcoholics Anonymous (AA) group in the community. If patients are determined to give up the use of alcohol, it can be done, and many have done it without the help of any program. It is a point of visceral realization—the "aha experience" or "hitting bottom"—when they realize that alcohol is a demon for them and that they need to abstain from it and keep away from those who would offer or persuade them to take that first drink.

AA is a nondenominational organization that calls upon a higher power to help those who acknowledge their powerlessness over alcohol, thereby breaking the cycle of denial. Standard

---

Box 14–1. Referral Resources for Alcoholic Patients and Their Families

- Alcoholics Anonymous
- Al-Anon, Alateen (support for family members)
- Inpatient detoxification unit of the hospital
- Alcoholism clinic
- Salvation Army (may offer rehabilitation services)
- Veterans Administration hospitals and clinics
- Physicians trained in dealing with addictions (detoxification and rehabilitation support)
- Alcoholism counselors
- Clergy and faith-based services (support and counseling)

reading is the "Big Book," and this can be recommended to patients on the ward. This is an inspirational book about how a physician and a businessman realized their common problem and began a fellowship that evolved into AA.

Other therapies, available for the nonspiritually inclined, have been successful in supporting efforts of alcohol-dependent individuals to take control of their problems and their lives.

Medications for Rehabilitation from Alcohol Dependence

The old standby disulfiram (Antabuse) can be effective in the motivated patient and used creatively in high-risk situations to prevent relapse. The usual dose is 250 mg per day. The patient must be warned about its interactions with alcohol, and liver function may need to be monitored.

Acamprosate (Campral) and naltrexone (ReVia) have been moderately successful in preventing relapse in alcohol-dependent patients. Acamprosate is given as 666 mg tid and is relatively free of side effects. It adds about 20% to the success rate (abstinence at 1 year). Naltrexone, an opioid blocker, has been found to reduce the craving for alcohol and the likelihood of a full-blown relapse. By blocking the opioid receptors, naltrexone blocks the unique euphoria that normally is triggered by alcohol in the dependence-prone alcoholic, thus reducing the reward that would ordinarily reinforce heavier drinking. The dosage of naltrexone should be titrated slowly because it has significant gastrointestinal side effects and also may contribute to elevation of liver enzymes. Therefore, it is prudent to monitor liver functions while the patient is taking naltrexone. Neither of these medications is recommended in the absence of a psychosocial program. Naltrexone is now available in a depot form, 150 mg IM monthly, and has been shown to be more effective than placebo.

Alcohol Intoxication

The legal blood level of intoxication is 0.08 to 0.10 gm/100 mL. Motor coordination and decision-making capacities are progressively impaired as the blood alcohol level rises (Table 14-2). The alcohol-intoxicated person may be overly talkative, belligerent, hostile, or agitated. At higher levels, as motor coordination decreases and sedation effects increase, the person is at risk for falls. At LD50 (lethal dose, 50%) blood levels of 0.40, the risk

Table 14–2

Stages of Alcohol Intoxication

BAL (gm/100 mL)/%	Effect on Body
0.01-0.05	Behavior appears normal; mild euphoria
0.08-0.10	Legally drunk; overly talkative, prolonged reaction time, impaired coordination
0.18-0.30	Reduced field of vision, ataxia, slurred speech, disorientation, dizziness, greater incoordination
0.35-0.50	Increased sedation and unresponsiveness; depressed reflexes; impairment of circulation and respiration; incontinence; significant risk of death in the alcohol-naïve individual with levels greater than 0.40 gm/100 mL

BAL, blood alcohol level.
*BAL by percentage, by mass, or mass by volume (gm/100mL) are roughly equivalent.

of coma, respiratory suppression, and death increases. The chronically dependent alcohol user may have a higher level of tolerance compared to an alcohol-naïve individual. It is important, therefore, to obtain a collateral history if the patient is unable to provide one.

Laboratory Findings

Aside from the high alcohol levels, there may be other indicators of abuse such as elevation of liver enzymes, anemia, and electrolyte abnormalities (Box 14-2).

Box 14–2. Laboratory Findings in Alcohol Abuse and Dependence

- Elevated liver enzymes (ALT, AST, GGT)
- Depressed platelet count
- Increased MCV
- Deficiencies in vitamin B_{12}, vitamin B_1, folic acid, and other micronutrients
- Decreased carbohydrate and transferrin levels

ALT, alanine aminotransferase; AST, aspartate transaminase; GGT, gamma-glutamyltransferase; MCV, mean corpuscular volume.

Complications

The most serious complications of alcohol intoxication include respiratory arrest and cardiovascular collapse. Aspiration, gastritis, and injury due to falls or aggressive behavior also lead to significant morbidity and suffering.

Treatment

Acute intoxication is an emergency and may require treatment in the ICU if the patient shows signs of decreasing alertness and respiratory suppression. Flumazenil does not reverse the alcohol intoxication but may reverse the effects of any benzodiazepines that may have been taken by the patient.

Close monitoring and respiratory support and protection of the airway from aspiration is warranted. For less severe intoxication, the patient may need to be placed in a quiet room and allowed to sober up while being monitored for emergence of withdrawal symptoms.

Delirium Tremens (Alcohol Withdrawal Delirium)

Early assessment and treatment is the best way to prevent delirium tremens. If the patient begins to hallucinate and lose orientation, the onset of delirium tremens is imminent. It is often marked by withdrawal seizures of a generalized, tonic-clonic nature. IM lorazepam may be given to control the seizures. Much higher doses of benzodiazepines may be needed for a period of 7 to 10 days in a setting of close supportive nursing care and avoidance of excessive auditory and visual stimuli for the patient. During this time more frequent monitoring of vital signs is necessary.

Other causes of seizures should be ruled out even though the seizures occur in the context of alcohol withdrawal syndrome. Untreated delirium tremens carries a mortality rate of about 15% and is an ominous development requiring transfer to the ICU for optimal management. It is one of the most serious of the emergencies related to the alcohol-dependent patient.

Further Reading

Cammarano WB, Pittet JF, Weitz S, et al: Acute withdrawal syndrome related to the administration of analgesic and sedative medications in adult intensive care unit patients. Crit Care Med 1998;26:676-684.

Dobrydnjov I, Axelsson K, Berggren L: Intrathecal and oral clonidine as prophylaxis for postoperative alcohol withdrawal syndrome: A randomized double-blinded study. Anesth Analg 2004;98:738-744.

Drummer OH, Gerostamoulos J, Batziris H: The incidence of drugs in drivers killed in Australian road traffic crashes. Forensic Sci Int 2003;134:154-162.

Jaeger TM, Lohr RH, Pankratz VS: Symptom-triggered therapy for alcohol withdrawal syndrome in medical inpatients. Mayo Clin Proc 2001;76:695-701.

Lenzenhuber E, Muller C, Rommelspacher H, Spies C: Gamma-hydroxybutyrate for treatment of alcohol withdrawal syndrome in intensive care patients. A comparison between two symptom-oriented therapeutic concepts. Anaesthesist 1999;48:89-96. [in German]

Mayo-Smith MF: Pharmacological management of alcohol withdrawal. A meta-analysis and evidence-based practice guideline. American Society of Addiction Medicine Working Group on Pharmacological Management of Alcohol Withdrawal. JAMA 1997;278:144-151.

Mravcik V, Zabransky T, Vorel F: Drugs and traffic accidents. Cas Lek Cesk 2005;144:550-555. [in Czech]

Mura P, Kintz P, Ludes B, et al: Comparison of the prevalence of alcohol, cannabis and other drugs between 900 injured drivers and 900 control subjects: Results of a French collaborative study. Forensic Sci Int 2003;133:79-85.

Spies CD, Dubisz N, Funk W, et al: Prophylaxis of alcohol withdrawal syndrome in alcohol-dependent patients admitted to the intensive care unit after tumour resection. Br J Anaesth 1995;75:734-739.

Spies CD, Otter HE, Huske B, et al: Alcohol withdrawal severity is decreased by symptom-orientated adjusted bolus therapy in the ICU. Intensive Care Med 2003;29:2230-2238.

Stanley KM, Amabile CM, Simpson KN, et al: Impact of an alcohol withdrawal syndrome practice guideline on surgical patient outcomes. Pharmacotherapy 2003;23:843-854.

Stanley KM, Worrall CL, Lunsford SL, et al: Department of Therapeutic Services, Medical University of South Carolina: Experience with an adult alcohol withdrawal syndrome practice guideline in internal medicine patients. Pharmacotherapy 2005;25:1073-1083.

C H A P T E R   1 5

The Drug-Abusing Patient and Related Emergencies

Tirath S. Gill, MD

KEY POINTS

- Epidemiologic studies indicate that drug abuse is two to three times more common among those with psychiatric illness than in the general population (Table 15-1).
- A mental health professional may be consulted to help deal with issues of intoxication, withdrawal, and rehabilitation. The various substances of abuse have individual patterns of intoxication and withdrawal (Table 15-2).
- Treatment of drug abuse is effective in a surprisingly high number of people. The emergency department (ED) may provide an opportunity for intervention at a time of crisis when patients may be receptive to offers of help.
- Negative attitudes toward this subset of the population hinder the provision of effective care and should be examined if they arise in the ED clinician.
- Urine drug screen testing on a routine basis in individuals with unusual behaviors is recommended. It almost doubles the detection rate of substance abuse compared with relying on the history alone (Table 15-3).
- Withdrawal symptoms are usually the opposite of the effects produced when a substance is ingested. The shorter the half-life of the drug or substance, the more intense and shorter the duration of the withdrawal symptoms.
- With most substances, onset of withdrawal symptoms is within hours; symptoms are much more noticeable on the second day, and by day 5, the patient usually has recovered.

Table 15–1

Comorbidity of Substance Abuse

	Incidence
General population	17%
Affective disorder	32%
Schizophrenia	47%

Table 15–2

Common Substances of Abuse and Associated Laboratory Abnormalities and Physical Findings

Substance	Laboratory Abnormalities	Physical Findings
Alcohol	Elevated ALT, AST, GGT levels, increased MCV, low platelet count; hyponatremia, hypokalemia, hypomagnesemia; megaloblastic anemia	Cirrhosis (ascites, pedal edema); gastritis (hematemesis, epigastric pain), esophageal varices, increased incidence of cancer of mouth and GI tract; malnutrition (low body weight); dementia (disorientation); cardiomyopathy (CHF); hypogonadism (impotence); increased rate of seborrheic dermatitis
Cocaine	Positive urine drug screen results	Underweight; at high risk for STDs; intoxication associated with seizures, angina, myocardial infarction, or stroke

Continued

Table 15–2

Common Substances of Abuse and Associated Laboratory Abnormalities and Physical Findings—cont'd

Substance	Laboratory Abnormalities	Physical Findings
Metham-phetamine	Positive urine drug screen results	Similar to above
LSD/ psychedelics	Not normally tested	May be associated with increased risk of psychosis; delayed mood and anxiety symptoms seen in some individuals
PCP	Positive urine drug screen results	May have vertical nystagmus; may present with agitated behaviors; may resemble psychotic disorder and manic syndromes
Cannabis	Positive urine drug screen results	Symptoms of cannabis amotivational syndrome

ALT, alanine aminotransferase; AST, aspartate transaminase; CHF, congestive heart failure; GGT, gamma-glutamyltransferase; GI, gastrointestinal; LSD, lysergic acid diethylamide; MCV, mean corpuscular volume; PCP, phencyclidine hydrochloride; STDs, sexually transmitted diseases.

Table 15–3

Screening Results for Various Substances of Abuse

Substance	Duration of Positive Screen
Alcohol	Depends on level of intoxication; may be detectable for 8 to 10 hours after last drink
Cocaine	Metabolites may be detectable for up to 3 days
Cannabis	May test positive for up to 4 weeks
PCP	9 days
Methadone	14 days
Oxycodone	4 days
Morphine	4 days
Barbiturates	3 days to 3 weeks

PCP, phencyclidine hydrochloride.

Overview (Fig. 15-1)

Substance abuse problems are rife in modern society and exact a heavy toll in terms of financial and emotional costs. Many different nations have deployed vast resources to stem this plague, and some limited success has been obtained. The real solution may lie in returning to a less hectic pace and restoring the fundamental values of a closely knit family and a spiritual base. The high rates of mental illness are directly linked to high rates of alcohol and substance abuse. An emotionally distraught individual is most likely to seek escape through chemicals.

The current worldwide political atmosphere is not conducive to a healthy family life. Until an honest man or woman of average education can support a family with a single job, stresses will mount, brewing despair with increased risk of drug abuse.

Another factor that has increased the risk of substance abuse is the development of synthetic analogues of naturally occurring drugs such as cocaine that are more addictive and have the ability to entrap an unwary individual even with one-time use. Often these dabblers are caught up in a vicious circle of psychological and physical dependence. They may not be able to get help until they present to the ED due to an acute crisis precipitated by their addiction.

Substance Abuse–Related Emergencies

Cocaine Intoxication

The word "cocaine" refers to the drug in both a powder (cocaine) and crystal (crack) form. It is made from the coca plant and causes a short-lived "high" that is immediately followed by opposite, intense feelings of depression and a craving for more of the drug. Cocaine may be snorted as a powder, converted to a liquid form for injection with a needle, or processed into a crystal form to be smoked.

Clinical Presentation

The patient may be referred to the ED because of acute agitation, paranoia, or severe depression during a "crash," or withdrawal. The high from smoking crack cocaine reaches peak

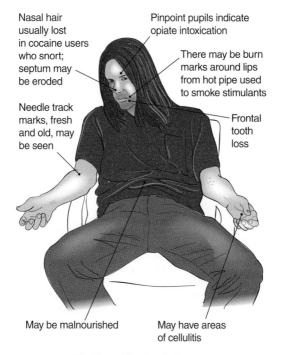

Nasal hair usually lost in cocaine users who snort; septum may be eroded

Pinpoint pupils indicate opiate intoxication

There may be burn marks around lips from hot pipe used to smoke stimulants

Needle track marks, fresh and old, may be seen

Frontal tooth loss

May be malnourished

May have areas of cellulitis

The Drug-Abusing Patient

- Patient may present with intoxication or withdrawal symptoms
- Stimulant intoxication may induce paranoia, delirium
- Opiate withdrawal marked by pupillary dilation, lacrimation, diarrhea, cramping
- Patient may present with physical pain symptoms and demand opiates for pain relief

FIGURE 15–1

The drug-abusing patient.

levels within seconds and has a short duration of action lasting 15 minutes to an hour. The crash is equally rapid in onset and intensity and may be marked by suicidal ideation.

Signs of acute intoxication include severe hypertension and vasospasm that can cause ischemia in vital organs resulting in angina or myocardial infarction. Transient and permanent brain strokes, subarachnoid hemorrhage, hyperthermia, and seizures have been reported as well. Because of the intense dopamine agonism during intoxication, psychotic symptoms may include delusions, formication, tics, and obsessive rituals. Some cases of marked hyperglycemia without a prior history of diabetes have also been reported with the use of stimulant drugs such as cocaine.

Management

The post-intoxication crash or acute dysphoria and depression tend to resolve in 24 to 48 hours but may last longer in some cases. Rest and supportive care are indicated. If the patient voices suicidal or homicidal thoughts, hospitalization for closer monitoring is recommended.

The patient often retains insight into any paranoid ideations related to the use of cocaine, and verbal reassurance and "talking down" may be helpful.

During intoxication, beta blockers may decrease the autonomic arousal and limit the risk of cardiovascular complications. Psychotic symptoms may be controlled with low doses of a sedating antipsychotic. The use of quetiapine, 50 to 100 mg, or chlorpromazine in similar doses may be helpful. However, if paranoia is severe, any antipsychotic may be titrated to achieve remission of the agitation and hallucinations. The use of potentially reinforcing medications such as intramuscular (IM) benzodiazepines should be avoided, as the short duration to peak effect may be reinforcing of addictive tendencies.

Rehabilitation

A structured 12-step program (e.g., AA, NA, CA) with sober living placement and removal from an environment that triggers cravings is recommended.

Various biological treatment options have been explored, but no specific treatment has been found to be successful. However, some success has been reported in reducing relapse risk with dopamine agonists such as bromocriptine and amantadine.

Other studies indicate some benefit with bupropion, disulfiram, and desipramine, but controlled trials are lacking.

Cocaine vaccine has been reported to be effective in reducing cravings by blunting the subjective high experienced by the user. It acts by binding to the cocaine molecule and making it unavailable for action at its usual target sites. This, however, has remained mostly in experimental use.

The success of any pharmacological intervention is strongly linked to the simultaneous provision of a psychosocial/spiritual approach that includes individual and group therapy, support groups, and a substance-free environment.

Methamphetamine and Related Stimulant Abuse

Methamphetamines and related stimulant abuse is noted to be more prevalent in certain geographical locations and among certain pockets of society. Such endemic abuse has deleterious effects on the individual and the society where he or she resides. Methamphetamines and related stimulants have systemic effects on the body and can affect many different organ systems. Some of these effects include an elevation of blood pressure, arrhythmias, decreased sleep, and increased incidence of myocardial infarction and stroke. Other less frequent but equally dangerous effects include seizures, muscle breakdown, and idiosyncratic liver necrosis. Psychiatric complications are legend in these individuals and include increased anxiety, paranoia, exacerbation or precipitation of mania, and a persisting delusional state in some patients. The cost to society is exacted in the form of increased theft, burglary, and related violent crimes. It is a rare individual that is able to maintain any semblance of a family life after becoming addicted to methamphetamines. Such psychosocial and psychiatric complications may be the direct proximate cause for consultation with the ED clinician.

Clinical Presentation

The patient may show acute anxiety and paranoia or loud and demanding behaviors marked by motor agitation. Stereotypic behaviors marked by sniffing, teeth clenching, purposeless searching, and picking of skin may also be evident. There may be evidence of needle marks, cellulitis, and skin excoriations from picking. Oftentimes, the pulse, blood pressure, and rate of respiration are elevated and the pupils show a distinct dilatation.

Withdrawal Signs and Symptoms

Early withdrawal is marked by acute depression and strong drug cravings. These are followed by a sense of physical exhaustion, fatigue, and a desire for sleep. The withdrawal may then be manifested by excessive sleeping and a voracious return of the appetite. Cravings tend to reemerge in cyclic fashion, often triggered by various cues during the early and late phases of the withdrawal. The acute withdrawal tends to last 2 to 3 days, but persisting anhedonia and joylessness may last for several weeks. A depressed mood state beyond 4 to 6 weeks may call for the consideration of a primary mood disorder in the patient and its treatment with the standard modalities (see also Chapter 7).

Treatment

The anxious intoxicated patient may benefit from "talking down" and from the use of medications such as lorazepam (Ativan), 1 to 2 mg, or temazepam (Restoril), 15 to 30 mg PO, for features of acute anxiety. If paranoia is a significant factor, haloperidol (Haldol) or fluphenazine (Prolixin), 5 mg, along with lorazepam, 2 mg, and diphenhydramine (Benadryl), 50 mg, may be a more suitable option. If there is evidence of increased muscle tone or rigidity, the use of potent antipsychotics such as haloperidol or fluphenazine should be avoided and the low-potency and more sedating antipsychotics such as quetiapine (Seroquel) or chlorpromazine (Thorazine), 50 to 100 mg, are preferred. Orthostatic hypotension marked by dizziness upon arising should be monitored for if the latter agents are used to control the psychiatric symptoms of intoxication. There is some anecdotal evidence that dopamine agonists such as amantadine and bromocriptine and antidepressants such as bupropion and desipramine are helpful for some patients with stimulant cravings. Patients with methamphetamine addiction can be famished and malnourished, and it may be prudent to rule out any syndromes related to nutritional deficiencies and medical conditions that have been neglected.

Long-term treatment is best provided in a structured rehabilitation program that is modeled on the 12-step program or other such program that breaks through the denial and links the individual to their higher power or motivation. Behavioral therapy may help with coping skills and gradual extinction of cues with abstinence. The involvement of the family is often helpful to the family members and the patient. Multimodal interventions have a way of acting synergistically to increase the success rate in achieving freedom from these powerful agents of addiction.

Opioid and Opiate Intoxication

Opioids are synthetic analogues; opiates are naturally occurring substances that act on the opiate receptors. Opioids include heroin, hydromorphone, oxycodone, fentanyl, buprenorphine, and methadone; opiates include codeine, morphine, and thebaine. The terms are often used synonymously. These substances induce analgesia and have a euphoric effect associated with reduction of anxiety and a generalized state of relaxation. The duration of effect ranges from a relatively short half-life of Dilaudid to the long half-life of methadone (Table 15-4).

The prevalence of opiate abuse and dependence tends to fluctuate and appears to be higher in the big metropolitan areas. More recently, considerable attention has been focused on the diversion of prescription opiates such as oxycodone into the Midwest and Appalachian areas of the United States, where it is crushed and injected intravenously. Its widespread abuse and associated dysfunction has earned it the infamous moniker of "hillbilly heroin" and has led to efforts to curb this unexpected epidemic.

Clinical Presentation

The patient may present to the ED in a state of intoxication or withdrawal. The intoxication may be inadvertent, caused by the use of an unusually potent and pure form of heroin, or may be intentional—for example the result of a suicide attempt by overdose.

Acute intoxication may be marked by sedation or euphoria progressing to unconsciousness. Physical signs include pinpoint pupils and depression of respiration and vital signs.

Symptoms of withdrawal include nausea, vomiting, chills, pupillary dilation, elevated vital signs, abdominal and muscular cramps, and insomnia. Other features may include a runny nose (rhinorrhea), tearing of the eyes (lacrimation), and generalized malaise. The dysphoria and physical discomfort may be intense but are not life-threatening in the normal adult without severe respiratory or cardiac disease.

Table 15–4

Morphine Equivalents of Commonly Used Drugs*

Drug	Morphine Equivalent	Comments
Codeine, 30 mg	10 mg PO	Codeine is converted to morphine by the P450 enzyme system; SSRIs inhibit this system, and 10% of the population that is deficient may not achieve adequate conversion and have an inadequate analgesic response
Methadone, 10 mg PO	20 to 30 mg PO	Methadone has a longer duration of action than morphine
Fentanyl, 25 mg/24 hr patch	50 to 75 mg PO	The patch is replaced every 72 hours
Oxycodone, 20 mg	30 mg PO	Metabolism of oxycodone is variable in different population subsets
Hydromorphone, 10 mg PO	30 mg PO	Parenteral dose is 1/3 to 1/4 of the oral hydromorphone dose

*Note: This table is only a rough guide; approximations are difficult due to the different pharmacokinetics of individual agents in different patient populations. Also note that the parenteral dose of morphine is one third of the oral dose.
PCP, phencyclidine hydrochloride; SSRIs, selective serotonin reuptake inhibitors.

Management

If the patient is conscious, obtain information about the amount taken and time of the last use of the opioid. Inquire about the use of alcohol or other drugs of abuse. Collateral information, if available, is useful.

To reverse acute intoxication, IM or intravenous (IV) naloxone, 2 mg, can be given. Although it may bring the patient rapidly out of a coma, be prepared to treat the onset of opioid withdrawal symptoms if the patient is a chronic user and opioid-dependent. The effects of naloxone last only about 1 hour, and repeated doses will need to be given until the opioid agent is cleared from the systemic circulation.

The treatment of opioid withdrawal has undergone a sea change over the last 10 years. Theoretically one can use any cross-tolerant opiate to treat opioid dependence, gradually tapering the dose. However, detoxification with methadone is allowed only in licensed methadone programs or facilities authorized for its use. Another legal opiate available for detoxification is buprenorphine, which can be dispensed from the office of a physician who is licensed and trained in its use. The office-based treatment of opioid intoxication has helped to destigmatize the treatment and allowed more clinicians to help more patients.

Buprenorphine can be used in doses of 2 to 24 mg/day, gradually tapered by 10% to 12% daily. It is usually given in divided bid doses. The formulation that contains naloxone prevents its diversion and abuse by the IV route; the opiate antagonist that is active when used parenterally is digested and broken down by the digestive enzymes when taken orally.

We have used sublingual (S/L) buprenorphine, 2 mg every 8 hours for 2 days, followed by 1 mg every 8 hours for 2 days, and have had very satisfactory results treating our patients with mild to moderate opioid dependence. A prn (as needed) dose of buprenorphine, 2 mg S/L every 6 hours, is also ordered per our protocol (for any breakthrough withdrawal symptoms), but it is rarely used by the patients.

Ongoing rehabilitation is needed to acquire refusal skills, build a support network, and obtain a sponsor to reduce risk of relapse.

Sedative Hypnotic Intoxication

Although benzodiazepines are one of the most commonly prescribed agents, problems related to dependence and abuse are infrequent. Some individuals who seek to abuse these agents may combine them with other sedating agents or alcohol.

Clinical Presentation

Patients taking benzodiazepines (alprazolam and diazepam appear to be particularly high-risk drugs for abuse), barbiturates, or other sedative hypnotics may present to the ED due to acute intoxication by overdose or to symptoms related to a withdrawal syndrome. Signs of intoxication include ataxia, slurred speech, disorientation, increasing sedation, and coma. When used with other sedating agents, they may cause suppression of respiration.

Management

Flumazenil can antagonize the intoxication caused by benzo-diazepines and may be used in a dose of 0.2 mg given intravenously every 15 seconds up to a dose of 1 to 2 mg. In view of the short half-life of this drug, the dose may need to be repeated every half-hour.

Because of the risk of inducing acute withdrawal symptoms, including seizures, IV lorazepam or diazepam should be available when flumazenil is being used. Withdrawal can be treated with cross-tolerant benzodiazepines with a long half-life, tapering the dose by 20% to 25% daily. Vital signs are elevated during withdrawal and serve as a good guide to the severity of withdrawal and adequacy of the tapering dose.

Barbiturates are life-threatening in overdose and may not respond to flumazenil therapy. Supportive measures such as assisted respiration and cardiovascular support may be needed during the acute intoxication phase. Withdrawal may be treated in a manner similar to the treatment of alcohol or benzodiazepine withdrawal.

Phencyclidine Hydrochloride (PCP)

PCP is sometimes used selectively by certain groups that glorify violence; it also is used as an adulterant to lace other substances of abuse such as cannabis, cocaine, and amphetamines. The exact incidence of PCP use is unknown and varies in different parts of the United States and worldwide.

Clinical Presentation

Patients with PCP intoxication may present to the ED with symptoms similar to those of manic and psychotic agitation. These patients are particularly prone to violence and may have analgesia and may exhibit great feats of strength, sometimes injuring themselves in the process.

Management

Verbal de-escalation and oral benzodiazepines are helpful. Dopamine-blocking agents such as conventional antipsychotics are contraindicated because they may increase muscle tone, resulting in muscle damage.

If psychotic symptoms are particularly severe, consider giving quetiapine, 50 to 100 mg PO, in view of its low liability to exacerbate rigidity. Physical restraints and seclusion may be used judiciously if the patient is acutely agitated and threatening toward others. Any restraint procedure carries a high risk of harm to the patient and the staff and should be used with great care.

A drug screen should be ordered to rule out the presence of other substances, and medical causes of agitation should be excluded.

Ongoing rehabilitation and lifestyle changes are a must in order to ensure lasting sobriety.

Cannabis Intoxication

The use of cannabis is widespread on a sporadic basis; its incidence and prevalence show a waxing and waning pattern over the decades. It is not a benign drug as portrayed at times and has been implicated in serious motor vehicle and train accidents.

Clinical Presentation
Cannabis tends to distort perception of time and may contribute to faulty judgment when operating machinery or vehicles. Its psychological effects are unpredictable. Although it may have a calming effect in some individuals, it may unmask psychotic and panic disorders and mood symptoms in others who may have a predisposition toward these disorders. Chronic use may be associated with lack of initiative or drive, leading some to give it the busy label of "cannabis amotivational syndrome."

Management
The acutely intoxicated patient who is anxious and agitated may be helped by verbal support and the use of benzodiazepines such as lorazepam, 1 to 2 mg. Chronic amotivational syndrome may resolve with ongoing abstinence. Treatment of underlying depression with serotonergic agents may also help in decreasing dependence and passivity in these patients.

Hallucinogen Intoxication

Hallucinogens such as lysergic acid diethylamide (LSD), peyote, mushrooms, and certain amphetamines can cause intoxication.

Clinical Presentation
The patient may present as floridly psychotic and disorganized in thinking and behavior or may have symptoms of acute panic. Vital signs tend to be elevated.

Management

Verbal reassurance and talking down helps most individuals who may find their psychedelic trip frightening. Lorazepam or other benzodiazepines may be used. Anticholinergics or stimulants are contraindicated because they can worsen the confusion and hallucinatory phenomena found in patients intoxicated with these drugs.

Further Reading

Breslow RE, Klinger BI, Erickson BJ: Acute intoxication and substance abuse among patients presenting to a psychiatric emergency service. Gen Hosp Psychiatry 1996;18:183-191.

Caton CL, Drake RE, Hasin DS, et al: Differences between early-phase primary psychotic disorders with concurrent substance use and substance-induced psychoses. Arch Gen Psychiatry 2005;62:137-145.

Dhossche DM: Aggression and recent substance abuse: Absence of association in psychiatric emergency room patients. Compr Psychiatry 1999;40:343-346.

Fine J, Miller NS: Evaluation and acute management of psychotic symptomatology in alcohol and drug addictions: J Addict Dis 1993;12:59-72.

Galanter M, Castaneda R, Ferman J: Substance abuse among general psychiatric patients: Place of presentation, diagnosis, and treatment. Am J Drug Alcohol Abuse 1988;14:211-235.

Johnson DA: Drug-induced psychiatric disorders. Drugs 1981;22:57-69.

Lambert MT, Griffith JM, Hendrickse W: Characteristics of patients with substance abuse diagnoses on a general psychiatry unit in a VA Medical Center. Psychiatr Serv 1996;47:1104-1107.

Regier DA, Farmer ME, Rae DS, et al: Comorbidity of disorders with alcohol and other drug abuse. Results from the Epidemiologic Catchment Area (ECA) Study. JAMA 1990;264:2511-2548.

Zealberg JJ, Brady KT: Substance abuse and emergency psychiatry. Psychiatr Clin North Am 1999;22:803-817.

CHAPTER 16

Psychiatric Aspects of Seizure Disorders

Tirath S. Gill, MD

KEY POINTS

- The incidence of seizure disorder is roughly equivalent to the incidence of schizophrenia in the general population, or about 1%.
- There is significant social stigma associated with epilepsy, similar to the stigma of mental illness.
- Medications that treat epilepsy can cause psychiatric symptoms.
- Primary lesions that cause epilepsy can cause psychiatric symptoms.
- Psychiatric problems in patients with epilepsy can be effectively treated.

Overview

Psychiatric symptoms are frequent in patients with seizure disorders. They are often not recognized and result in significant morbidity, mortality, and overall reduction in the quality of life for the patient. This chapter reviews the epidemiology, classification, and treatment of seizures and their emergent side effects.

Definition

Epilepsy. A chronic disorder of the brain marked by recurrent unprovoked seizures.

Classification of Seizures

The epileptic phenomenon can be classified as generalized, partial, and partial complex seizures (Box 16-1). Seizures that arise without a specific locus are classified as generalized seizures.

Box 16–1. Classification of Seizures

Generalized Seizures
Generalized tonic-clonic seizure (grand mal)
Absence seizure (petit mal)
Myoclonus seizure
Infantile spasms
Clonic seizure
Tonic seizure
Akinetic seizure

Partial Seizures
With motor symptoms
With sensory symptoms
With autonomic symptoms
Compound forms

Partial Complex Seizures
With alteration of consciousness
With affective symptoms
With psychosensory symptoms
Compound forms

The seizure event is marked by rapid firing of a group of neurons. When the focal discharge remains localized, consciousness is usually not impaired and the event is classified as a partial seizure. When the localized discharge spreads to other parts of the brain, the event is labeled as a complex partial seizure and is often associated with alteration of awareness or loss of consciousness.

The ictal or seizure event may be preceded by an aura or symptoms that the patient learns to recognize. The seizure event itself may have a distinct pattern, and the period of recovery from the seizure or the postictal period may have features of mild delirium.

True seizures should be distinguished from pseudoseizures, keeping in mind that patients with true seizures may manifest pseudoseizures as well (Table 16-1; also see Table 16-3).

Nonconvulsive status epilepticus (NCSE) may present with psychiatric symptoms. NCSE may be associated with behavioral changes as well. This may manifest as dissociative, anxiety, or mood symptoms in adolescents and adults, and the underlying

Table 16–1

Differentiating True Seizures from Pseudoseizures

Clinical Features	True Seizures	Pseudoseizures
Etiology	Neurologic disorder, sometimes of unknown etiology	Nonverbal expression of distress
EEG findings	Postictal slowing; EEG abnormalities during the true ictal event	Normal EEG findings
Babinski sign	Present	Absent
Prolactin level	Elevated during postictal phase	Normal
Injuries	Frequent	Rare
Incontinence	Frequent	Absent
Postictal confusion and dysphoria	Present	Absent; patient attains full alertness fairly quickly
Stereotypical seizure activity	Present with tonic-clonic phase or a more classic pattern of seizure activity	Usually atypical flailing of extremities without consistent pattern

illness may be unrecognized. NCSE may also present as episodes of confusion in the elderly. Phenytoin and carbamazepine have been implicated in some cases with precipitating or worsening of this condition.

Comorbid Psychiatric Illnesses

About 30% of epileptic patients may develop signs of depression. Significant anxiety and phobia about the next seizure may develop and lead to social withdrawal. Certain distinctive personality traits labeled as epileptoid personality have been historically described (Box 16-2). At times the patient may manifest psychotic symptoms.

Cases of abdominal pain associated with epileptic seizures have been reported. Sometimes, phenobarbital used in the treatment of seizure disorders may precipitate an episode of acute intermittent porphyria.

Box 16–2. Epileptoid Personality Traits

Viscosity of thought
Digressive and circumstantial speech
Hyperreligiosity
Increased concern with issues of morality and right and wrong
Hypergraphia
Decreased or increased sexuality

Symptom Patterns of Seizures

Preictal Symptoms

These symptoms are called auras and in some cases make individuals aware of the onset of a seizure. The aura is sometimes related to the autonomic system, and the individual may experience symptoms such as a sense of fullness of the stomach, involuntary blushing, or a change in the heart rate or respiratory pattern.

At times the preictal sensation can have a surreal cognitive quality, such as feeling of being in a familiar place (déjà vu) or feeling alienated from common surroundings (jamais vu), forced thinking, and dreamlike states. The most remarkable symptom pattern is related to intense emotional states such as intense fear or dread, panic, foreboding, depression, or sense of elation.

Other preictal states are accompanied by automatisms (automatic motor behaviors) such as automatic chewing, blinking, rubbing oneself, and lip smacking.

Ictal Symptoms

These may be manifested as sensory or motor symptoms that radiate from one site (Jacksonian march) and spread to the opposite side. The seizures may become generalized and present with a typical tonic phase followed by a clonic phase (generalized tonic-clonic seizure). Incontinence may occur during the seizure. Complications related to the ictal event include injuries from falls, tongue biting, and aspiration of blood or food contents.

Postictal Symptoms

The individual is often in a state of mild delirium after a seizure and may be amnestic for the event.

Interictal Symptoms

The patient with epilepsy is vulnerable to the development of a syndrome characterized by interictal symptoms and personality features that are as unique as they are fascinating, including the following:

- Hyperreligiosity
- A change in the quality of thought and emotions that is described as viscous
- A change in sexual patterns
- An unusual concern for moral or ethical issues and preoccupation with right and wrong
- Heightened concern with philosophical dilemmas and global problems

The presence of all the symptoms is uncommon. Psychotic symptoms can develop in 10% of such individuals. Certain features such as a temporal lobe focus or early age of onset may increase the risk for developing this syndrome. About one third of the patients develop symptoms related to depressive clinical states and anxiety syndromes.

Diagnosing Epilepsy

The emergency department (ED) clinician should maintain a high level of suspicion, especially when symptoms are noted in a new patient presenting with psychosis, depression, or symptoms of panic or anxiety. This is especially wise if the onset of symptoms is abrupt in a previously healthy person or if there is a history of unexplained falls or fainting or there is an abrupt onset of a rapidly resolving delirium lacking an identified cause. Adult onset absence seizures may also present as episodic psychiatric episodes.

Although electroencephalography (EEG) studies may be positive in 25% to 50% of patients, a negative study does not rule out the presence of a seizure disorder. Sleep-deprived EEG with sphenoidal leads and photic stimulation is sometimes used to increase the chances of detection. However, use of sphenoidal leads is considered by some to be an unnecessary discomfort for the patient, as they do not significantly add to the detection rates of an ictal event. Hospitalization with video and EEG monitoring for 24 to 72 hours may help to clarify the nature of the disorder.

Treatment of Seizures

Adequate treatment of the epileptic disorder is thought to limit psychiatric comorbidity. Some medications efficacious in the treatment of epileptic seizures are shown in Box 16-3. Some of the medications may lead to confusion, agitation, and psychosis. A neurological consultation to explore an alternative therapeutic agent is often useful. Psychiatric support and follow-up should also be provided for these patients.

Problems Associated with Anticonvulsant Medication

Certain medications may increase the risk of seizure and should be avoided when treating patients with epilepsy. These include clozapine, Wellbutrin, amoxapine, and maprotiline. Some agents can cause mild to moderate impairment of cognitive function, and a dosage adjustment may be indicated to diminish such side effects. Topiramate is especially noted for causing a dulling of the cognitive faculties. Table 16-2 lists some common side effects of antiepileptic drugs.

Valproic acid may raise ammonia levels in some patients due to deficiency of the mitochondrial isoenzymes involved in the metabolism of carnitine. This may lead to lethargy, which may be interpreted as an antimanic response to the divalproic acid. A high index of suspicion, especially in the case of women, is needed to prevent complications of worsening mental status and the development of coma. Thus, patients taking this agent should be monitored for a sudden change in mental status.

 Levetiracetam can cause paranoia and agitation; a dosage adjustment downward, along with the use of antipsychotic agents, is helpful in managing these symptoms. One of the problems occurring with drugs such as phenobarbital, carbamazepine, and phenytoin is the induction of the metabolic enzyme system, which leads to lowering of the levels of other prescribed agents being taken by the individual.

Failure of contraceptive agents can result in pregnancy. Pregnancy in an epileptic woman should be carefully planned, in view of the serious teratogenic risk to the unborn child. Defects related to neural tube development including spinal bifida tend to occur more frequently. Supplementation with folic acid and

Box 16–3. Medications Efficacious in Treatment of Epileptic Seizures

Generalized Seizures
Carbamazepine
Phenobarbital
Tiagabine
Zonisamide
Valproic acid

Generalized Tonic-Clonic Seizures
Carbamazepine
Phenytoin
Valproic acid

Partial Seizures
Carbamazepine
Oxcarbazepine
Phenobarbital
Phenytoin
Primidone

Partial Complex Seizures
Levetiracetam
Topamax

Atypical Myoclonic Seizure
Clonazepam

Petit Mal (Absence Seizure)
Ethosuximide
Valproic acid
Lamotrigine

Lennox-Gastaut Seizure
Lamotrigine

avoidance of polypharmacy may help to reduce the risk for such defects.

Lamotrigine is considered to be less teratogenic than other agents. The use of clonazepam should be avoided in conjunction with Depakote, as it may result in worsening of absence seizures.

Table 16-2

Some Common Side Effects of Antiepileptic Drugs

Anticonvulsant	Prominent Side Effect(s)
Vigabatrin	May exacerbate psychosis
Levetiracetam	May exacerbate psychosis
Lamotrigine	Potential for serious rash, Stevens-Johnson syndrome; slow titration; less teratogenic than others; preferred in pregnant patients for seizure control
Phenytoin	Gingival hyperplasia, decreased folate levels; depression and mania reported in some cases
Carbamazepine	Hyponatremia, self-induction and induction of metabolic enzymes affect levels of other medications; rare cases of agranulocytosis; teratogenic risk
Divalproic acid	Weight gain, polycystic ovary syndrome, hair loss; teratogenic risk; risk of hyperammonemia in some patients; may exacerbate hepatitis; rare cases of acute pancreatitis
Topiramate	Cognitive dulling, paresthesias, kidney stones
Oxcarbazepine	May induce hyponatremia due to SIADH
Phenobarbital	Depression and increased irritability and disruptive behaviors in developmentally disabled populations; potential for enzyme induction; may precipitate interactions due to vulnerability for porphyria

SIADH, syndrome of inappropriate antidiuretic hormone.

Treatment of Associated Psychiatric Symptoms

The treatment of psychiatric symptoms with conventional agents is effective but certain caveats are in order. Psychotic symptoms are effectively treated with atypical agents such as risperidone, quetiapine, ziprasidone, and olanzapine. The development of a metabolic syndrome associated with weight gain, hyperlipidemia, and insulin resistance may occur in some patients while on these agents.

Conventional antipsychotics such as haloperidol, fluphenazine, perphenazine, trifluoperazine, and thiothixene also are effective. It is important to monitor for side effects such as parkinsonism, akathisia, and tardive dyskinesia with greater alacrity when using these agents.

Antianxiety agents such as the benzodiazepines are helpful with anxiety symptoms. Clonazepam is preferable in view of its augmenting anticonvulsant effects in addition to the anxiolytic action. Clonazepam and the long-acting benzodiazepines have a risk of cumulative toxicity because steady state levels may not stabilize until after 10 to 14 days. The increasing sedation may lead to risks for falls and other hazards in some patients.

For depressive symptoms, selective serotonin reuptake inhibitors (SSRIs) such as sertraline, mirtazapine, venlafaxine, citalopram, and escitalopram, which do not raise the levels of other medications, are preferred. However, there have been some reports that citalopram causes elevation of other drugs, and caution is advised when using this agent.

The tricyclics can be used as well for severe depressive syndromes. There is, however, a risk of a lethal overdose with tricyclic agents when dispensed to a depressed patient, and close monitoring is warranted.

Monoamine oxidase inhibitors (MAOIs) should be avoided in view of their serious noradrenergic and serotonergic interactions. Wellbutrin is contraindicated because of its tendency to lower the seizure threshold.

For the epileptic patient with manic symptoms, lithium may be a suitable option as well. Other options include valproic acid and carbamazepine in this population.

It is being increasingly realized that psychosocial interventions are of major importance in bringing about a good outcome for these patients. Programs aimed at substance abuse counseling and prevention may limit complications if such problems are noted.

Family education and support measures also afford a measure of protection against depressive symptoms in patients and family members. Individual therapy and group therapy have been found to help individuals cope with the psychosocial difficulties associated with a disabling lifelong illness.

Patients with epilepsy often have literary and other artistic talents. They should be encouraged to pursue their interests, as success in these areas may protect against depressive symptoms.

Frontal Lobe Seizures

Clinical Presentation

Frontal lobe seizures can present in a myriad of ways, ranging from clonic symptoms to bizarre behavioral features. Because of the odd presentations, they can sometimes be confused with pseudoseizures or malingering (Table 16-3).

The distinguishing features of frontal lobe seizures are the preservation of consciousness in most cases, duration of less than one minute, and early postictal recovery. Other distinguishing features include a tendency to occur in clusters and to occur at nighttime.

Aura is not a regular feature of frontal lobe seizures; although some patients may report having odd somatosensory symptoms in the head area. Bizarre automatisms involving pelvic thrusting, sexualized movements, mutism, or loud stereotypical vocal outbursts, including grunting and various odd noises, may be noted.

The orbitofrontal and medial frontal lobe areas are implicated as sites of origin, but the symptoms may be related to the spread of the seizure to different areas. The postictal recovery period is brief, and EEG findings may be absent, leading at times to mislabeling these phenomena as psychogenic.

Theological accounts of exorcisms and demon possession may have been dealing with cases of frontal lobe seizures.

Brief tonic seizures lasting 20 to 30 seconds may occur at night, are often asymmetric, and involve the extension of a limb while consciousness is maintained. Another manifestation of frontal lobe seizures is "frontal spike stupor" (i.e., EEG findings in the frontal lobe area with an irregular spiking pattern and a trance-like state of confusion and stupor in which the patient does not understand or makes illogical responses to questions.

A strong genetic predisposition, with an autosomal-dominant inheritance pattern, for frontal lobe epilepsy is noted in certain families. Local pathology due to infection, infarcts, and rare autoimmune diseases of the brain such as Rasmussen's disease are also associated with the development of frontal lobe seizures.

Treatment

Therapy often includes anticonvulsant medications. Anticonvulsant agents such as divalproic acid and phenytoin and newer agents such as lamotrigine, topiramate, zonisamide, and levetiracetam may be effective. Polypharmacy is discouraged, but it may be needed for some patients.

If the seizures are refractory to antiepileptic pharmaceuticals, psychosurgery with resection of the site of the seizure and, at times, an anterior cingulotomy can help to eliminate or greatly

Table 16–3

Frontal Lobe Seizures Compared with Focal Seizures and Pseudoseizures

Clinical Feature	Focal Seizures	Pseudoseizures	Frontal Lobe Seizures
Duration	1 to 3 minutes	Variable	Less than 60 seconds
Time of day	Usually during day	Usually during day	May occur at night
Frequency	Usually one	Variable	May occur in clusters
Motor	Classic: tonic, atonic, and clonic patterns	Variable; flailing, jerking, atypical motor movements	May be bizarre; tend to be stereotyped
Speech	May be high-pitched shriek at beginning of seizure	Slurred; variable	Explosive verbalization or speech arrest
Consciousness	May be altered or lost	Waxing and waning	Often preserved
Postictal	Confusion and amnesia	May recall event; variable	Brief postictal period; may be recall if no LOC
Incontinence	Usually present with LOC	Not usually seen	Uncommon

LOC, loss of consciousness.

reduce the frequency of the ictal events. In case of autoimmune and inflammatory phenomena, the use of corticosteroids may be of some benefit as well.

Further Reading

Barraclough B: Suicide and epilepsy. In Trimble MR, Reynolds EH (eds): Epilepsy and Psychiatry. New York, Churchill Livingstone, 1981, pp 72-76.

Benson DF, Hermann B: Personality disorders. In Engel J, Pedley TA (eds): Epilepsy: A Comprehensive Textbook. Philadelphia, Lippincott-Raven, 1997, pp 2065-2070.

Mai R, Sartori I, Francione S, et al: Sleep-related hyperkinetic seizures: Always a frontal onset? Neurol Sci 2005;26:s220-s224.

Rheims S, Demarquay G, Isnard J, et al: Ipsilateral head deviation in frontal lobe seizures. Epilepsia 2005;46:1750-1753.

Tinuper P, Provini F, Bisulli F, Lugaresi E: Hyperkinetic manifestations in nocturnal frontal lobe epilepsy. Semeiological features and physiopathological hypothesis. Neurol Sci 2005;26:s210-214.

Turnbull J, Lohi H, Kearney JA, et al: Sacred disease secrets revealed: The genetics of human epilepsy. Hum Mol Genet 2005;14 Spec No. 2:2491-2500.

Waxman SG, Geschwind N: The interictal behavior syndrome of temporal lobe epilepsy. Arch Gen Psychiatry 1975 Dec; 32(12):1580-1586.

Williams D: The structure of emotions reflected in epileptic experiences. Brain 1956;79:26-67.

Wolf P: Acute behavioral symptomatology at disappearance of epileptiform EEG abnormality: Paradoxical or forced normalization. In Smith D, Treiman D, Trimble MR (eds): Neurobehavioral Problems in Epilepsy: Advances in Neurology, vol 55. New York: Raven Press, 1991, p 127.

Zucconi M, Manconi M, Bizzozero D, et al: EEG synchronisation during sleep-related epileptic seizures as a new tool to discriminate confusional arousals from paroxysmal arousals: Preliminary findings. Neurol Sci 2005;26:s199-204.

CHAPTER 17

The Geriatric Patient

Hani R. Khouzam, MD, MPH, FAPA

KEY POINTS

- Evaluating and treating psychiatric emergencies in the elderly is challenging due to the coexistence of other medical and psychiatric conditions.
- The four Ds (delirium, dementia, depression, and drugs/medications) are usually the main underlying causes of most geriatric psychiatric emergencies.
- The coexistence of medical illnesses in the elderly may mimic or worsen preexisting psychiatric conditions.
- Geriatric psychiatric emergencies may be associated to a greater degree with delirium, dementia, severe depression, adverse effects of medications, anxiety disorders, and persistent sleep difficulties.
- Geriatric psychiatric emergencies may be associated to a lesser degree with psychotic disorders, substance abuse disorders, and bipolar disorder.

Epidemiology

With the increased life expectancy of the U.S. population, more elderly patients will be suffering from mental illness, leading to an expected increase in the incidence of geriatric psychiatric conditions. More than 50% of the U.S. population now reaches age 75, and 25% live until age 85.

Elderly patients, defined as those who are 65 years and older, represent approximately 13% of the U.S. population; this percentage is expected to increase to 20% by the year 2035.

Geriatric patients account for medical emergencies, including psychiatric emergencies, at a greater rate than the general population, accounting for 13% to 20% of emergency department (ED) visits.

The Four Ds of Geriatric Psychiatric Emergencies

 The four Ds of geriatric psychiatric emergencies are delirium, dementia, depression, and drugs/medications. They are discussed in detail here.

THE FIRST D = DELIRIUM

Overview

Emergency Department (ED) Delirium Pearls

Delirium is often underdiagnosed by ED personnel. The under-diagnosis of this potentially reversible condition may be due to overlap in symptoms of delirium with those of other conditions, especially dementia.

Because delirious patients often are confused and unable to provide accurate information, getting a detailed history from collateral sources, including family, caregivers, and nursing staff, is of paramount importance.

Reviewing prior clinical documentation of episodes of dis-orientation, abnormal behavior, and hallucinations can provide a relevant explanation of the emergency condition of a delirious patient.

Delirium should always be suspected when an acute deteri-oration in behavior, cognition, or perception occurs in the elderly, especially in patients who have dementia, patients maintained on multiple medications, and patients with depression.

Although patients with dementia have a high risk for devel-oping delirium, dementia cannot be diagnosed with certainty in the presence of delirium. The differentiating features of delirium and dementia are summarized in Table 17-1 (also see Chapter 5).

Patients with hypoactive withdrawn delirium may be mis-diagnosed as being depressed; however, although depressed patients may present with impaired cognitive functioning, they usually have a normal level of consciousness that is less prone to fluctuation.

Assessment of Delirium

The diagnosis of delirium is based on clinical presentation of the patient, and with the exception of electroencephalography

Table 17–1

Features Differentiating Delirium and Dementia

Feature	Delirium	Dementia
Onset	Acute and sudden	Insidious and gradual
Course	Fluctuating, usually reversed with treatment; may be superimposed on dementia	Progressive, usually downward deterioration if irreversible; risk factor for delirium
Duration	Short (a few days)	Months to years
Sensorium	Altered consciousness	Clear; no alteration in consciousness
Attention	Impaired	Normal, except for severe dementia
Concentration	Altered	Altered
Psychomotor activities	Increased or decreased; agitation may occur	Often normal, may worsen at night; agitation may occur
Reversibility	Usual; resolution of symptoms may take longer in patients with poor premorbid cognitive functioning	Rare; may be reversible if secondary to treatable medical, neurologic, and surgical conditions

Compiled from Alagiakrishnan K, Wiens CA: An approach to drug-induced delirium in the elderly. Postgrad Med 2004;80:388-393.

(EEG), no single test is fully successful in making an accurate diagnosis. A careful, systematic assessment in the ED can avoid the common underdiagnosis or misdiagnosis of delirium.

Several diagnostic and screening instruments can be used. One screening instrument is the Confusion Assessment Method (CAM), summarized in Table 17-2.

The devised mnemonic DELIRIUM can help the ED clinician recall the diagnostic criteria for delirium:

D = Disorientation and clouded sensorium

E = Evidence of acute changes and fluctuation in mental status

L = Level of consciousness altered

I = Inattention, easy distractibility with disorganized thinking

R = Rhythm of sleep shows disruption in sleep-wake cycle

Table 17–2

The Confusion Assessment Method (CAM)*

Feature	Description	Characteristics
Feature 1	Acute onset and fluctuating course	Obtained from a family member or people who witnessed the presenting patient by asking for evidence of an acute change in mental status from the patient's baseline, as well as fluctuation of abnormal behaviors during the day, including increase and decrease in severity.
Feature 2	Inattention	Elicited by obtaining information about the patient's difficulty in focusing attention, easy distractibility, or difficulty keeping track of what was being said.
Feature 3	Disorganized thinking	Manifested by incoherence, illogical flow of ideas, unclear or unpredictable switching
Feature 4	Altered level of consciousness	Shown by rating the patient's level of consciousness as alert, vigilant, lethargic, stuporous, or comatose

*The diagnosis of delirium by CAM requires the presence of features 1 and 2 and either 3 or 4.
Compiled from Segatore M, Adams D: Managing delirium and agitation in elderly hospitalized orthopaedic patients: Part 1—Theoretical aspects. Orthop Nurs 2001;20:31-45.

I = Illusions, and/or hallucinations may be prominent due to extreme inability to perceive stimuli and to differentiate between internal and external reality

U = Unstable level of psychomotor activity reflecting hyperactive or hypoactive variant of delirium

M = Mood fluctuation with rapid changes in prevailing mood, e.g., crying for no apparent reason

The ED clinicians could use a different version of this mnemonic to identify potential causes of delirium, as shown in Table 17-3.

Table 17–3

The Mnemonic DELIRIUM for Identifying Potential Causes of Delirium

D = Drugs	Alcohol, antibiotics, anticancer drugs (chemotherapy), anticholinergics, anticonvulsants, antidepressants, antihypertensives, antiparkinsonian agents, antipsychotics, cardiac glycosides, cimetidine, clonidine, corticosteroids, disulfiram, insulin, lithium, NSAIDs, opiates, ranitidine, salicylates and sedatives/hypnotics
Delirium tremens	Occurs during alcohol withdrawal after prolonged or heavy consumption; symptoms also occur with benzodiazepine and barbiturate withdrawal
Deficiency states	Folate, nicotinic acid, thiamine, vitamin B_{12}
E = Endocrine	Hypofunction or hyperfunction of adrenal, pancreatic, parathyroid, pituitary, or thyroid glands
L = Liver	Liver diseases, hepatitis, cirrhosis, hepatic encephalopathy, and cancer.
I = Infections	CNS infections, encephalitis, meningitis, brain abscess, urinary tract infections, systemic infections with fever and sepsis
R = Respiratory	Hypercapnia, hypoxia
I = Intoxication	Alcohol, illicit drugs (cannabis, LSD, and other hallucinogens, amphetamines, cocaine, opiates including heroin and morphine, PCP, inhalants).
Toxic encephalopathy	Carbon monoxide, heavy metals (lead, mercury, arsenic), industrial poisons (gasoline, kerosene, turpentine, benzene, refrigerants [Freon]), insecticides (Parathion, Sevin), mushrooms (*Amanita* spp), plants like jimsonweed (*Datura stramonium*), morning glory (*Ipomoea* spp), and animal venoms

Continued

Table 17–3

The Mnemonic DELIRIUM for Identifying Potential Causes of Delirium—cont'd

Uremic encephalopathy	Uremia is a systemic intoxication due to renal insufficiency resulting in disturbances in tubular and endocrine functions of the kidney, production of toxic metabolites, changes in volume and electrolyte composition of the body fluids, and excess or deficiency of various hormones
U = Unmet needs	Fluid and electrolyte imbalances, severe dehydration, sensory deprivation, sleep deprivation, fecal impaction, urinary retention, change of environment
M = Miscellaneous	Diabetes mellitus (hypoglycemia, hyperglycemia), trauma (head or general), seizures and postictal states, hyperthermia, neoplasia, vascular disorders (arrhythmias, cardiac failure, hypertensive encephalopathy, hypotension), surgery-related complications (preoperative, intraoperative, postoperative)

CNS, central nervous system; LSD, lysergic acid diethylamide; NSAIDs, nonsteroidal anti-inflammatory drugs; PCP, phencyclidine.

Medical Evaluation of Delirium

Although preexisting cognitive impairment is a predisposing risk factor for delirium, most often it is difficult to identify a delirious patient as being in the preclinical phase of dementia. Also the development of delirium may unmask or worsen an underlying global cognitive deterioration; thus an emergency psychiatric evaluation of delirium will require a comprehensive medical assessment for the detection of underlying medical conditions.

Almost any medical illness, intoxication, or medication can cause delirium. Often, delirium is due to multiple factors, and the ED clinician treating the delirium should investigate each cause contributing to it. A careful and complete physical examination is necessary, including the following:

Physical Status
- History
- Physical and neurologic examination
- Review of vital signs (i.e., temperature, pulse, blood pressure, and respiratory rate) and anesthesia record if postoperative
- Review of general medical records
- Careful review of medications and any correlation with behavioral changes
- Pulse oximetry to detect hypoxia

Mental Status
- Psychiatric interview
- Cognitive tests during periods of clear sensorium such as the Mini-Mental State Examination (MMSE) (see Table 17-7) and trail making, clock drawing, and digit span tests

Basic Laboratory Tests
- Blood chemistries (electrolytes, glucose, calcium, albumin, urea nitrogen, creatinine, aspartate transaminase [AST], alanine transaminase [ALT], bilirubin, alkaline phosphatase, magnesium, and phosphate) to detect electrolyte abnormalities, assess liver and kidney functioning, and diagnose hypoglycemia, diabetic ketoacidosis, and hyperosmolar nonketotic states
- Complete blood count (CBC) to diagnose infection and anemia
- Thyroid function tests to rule out hypothyroidism
- Electrocardiography (ECG) to diagnose ischemic and arrhythmic causes
- Chest x-ray to diagnose pneumonia or congestive heart failure if indicated by physical examination
- Arterial blood gases (ABGs) or oxygen saturation
- Urinalysis for urinary tract infection

Additional Laboratory Tests
As indicated by individual clinical conditions, the following tests may be necessary:

- Urine culture and sensitivity
- Serum and urine drug screen
- Urine heavy metal screen
- Blood tests: Venereal Disease Reference Laboratory (VDRL) test; test for human immunodeficiency virus (HIV)
- Thyroid function tests to rule out hypothyroidism or hyperthyroidism
- Thiamine folate and vitamin B_{12} levels to detect deficiency states of these vitamins
- Blood cultures
- Antinuclear antibody (ANA) test, urine porphyrins, and serum ammonia level
- Serum drug levels (e.g., digoxin, lithium, theophylline, phenobarbital, cyclosporine)
- Lumbar puncture, when central nervous system (CNS) infection is suspected as a cause of delirium or when the source for the systemic infection cannot be determined
- Computed tomography (CT) or magnetic resonance imaging (MRI) of the brain to diagnose stroke, hemorrhage, and structural lesions
- EEG
  - In patients with delirium, slowing of the posterior dominant rhythm and increased generalized slow-wave activity are usually observed.
  - In patients with delirium resulting from alcohol/sedative withdrawal, increased fast-wave activity occurs.
  - In patients with hepatic encephalopathy, diffuse slowing of activity occurs.
  - Triphasic waves are seen in cases of toxicity or metabolic derangement, continuous discharges in patients with nonconvulsive status epilepticus, and localized delta activity in patients with focal lesions.

Causes of Delirium

There are a large number of possible causes of delirium. Metabolic disorders, termed "metabolic encephalopathy," resulting from organ failure, including liver or kidney failure, are the single most common cause of delirium, accounting for 20% to 40% of all cases. Drug intoxication ("intoxication confusional state") resulting from side effects, exposure to toxins, accidental overdose, or deliberate ingestion is responsible for up to 20% of delirium cases.

Treatment of Delirium

When delirium is diagnosed or suspected, the underlying causes should be sought and reversed, if possible. Despite every effort, no cause for delirium can be found in approximately 16% of patients. Components of delirium management in the ED setting include general supportive therapy, pharmacological treatment, and environmental interventions.

ED clinicians caring for delirious patients with agitation, confusion, combativeness, or apathy must ensure the safety of both the patient and the staff while attending to issues of airway protection and immediate recognition and treatment of rapidly reversible problems (e.g., hypoxia, hypoglycemia, narcotic overdose).

Fluid and nutrition should be given to correct any dehydration, electrolyte, and metabolic abnormalities; they need to be carefully administered with close monitoring of intake, especially when delirious patients are unwilling or physically unable to comply.

Supplemental oxygen is usually provided unless oxygen saturation is above 93% on room air. If carbon monoxide poisoning is suspected, administer 100% oxygen until normal carboxyhemoglobin levels are reached.

In cases of airway compromise, coma, or poor gag reflex, intubation may be necessary. Rapid sequence intubation in the setting of possible head trauma or combativeness may be necessary to facilitate imaging studies.

Some patients with life-threatening overdoses of oral medications as the cause of their delirium who are uncooperative may require sedation and intubation prior to gastric lavage. However, the practice of gastric lavage is controversial and is only indicated in recent (less than 1 hour) and potentially severe or fatal ingestion for which less invasive therapy (e.g., activated charcoal or specific antidote) is unavailable or unlikely to help.

Behavioral control of a patient with delirium who is agitated and combative should be primarily medication-based, with physical restraint kept to a minimum.

Specific Pharmacological Treatment of Delirium

Two types of delirium require specific pharmacological treatment. The first type is delirium due to alcohol or sedatives or hypnotics such as benzodiazepines or barbiturate withdrawal. The second type is delirium caused by centrally acting anticholinergic agents.

Delirium Due to Alcohol or Sedative/Hypnotic Withdrawal

Symptoms of withdrawal from alcohol, barbiturates, and other sedatives/hypnotics (including benzodiazepines) are similar clinically. When symptoms are severe, treatment in a hospital is safest and is mandatory if the patient is febrile (>38.3° C [>101° F]), cannot hold down fluids, or has a severe underlying physical disorder. Withdrawal syndromes, which can be life-threatening and can be associated with seizures, are manifested by a cluster of symptoms in persons who abruptly stop drinking alcohol or stop using sedatives/hypnotics following continuous and heavy consumption. Milder forms of the syndrome include tremulousness and hallucinations, typically occurring within 6 to 48 hours after the last drink or last intake of the sedative/hypnotic.

A more serious syndrome, delirium tremens (DT), involves profound confusion, hallucinations, and severe autonomic nervous system overactivity, which starts within 7 days of withdrawal (usually within 24 to 72 hours). DT is a medical emergency and should be treated in an intensive care unit (ICU) rather than in the ED (details related to DT are discussed in Chapters 4 and 15).

Benzodiazepines are the mainstay in treatment of withdrawal syndromes and are associated with alcohol, and the sedative/hypnotics, including the benzodiazepines and the barbiturates. The choice among the different various benzodiazepines is usually guided by duration of action, rapidity of onset, and cost. Dosage should be individualized, based on withdrawal severity measured by withdrawal scales, comorbid illness, and history of withdrawal seizures. Benzodiazepines can be administered by the intramuscular (IM) route for rapid symptom control and then changed to oral administration. Although there is no difference in the efficacy of long-acting versus short-acting benzodiazepines, some experts recommend shorter-acting benzodiazepines for elderly patients, especially lorazepam; because of its lack of active metabolites, it has the most reliable absorption following IM administration and offers an advantage in patients with impaired liver functioning. Longer-acting benzodiazepines can cause prolonged and excessive sedation because of changes related to aging.

Concomitant treatment during detoxification includes thiamine and other vitamin supplementation, correction of electrolyte disturbances, and general supportive care. Beta blockers, clonidine, carbamazepine, and antipsychotics may be used as adjunctive therapy but are not recommended as monotherapy because they cannot prevent alcohol withdrawal seizures.

Box 17-1 describes several protocols for pharmacological therapy interventions for delirium resulting from withdrawal.

Box 17–1. Pharmacological Therapy Management Protocols for Delirium

I. Management: Mild Withdrawal Protocol

A. General protocol
   1. Diazepam, 5-10 mg PO as needed (prn) or
   2. Lorazepam 1-2 mg PO q4-6h prn for 1-3 days
B. Defining criteria and additional medication indications
   1. Systolic blood pressure >150 mmHg
   2. Diastolic blood pressure >90 mmHg
   3. Heart rate >100 bpm
   4. Temperature >37.7° C (100° F)
   5. Tremulousness, insomnia, agitation

II. Management: Moderate Withdrawal Protocol
   (Usually-triggered by symptoms/events)

A. General protocol
   1. Diazepam
      a. Day 1: 15 to 20 mg PO qid
      b. Day 2: 10 to 20 mg PO qid
      c. Day 3: 5 to 15 mg PO qid
      d. Day 4: 10 mg PO qid
      e. Day 5: 5 mg PO qid
   2. Lorazepam
      a. Days 1-2: 2-4 mg PO qid
      b. Days 3-4: 1-2 mg PO qid
      c. Day 5: 1 mg PO bid
   3. Chlordiazepoxide, 25-50 mg PO qid (decrease by 20% per day)
B. Defining criteria and additional medication indications
   1. Systolic blood pressure 150-200 mmHg
   2. Diastolic blood pressure 100-140 mmHg
   3. Heart rate 110-140 bpm
   4. Temperature 37.7° to 38.3° C (100° to 101° F)
   5. Tremulousness, insomnia, agitation

Continued

> ### Box 17–1. Pharmacological Therapy
> ### Management Protocols for Delirium—cont'd
>
> **III. Management: Severe Withdrawal Protocol**
>   (Indicated for delirium tremens)
> A. General protocol (requires ICU observation)
>   1. Diazepam
>   a. Dose: 10-25 mg PO q1h prn while awake
>   b. End point: until adequate sedation
>   2. Lorazepam
>   a. Dose: 1-2 mg IV q1h prn while awake, for 3-5 days
>   b. End point: until adequate sedation
>   3. Chlordiazepoxide
>   a. Dose: 50 to 100 mg PO/IM/IV q4h (max: 300 mg/day)
>   b. End point: until adequate sedation
> B. Defining criteria and additional medication indications
>   1. Systolic blood pressure >200 mmHg
>   2. Diastolic blood pressure >140 mmHg
>   3. Heart rate >140 bpm
>   4. Temperature >38.3° C (101° F)
>   5. Tremulousness, insomnia, agitation

Delirium Due to Centrally Acting Anticholinergic Agents

The antidote for anticholinergic toxicity is physostigmine salicylate. Physostigmine is the only reversible acetylcholinesterase inhibitor capable of directly antagonizing the CNS manifestations of anticholinergic toxicity.

The typical dose of physostigmine is 2 mg given by the IM route or via slow intravenous (IV) push. Because of physostigmine's short duration of action (about 60 minutes), repeated doses may be necessary to counteract the effects of the somewhat longer-acting anticholinergic agents.

The most common adverse effects of physostigmine are peripheral cholinergic manifestations (e.g., vomiting, diarrhea, abdominal cramps, diaphoresis). Physostigmine also may produce seizures, a complication frequently reported when administered to individuals with tricyclic antidepressant (TCA) overdose. Rarely, physostigmine may produce bradyasystole; this complication occurred when physostigmine was administered to patients with severe TCA overdose.

Most patients can be treated successfully without physostigmine, but it is recommended when at least one of the following aberrations is present: tachyarrhythmias with subsequent hemodynamic compromise, intractable seizures, or severe agitation. It is also recommended for patients with psychosis who are considered a threat to self or others.

Although benzodiazepines have been suggested as first-line agents for the control of agitation associated with anticholinergic toxicity, physostigmine is significantly more effective and no less safe for use in the ED setting. Physostigmine is contraindicated in patients with cardiac conduction disturbances, such as prolonged PR and QRS intervals.

Nonspecific Pharmacological Treatment of Delirium

Some cases of delirium, especially in the elderly, are protracted and may take weeks to clear. Subclinical delirium lasting months has been associated with hepatic encephalopathy. Specific pharmacological intervention may be necessary to help reduce the intensity and duration of prolonged delirium. The medications that have been most used in an emergency setting are the low-dose, high-potency antipsychotics. Multiple studies have demonstrated the safety and efficacy of antipsychotics in treating agitation and psychotic symptoms in delirium. Although there has been a recent increase in the use of atypical antipsychotics such as risperidone, olanzapine, and ziprasidone in the treatment of delirium, most ED clinicians still prefer the use of haloperidol.

Haloperidol

Among antipsychotics, haloperidol is the most frequently studied and used medication. It is relatively safe in the elderly population and has few or no anticholinergic side effects, minimal cardiovascular effects, few sedating side effects, and few active metabolites.

No optimal dose for haloperidol has been established for the treatment of delirium. In general, scheduled low doses are preferable to larger doses administered on an as-needed basis. Several studies have recommended doses as low as 0.25 and 0.5 mg every 4 hours for elderly patients, but the average dose is in the range of 1 to 2 mg every 4 hours. Severely agitated patients may require higher doses; in such cases, special attention must be paid to potential adverse cardiac effects, especially QTc prolongation. Prolongation of the QTc interval to greater than 450 msec or to greater than 25% of that seen on previous ECGs may warrant discontinuation.

Haloperidol is available in oral, IM, and IV formulations. (The IV form is not approved by the Federal Drug Administration [FDA].) Although the use of haloperidol is associated with neurologic effects, especially extrapyramidal symptom (EPS) side effects, these are rarely observed when the medication is administered intravenously. However, the ED clinician should keep in mind that the IV form of haloperidol is twice as potent as the oral form.

Atypical Antipsychotics

Several studies have documented the benefit of atypical antipsychotics in the management of delirium, especially with the recent availability of the parenteral forms of ziprasidone and olanzapine. Atypical antipsychotics have a lower incidence of anticholinergic and EPS side effects and do not require the adjunctive use of benzodiazepines for the control of agitation. Risperidone, olanzapine, and quetiapine have been used in the management of delirium.

Risperidone is available in oral tablets, rapidly disintegrating tablets, and solution formulations; the IM long-acting form (Risperdal Consta) is recommended only for maintenance treatment of schizophrenia. The oral or IM recommended starting dose is 0.25-0.5 mg given twice daily for mild to severe agitation. This may be increased up to 4 mg/day if symptoms initially fail to clear. "As-needed" risperidone may also be effective at 0.25-0.5 mg given every 4 hours for agitation or increased delirium symptoms.

Olanzapine is available in oral tablets, rapidly disintegrating tablets, and IM formulations. The recommended oral or IM starting dose is 2.5-5.0 mg given at bedtime for mild to severe agitation. This may be increased to 20 mg/day if symptoms fail to clear. As-needed olanzapine may also be used; clinical experience has not shown greater efficacy at higher doses.

Quetiapine is only available orally; 25-50 mg twice a day is a reasonable starting dose. This may be increased every 1 to 2 days in increments of 100 mg twice a day if it is well tolerated. Up to 600 mg/day may be used. As-needed quetiapine may also be effective, given at 25-50 mg every 4 hours for agitation or increased delirium symptoms.

Risperidone, olanzapine, and quetiapine may be discontinued without difficulty 7 to 10 days after the patient's functioning returns to baseline, with cleared sensorium and alleviation of delirium symptoms, particularly after reorganization of the sleep-wake cycle.

There is a paucity of data on the use of the atypical antipsychotics ziprasidone and aripiprazole in the management of delirium. It was reported, however, that delirium developed with severe agitation and psychotic symptoms in three patients after withdrawal of the atypical antipsychotic clozapine.

The ED clinician should be aware that the FDA has determined that the treatment of behavioral disorders in elderly patients with dementia with atypical (second-generation) antipsychotic medications is associated with increased mortality.

Environmental Interventions

Environmental interventions can be very useful in the overall management of delirium (Table 17-4).Their main objective is to reduce environmental factors that exacerbate delirium, confusion, and misperception while providing familiarity and a tolerable level of environmental stimulation. For example,

Table 17–4
Environmental Interventions for Delirious Patients

Presenting Problem	Intervention
Disorientation	Frequent reorientation; memory cues such as a calendar, clocks, and family photos may be helpful
Environmental distraction	A stable, quiet, well-lit environment
Unfamiliar surroundings	Support from a familiar nurse and family should be encouraged; family members and staff should explain proceedings at every opportunity, reinforce orientation, and reassure the patient
Sensory deficits	Correct, if necessary, with eyeglasses and hearing aid
High risk for elopement and leaving against medical advice	Precautions must be taken to prevent patients from leaving the facility and becoming lost or injured

Adapted from Volicer L: Dementia and personality. In Mahoney L, Volicer L, Hurley AC (eds): Management of Challenging Behaviors in Dementia. Baltimore, Health Professions Press, 2000, pp 11-28.

"timelessness" in the ED setting, in which there are often no indicators to distinguish day from night, can contribute to disorientation, sleep disturbance, and nighttime agitation. Delirious patients may benefit from repeated, gentle reorientation by nurses, companions, or family members several times throughout the course of the day; reorientation should be practiced in a nonconfrontational manner and should include reminders that the patient's symptoms are temporary and reversible.

The confused patient can be overstimulated by excessive noise from IV equipment, beepers, overhead pagers, alarms, and so forth, and some patients may need to be placed in a room without a roommate or in a room that is distant from a noisy nurses' station.

Delirium can also be exacerbated by sensory impairment, such as poor vision or hearing. Every effort should be made to ensure that the patient has appropriate access to glasses or hearing aids. Lack of comprehension can contribute to fear, paranoia, and agitation, especially in patients who are already agitated.

The bedside presence of family members or familiar items from the patient's home may be calming and reassuring to the delirious patient.

Physical restraints should be avoided if at all possible in delirious patients, who usually will not comprehend the reasons for being restrained. However, such restraints occasionally are necessary for safety reasons. Delirious patients may pull out IV lines and climb out of bed. Perceptual problems may lead to agitation, fear, combative behavior, and wandering. Severely delirious patients benefit from constant one-on-one observation (sitters); this provides assurance of safety, and despite its associated cost, it is a long-term cost-effective intervention.

Patient Education

Families, primary caregivers, and patients should be educated about the etiology and course of the illness and informed about future risk factors.

The ED clinician should reassure families and patients that the delirium often is temporary and can be the result of a reversible medical condition.

Suggest that family members and friends visit one at a time, thus providing a calm and structured environment. Ask visitors to bring some familiar objects, such as photos, to help with reorientation.

Prognosis

Resolution of symptoms may take longer in patients with poor premorbid cognitive function, incorrect or incomplete diagnosis of contributing factors, and structural brain diseases treated with large doses of psychoactive medications prior to the onset of acute medical illness.

In some patients, the cognitive effects of delirium may resolve slowly or not at all.

THE SECOND D = DEMENTIA

Overview

Dementia is present in approximately 10% of the U.S. population older than 65 years; by age 85, approximately 30% to 40% will have developed dementia.

The dementias are a devastating and debilitating group of disorders with major psychosocial and economic repercussions for patients, caregivers, and society at large. The consequences of overlooking dementia in elderly patients can be catastrophic. Nevertheless, in many, if not most, cases it may not be recognized by patients, families, or physicians. Patients often are unaware of their cognitive impairment. Families may dismiss it as part of the normal aging process.

In general, up to 40% of the geriatric population presenting to the ED will show some evidence of cognitive difficulties, usually in the form of dementia or dementia with superimposed delirium. However, dementia in approximately half of these patients is unrecognized in the ED. Also, often patients with recognized dementia are discharged from the ED without any follow-up plan or recommendations to address their cognitive impairment. Thus, when an elderly patient presents to the ED, the responsibility of recognizing dementia ultimately rests with the ED clinician (see Chapter 4). The mnemonic DEMENTIA described in Table 17-5 can aid the ED clinician in recalling the diagnostic criteria for dementia.

ED management of patients with dementia requires an appropriate workup to confirm the diagnosis, identify reversible causes, make pharmacological and psychosocial interventions for the management of disturbing behaviors, and coordinate proper disposition with family members, caregivers, and available resources and agencies. Lengthy delays between diagnosis

Table 17–5

The Mnemonic DEMENTIA to Aid in Recalling Dementia Diagnostic Criteria

D = Disturbances in cognition	One or more of these cognitive disturbances may occur: aphasia, apraxia, agnosia
E = Executive functioning	Impairment in planning, organizing, sequencing, abstraction
M = Memory	Impaired ability to learn new information or to recall previously learned information
E = Exclusive	Exclusively not occurring during the course of delirium, although delirium can be superimposed on dementia.
N = Not due to other causes	Other neurologic, cardiovascular, and systemic conditions of cognitive decline have been ruled out
T = Time of onset	Gradual onset and continuous cognitive decline
I = Impaired functioning	Significant decline in social and occupational functioning
A = Activities of daily living	Dressing, eating, toileting, bathing, and so forth, are impaired

Compiled from American Psychiatric Association: Diagnostic and Statistical Manual of Mental Disorders, 4th ed, Text Revision. Washington, DC, American Psychiatric Association, 2000, pp 135-180.

and treatment can deprive patients and their caregivers of potentially beneficial interventions; they also deny patients and caregivers the chance to make appropriate plans that will result in improved quality of life for all involved.

Differential Diagnosis of Dementia

Mild Cognitive Impairment (MCI)
Dementia needs to be differentiated from age-related forgetfulness and from memory difficulties related to MCI. Many older people have mild memory problems such as difficulty in recalling names and slowed information retrieval but have normal day-to-day functioning. MCI has had many names over the years, including benign senescence and minimal cognitive impairment and age-associated memory decline. Patients with MCI usually have only minimal impairment, but in some patients the impairment may progress to Alzheimer's disease

(AD). Because little is known about the risk for progression, any patient presenting to the ED with memory complaints should be referred for regular follow-up care.

Signs and symptoms that suggest dementia rather than MCI include the following:

- Inability to follow a complex train of thought, balance checkbook, or cook a meal
- Loss of ability to formulate problem-solving plans
- Difficulty in driving a car, finding one's way in familiar places
- Hardship in finding words to express oneself or follow conversations
- Increased passivity and unresponsiveness to environmental surroundings
- Increased irritability and/or suspiciousness
- Misinterpretation of visual and/or auditory stimuli

Reversible vs. Irreversible Causes of Dementia

Because dementia may be due to multiple causes, the ED clinician needs to differentiate the various medical conditions that can present with a clinical picture of a dementia. It is important to distinguish reversible causes from irreversible causes of dementia. AD and vascular dementias (VD) are probably the two most common types of dementia, accounting for up to 90% of cases of established dementia, with a ratio of 2 AD to 1 VD. Dementias are often divided into those with cortical presentation, of which AD is the prototype, and those with subcortical presentation, of which vascular dementia is the prototype. The division between cortical and subcortical dementias may be imprecise; many cases can be confirmed only by postmortem pathologic examination, which usually is not performed. Moreover, mixed dementias are common.

Selected Causes of Irreversible Dementia
Alzheimer's Disease (AD)

AD, or dementia of the Alzheimer type (DAT), is the most common cause of dementia. Typically, the course is one of progressive decline, with survival averaging 2 to 10 years after diagnosis. Diagnosis is confirmed by progressive worsening in memory and at least one other intellectual function that occurs in the absence of delirium, as evidenced by clinical examination and documented by MMSE. These findings may be confirmed by neuropsychological testing. Onset of AD usually is between ages 40 and 90. As the disease progresses, the patient manifests impaired activities of daily living (ADLs), aphasia, apraxia, and agnosia. Early in the disease, patients often worry about their cognition and try to cover for their deficits. Depression is common. Those with prominent frontal lobe involvement may also show poor judgment. Caregivers begin to notice subtle changes in personality.

 Risk Factors for AD

Factors that may increase the risk for AD include:

- *Age*: The risk of developing AD increases with age. According to the Alzheimer's Association, 10% of all people over age 65 have AD, and as many as 50% of those people over age 85 have AD.
- *Gender*: AD affects women more frequently than men.
- *Family history*: A positive family history increases the risk for AD.
- *Down syndrome*: People with Down syndrome (trisomy 21) often develop AD in their 30s and 40s, although the exact reason is not known. Down syndrome has neuropathologic and cognitive features similar to those of AD.
- *Head injury*: Some studies have shown a link between significant head injury with loss of consciousness and retrograde amnesia and increased risk of AD in later life.
- *Environmental toxins*: Some researchers suspect that increased exposure to certain substances, such as aluminum, may make a person more susceptible to AD; however, this finding has not been proved.
- *Low education level*: Although the reason is not clearly understood, some studies have shown that low education levels may be related to an increased risk for AD.
- *Smoking*: Both positive and negative associations have been found.
- *Alcohol*: Alcohol dependence may increase the risk in some patients.
- *Diet*: Some studies suggest a lower incidence in people eating a vegetarian diet compared with a heavy meat diet.
- *Thyroid disease*: Unconfirmed association.
- *Maternal age*: Late maternal age may increase the risk for AD in offspring.
- *Estrogen deficiency*: May increase the risks in postmenopausal women, not maintained on estrogen supplements.

- *Other factors*: Recent research suggests that high cholesterol levels and high blood pressure, factors linked to heart disease, stroke, and diabetes, may also increase the risk for AD.

Pick's Disease and Other Frontal Lobe Dementias

Pick's disease, a frontal lobe dementia, is typically diagnosed before age 65 but may occur as late as after age 80. The first phase of Pick's disease and other frontal lobe dementias is notable for personality changes and alterations in behavior. Patients manifest a striking lack of insight and judgment. They frequently exhibit social neglect and impaired personal hygiene and may be impulsive and disinhibited, with sexually inappropriate behaviors. As time goes by, patients often become apathetic. Language disorders such as perseveration occur early and progress to marked reticence. Depression and anxiety with or without delusions may occur as well. Hyperphagia and obsessive-compulsive activities may develop.

Lewy Body Dementia (LBD)

The course of LBD usually is rapidly progressive and is associated with prominent parkinsonian motor features such as resting tremor, limb rigidity, bradykinesia, and loss of righting reflexes. Patients may have slowed cognition and marked recall deficits, yet have relatively well-preserved recognition abilities. Executive function, abstraction, and judgment are significantly affected early in the disease. Depression, delusions, and visual hallucinations are common. Treatment with levodopa and other dopaminergics often results in new or worsened psychosis and delusions. Treatment with antipsychotics worsens the motor symptoms. Treatment with cholinesterase inhibitors may improve cognitive functioning.

Parkinson's Disease Dementia (PDD)

PDD develops late in the course of Parkinson's disease, and as it progresses it has features similar to those of AD. It is estimated that approximately 20% to 40% of patients with Parkinson's disease develop dementia at some time during the course of their disease. In fact, patients with Parkinson's disease have a sixfold increase in the risk of developing dementia compared with elderly patients without the disease. In addition to the cognitive impairment seen in many patients with PDD, neuropsychiatric symptoms are highly prevalent, particularly depression, hallucinations, delusions, anxiety, and apathy. These symptoms are important determinants of mortality and disease progression, as well as of the patient's quality of life, caregiver distress, and nursing home admission. It has been shown that some psychotic symptoms are strongly associated with cognitive impairment. As the cognitive impairment increases, delusional interpretations of the patient's experiences are more likely to occur, leading to increasingly severe behavioral disturbances.

Vascular Dementia (VD)

VD accounts for 10% to 20% of all dementias and in another 10% to 15% of cases, it coexists with AD. The infarctions of vascular dementia can be associated with small-, medium-, or large-vessel disease. Although multiple small infarcts from atherosclerotic disease are the most common form, other causes, which require different treatment strategies, include infectious vasculitis, granulomatous vasculitis, amyloid angiopathy, and embolic disease resulting from endocarditis.

Selected Causes of Reversible Dementias

Diseases and conditions commonly associated with reversible dementias are shown in Table 17-6. Treatment of these underlying disorders can result in amelioration of most or all of the symptoms and signs of dementia. The two most common causes of reversible dementia are depression and adverse reactions to medications (these are covered in detail in other sections of this chapter). Any medication that affects homeostasis (e.g., diuretics) or the CNS (e.g., sedative hypnotics) should be reassessed and evaluated for its effects on cognitive functioning. Suspected medications should be decreased, changed, or systematically withdrawn in order to identify the offending agent.

Assessment for Dementia

The standard medical workup for dementia, including AD, includes a medical history and physical examination, as well as laboratory tests, radiology with brain imaging, rating scales, and neuropsychological testing.

Physical Examination

The physical examination should focus on cognitive, emotional, and neurologic findings but also must be thorough, looking

Table 17–6

Causes of Potentially Reversible Dementia

Type of Disorder	Conditions
Metabolic disorders	Thyroid disease (hypo- and hyperthyroidism), renal failure, uremic encephalopathy, dialysis, liver failure, Wilson's disease, anoxic and postanoxic dementia, chronic electrolyte disturbances
Adverse medication reactions	Sedatives/hypnotics, barbiturates, anticholinergics; many others
Autoimmune disorders	Vasculitis, lupus erythematosus
Infections	AIDS encephalopathy, Lyme encephalitis, syphilitic meningoencephalitis
Tumors	Intracranial tumors (primary or metastatic), metastasis
Poisoning	Insecticides, alcohol, aluminum, heavy metals (arsenic, lead, mercury, manganese)
Nutritional deficiencies	Vitamin B_{12}, vitamin B_6 (pellagra), thiamine, folate, Wernicke's encephalopathy
Psychiatric disorders	Depression
Other	Normal pressure hydrocephalus, head trauma (post-traumatic encephalopathy), subdural hematoma

AIDS, acquired immunodeficiency syndrome.
Compiled from Fago JP: Dementia: Causes, evaluation, and management.
Hosp Pract (Minneap) 2001;36:59-66, 69.

for signs of diseases such as hypothyroidism, congestive heart failure, and diabetes. Diagnostic evaluation should focus on underlying reversible causes of dementia.

Standard Laboratory Tests

Currently no laboratory tests can diagnose AD with greater accuracy than can be attained by a standard clinical examination.

Laboratory tests employed in the standard workup are intended to rule out causes of dementia such as nutritional deficiencies, infection, metabolic disorders, and drug effects. These tests may include:

- Urinalysis and urine microscopy
- CBC to investigate anemia, infection
- Serum electrolyte levels to investigate metabolic disease
- Serum chemistry panel including liver function tests
- Thyroid panel to rule out hypothyroidism
- Serum vitamin B_{12} and folic acid levels to rule out deficiency
- Neurosyphilis serology if indicated
- Urine toxicology for illicit drugs, alcohol, and heavy metals if indicated
- Serum toxicology for alcohol, medications, and illicit drugs
- Erythrocyte sedimentation rate (ESR), screens for connective tissue disease
- HIV titer if indicated
- ECG and EEG if indicated by the history and physical examination

Other Tests
Lumbar Puncture
Cerebrospinal fluid (CSF) analysis is not usually recommended unless CNS infection is suspected.

Radiologic Studies
Chest and head radiography are not necessary unless indicated by the physical examination.

Brain Imaging
Brain imaging tests such as CT, MRI, positron emission tomography (PET), and single photon emission computed tomography (SPECT) may be ordered to rule out conditions such as tumors, infarcts, and hydrocephalus. MRI can reveal brain tissue loss patterns characteristic of later-stage AD and may be a useful adjunct to standard methods. MRI can also provide some structural findings that could help to differentiate AD from other types of dementia, particularly frontal lobe dementia. Recent research has suggested that high-resolution structure imaging and functional imaging (fMRI, PET) can detect changes that are predictive of AD.

Many clinicians recommend a neuroimaging examination in all patients with dementia unless the dementia is advanced or the course is characteristic and classic. Others feel that imaging studies should be reserved for those with an atypical presentation, rapid decline, or focal neurologic findings.

Tests for Assessment of Cognitive Status

Neuropsychological tests, although not performed in the ED, can help clinicians analyze patients' cognitive status, as well as emotional, psychological, motor, and sensory functions. They may be performed to:

- Confirm a clinical diagnosis of AD
- Rule out other types of dementia
- Provide documentation of the progression of the disease
- Identify depression or suicidal ideation, which could be missed in the initial stage of clinical assessment.

In addition to neuropsychological tests, several screening tests and assessment scales are useful for assessing cognitive status, because early diagnosis rests on recognition of the subtle signs of multifocal cognitive losses associated with visuospatial or personality changes.

The test most commonly used in clinical practice is the MMSE, shown in Table 17-7. The MMSE is a useful tool for assessing cognitive function related to memory, orientation, attention, and language skills and for documenting subsequent decline. Scores of 26 or higher are generally considered normal; lower scores are considered abnormal in a high school graduate, whereas a score of 27 to 30 with evidence of cognitive decline should prompt more neuropsychological testing.

The Short Portable Mental Status Questionnaire (SPMSQ) (Table 17-8) is also useful for detecting cognitive dysfunction. The clock test has been shown to be sensitive in identifying early stages of dementia. The rating scores of the ADLs (Box 17-2) and instrumental activities of daily living (IADLs) (Box 17-3) help to determine the level of assistance needed for performing ADLs.

Management of Dementia

Once the diagnosis of delirium, depression, or reversible dementia has been made, the underlying disorder(s) should be treated. If the problem is caused by one or more specific medications, the patient should be switched to other medications that are less likely to cause cognitive dysfunction in the elderly. Depression should be treated appropriately. Treatment of depression and the reversal of delirium may result in improved cognitive functioning in patients with dementia. Treatment of associated behavioral problems may need to be initiated by the ED

Text continues on page 336.

Table 17–7

Mini-Mental State Examination (MMSE)

Area	Question	Point Score
Orientation	What is the day?	1 point
	What is the date?	1 point
	What is the month?	1 point
	What is the year?	1 point
	What is the season?	1 point
	What is the city?	1 point
	What is the state?	1 point
	What is the county?	1 point
	What is the building?	1 point
	What is the floor?	1 point
Immediate memory	Name three objects, with 1 second to say each; then ask patient to repeat the names of all three objects.	1 point for each correct answer (3 points possible)
Attention and calculation	Use either of these but not both: Serial 7's: Ask patient to count backward from 100 by 7's. Spell W-O-R-L-D backward.	1 point for each correct answer (5 points possible)
Recall	After 2 minutes, ask patient to repeat the names of the three objects in the immediate memory question.	1 point for each correct answer (3 points possible)
Language	Point to a pencil and a watch and ask patient to name them.	1 point for each correct answer (2 points possible)
	Ask patient to repeat: "NO IFS, ANDS, OR BUTS."	1 point
	Ask patient to perform a 3-step command: "Take this piece of paper, fold it in half, give it back to me."	1 point for each correct step (3 points possible)
	Read & Do, "CLOSE YOUR EYES."	1 point
	Write a sentence (must contain a noun and verb and make sense).	1 point

Continued

Table 17–7

Mini-Mental State Examination (MMSE)—cont'd

Area	Question	Point Score
Other	Draw an interlocking pentagon.	1 point

Compiled from Folstein MF, Folstein SE, McHugh PR: "Mini-mental state."
A practical method for grading the cognitive state of patients for the clinician.
J Psychiatr Res 1975;12:189-198.

Table 17–8

 ## The Short Portable Mental Status Questionnaire (SPMSQ)*

Question	Response	Incorrect Responses
1. What are the date, month, and year?		
2. What is the day of the week?		
3. What is the name of this place?		
4. What is your phone number?		
5. How old are you?		
6. When were you born?		
7. Who is the current president?		
8. Who was the president before him?		
9. What was your mother's maiden name?		
10. Can you count backward from 20 by 3's?		

*Scoring: 0-2 errors, normal mental functioning; 3-4 errors, mild cognitive impairment; 5-7 errors, moderate cognitive impairment; 8 or more errors, severe cognitive impairment. One more error is allowed in the scoring if a patient has had a grade school education or less. One less error is allowed if the patient has had education beyond the high school level.

Compiled from Pfeiffer E: A short portable mental status questionnaire for the assessment of organic brain deficit in elderly patients. J Am Geriatr Soc 1975;23:433-441.

Box 17–2. Activities of Daily Living (ADLs)

Instructions: Indicate the level of assistance needed with the following six ADLs by circling the score that most closely describes the patient.

1. Bathing (sponge bath, tub bath, or shower)

   Receives no assistance (gets in and out of tub by self if tub is usual means of bathing (3)

   Receives assistance in bathing only one part of body, such as the back or leg (2)

   Receives assistance in bathing more than one part of body or is not bathed (1)

2. Continence

   Controls urination and bowel movement completely by self (3)

   Has occasional "accidents" (2)

   Needs supervision to maintain urine or bowel control, uses catheter, or is incontinent (1)

3. Dressing (gets clothes from closets and drawers, including underwear/outer garments; uses fasteners, including braces, if worn)

   Gets clothes and gets completely dressed without assistance (3)

   Gets clothes and gets dressed without assistance except in tying shoes (2)

   Receives assistance in getting clothes or getting dressed or stays partly or completely undressed (1)

4. Feeding

   Feeds self without assistance (3)

   Feeds self except for assistance in cutting meat or buttering bread (2)

   Receives assistance in feeding or is fed partly or completely by nasogastric or gastric tubes or intravenous fluids (1)

5. Toileting (going to the "toilet room" for bowel and urine elimination, cleaning self after elimination and arranging clothes)

   Goes to "toilet room," cleans self, and arranges clothes without assistance (may use object for support, such as cane, walker, or wheelchair, and may manage night bedpan or commode, emptying same in morning) (3)

   Receives assistance in going to "toilet room," cleaning self, or arranging clothes after elimination or receives assistance in using night bedpan or commode (2)

   Does not go to "toilet room" for the elimination process (1)

Continued

Box 17–2. Activities of Daily Living (ADLs)—cont'd

6. Transferring

   Moves in and out of bed or chair without assistance (may use object for support such as cane or walker) (3)

   Moves in and out of bed or chair with assistance (2)

   Does not get out of bed (1)

Total score_____

Adapted with permission from Pfeffer RI, Kurosaki TT, Harrah CH Jr, et al: Measurement of functional activities of older adults in the community. J Gerontol 1982;37:323-329.

Box 17–3. Instrumental Activities of Daily Living (IADLs)

Instructions: For the following seven categories, indicate the patient's level of function, as independent = I, needs assistance = A, or dependent = D; then sum the number of activities in each function level.

1. Telephone
   - I. Able to look up numbers and dial, receive, and make calls without help
   - A. Able to answer phone or dial operator in an emergency but needs special phone or help in getting number or dialing
   - D. Unable to use telephone

2. Traveling
   - I. Able to drive own car or travel alone on bus or taxi
   - A. Able to travel but not alone
   - D. Unable to travel

3. Shopping
   - I. Able to take care of all shopping with transportation provided
   - A. Able to shop but not alone
   - D. Unable to shop

4. Preparing meals
   - I. Able to plan and cook full meals
   - A. Able to prepare light foods but unable to cook full meals alone
   - D. Unable to prepare any meals

Continued

> ## Box 17–3. Instrumental Activities of Daily Living (IADLs)—cont'd
>
> 5. Housework
>   - I. Able to do heavy housework (e.g., scrub floors)
>   - A. Able to do light housework but needs help with heavy tasks
>   - D. Unable to do any housework
> 6. Medication
>   - I. Able to take medications in the right dose at the right time
>   - A. Able to take medications but needs reminding or someone to prepare them
>   - D. Unable to take medications
> 7. Money
>   - I. Able to manage buying needs; writes checks, pays bills
>   - A. Able to manage daily buying needs but needs help managing checkbook, paying bills
>   - D. Unable to manage money
>
> **Total number of IADs rated as**:
> ____ Independent
> ____ Assistance needed
> ____ Dependent

Adapted with permission from Pfeffer RI, Kurosaki TT, Harrah CH Jr, et al: Measurement of functional activities of older adults in the community. J Gerontol 1982;37:323-329.

clinician with plans for ongoing follow-up care. Fortunately, nonpharmacological and pharmacological therapies are often effective and can dramatically improve the quality of life for patients as well as their families. However, treatment is rarely successful immediately. The old treatment adage "start low and go slow" is the key to ED intervention and success. The ED clinician needs to consider the following factors.

Demented patients may behave unpredictably. Typical modes include anxiety, aggression, and repetitive questions or gestures. Often these behaviors occur in combination, making it difficult to distinguish one from another.

Causes of behavioral disturbances in patients with dementia have been attributed to four models:

I. *The diminished adaptive capacity model* refers to the frustration imposed by the dementing illness, primarily the loss of functional capacity.

II. *The stress model* focuses on the multiple stressors faced by elderly patients with dementia, such as loss of autonomy and the limitations of a new living environment when institutionalized.

III. *The character model* deals with discovering the character of the individual, including basic personality traits and social skills that may be lost in elderly patients with dementia, leaving them vulnerable and prone to behavioral disturbances.

IV. *The neurobiological model* deals with the neurobiological and neurochemical bases of behavioral changes in the elderly patient with dementia. This model is useful in exploring pharmacological options to manage these behaviors.

Behavioral problems may appear slowly and change as dementia progresses. The most common problematic behavior disturbances include agitation, aggression and combativeness, suspiciousness and paranoia, delusions and hallucinations, and insomnia and wandering.

Nonpharmacological Treatment of Behavioral Disturbances

The initiation of nonpharmacological treatment may relieve depression, agitation, and wandering. Some of these interventions are similar to the techniques used earlier in this chapter for the management of delirium, including:

- Modifying the environment with lighting, color, and noise. Dim lighting may increase uneasiness and confusion; loud or erratic noises often cause confusion and frustration.
- Keeping familiar personal possessions visible.
- Planned activities and daily routines such as bathing, dressing, cooking, cleaning, and laundry.
- Exploring creative and leisure activities such as singing, playing a musical instrument, painting, walking, playing with a pet, and reading.

Pharmacological Treatment of Behavioral Disturbances

Numerous neurochemical alterations have been described in patients with dementia and aggressive behaviors. The cholinergic system is the most well studied, particularly in patients with dementia, but alterations in serotonergic (serotonin; 5-hydroxytryptamine), noradrenergic (norepinephrine), dopaminergic (dopamine), and gamma-aminobutyric acid (GABA) neurotransmitter systems have also been described. It is the alteration of these multiple neurotransmitter systems that usually guides pharmacological interventions in patients with dementia. Melatonin dysregulation and circadian rhythm alteration have also been implicated. The alteration in the cholinergic system is discussed later in the section on the pharmacological treatment of cognitive dysfunction.

The use of pharmacological agents in treating behavioral disturbances in dementia usually is geared toward the management of agitation and aggression.

The mnemonic AGITATION is a useful guide to help the ED clinician to recall comorbid conditions predisposing to agitation and aggression:

A = *Alcohol:* Alcohol dependence, intoxication, or withdrawal can lead to agitation even when obvious signs or symptoms of alcohol use are not present.

G = *Genetic diseases:* Patients with dementia may have congenital diseases such as Huntington's disease and may present with Huntington's chorea and psychotic symptoms.

I = *Infections:* Abnormal vital signs, especially fever or sweating, may be present; general achiness may indicate meningitis, a viral infection prodrome, or tetanus infection.

T = *Tumors:* Family history of cancer; unexplained pain that cannot be adequately controlled.

A = *Akathisia:* Inner restlessness and inability to stay still; may be due to illicit drugs or medications.

T = *Trauma:* Elderly patients with current undetected bone or skull fractures; and patients with a history of a head injury.

I = *Illicit drug use:* Patients with dementia may accidentally take, or may be tricked into taking, drugs such as stimulants, anabolic steroids, ketamine, phencyclidine (PCP), methylene dioxymethamphetamine (MDMA, or Ecstasy), and gamma hydroxybutyrate (GHB).

O = *Other predisposing medical factors:* Chronic pain, respiratory distress, endocrine and metabolic abnormalities.

N = *Neuropsychiatric conditions:* Parkinson's disease, multiple sclerosis, Tourette's syndrome, pervasive developmental disorder, Wilson's disease.

Table 17–9

Pharmacological Management of Agitated/Aggressive Behaviors in Dementia

Behavior	Possible Pharmacological Agent
Psychotic symptoms	Antipsychotics
Mood symptoms, mania	Anticonvulsants, lithium, antipsychotics
Depression	Antidepressants, lithium
Anxiety features	Antidepressants, anxiolytics, anticonvulsants
Nonspecific episodic aggression	Antipsychotics, anticonvulsants, lithium, beta blockers
Nonspecific nonepisodic aggression	Nonantipsychotic agents can be used like alpha adrenergic agents and calcium channel blockers

The rationale for using pharmacological agents for the treatment of agitation and aggression are summarized in Table 17-9. Antipsychotic medications can be used in patients with distressing levels of paranoia or violent outbursts unresponsive to treatment of underlying conditions or to environmental approaches. Atypical antipsychotics (Table 17-10) have a lower incidence of extrapyramidal side effects compared with conventional antipsychotics (Table 17-11) and thus, despite their higher cost, are the medications of choice. Unless the patient is experiencing a dangerous level of psychosis, starting doses should be low and titrated upward slowly, depending on effect. Once the psychosis is under control, attempts to lower the dose or discontinue the medication are warranted because of possibly serious long-term side effects of antipsychotics.

Pharmacological Treatment of Cognitive Dysfunction

Table 17-12 summarizes the characteristics of pharmacological agents used for the management of cognitive decline in AD.

The Cholinesterase Inhibitors

Because the main deficit in neurotransmission in dementia appears to involve acetylcholine, various strategies have evolved to boost the cholinergic system, particularly in AD. A number of cholinesterase (ChE) inhibitors have been examined for their ability to alleviate the symptoms of dementia. ChE inhibitor

Text continues on page 345.

Table 17-10

Atypical Antipsychotic Agents Used for Behavioral Disturbances in Patients with Dementia

Medication	Initial Daily Dose	Properties	Dosage Forms
Clozapine (Clozaril)	6.25 mg	Sedation, orthostasis, agranulocytosis, weight gain, sialorrhea	Oral tablets: 25 and 100 mg
Risperidone (Risperdal, Consta)	0.25 mg	High risk for EPS, orthostasis; may have a therapeutic window	Oral tablets: 0.25, 0.5, and 1 to 4 mg; oral solution for immediate action: 1 mg/mL; Consta is IM long-acting formulation
Olanzapine (Zyprexa Zydis, Zyprexa Intramuscular)	2.5 mg	Weight gain, orthostasis, sedation; can be used in emergency situation	Oral tablets: 2.5, 5, 7.5, and 10 mg; orally disintegrating tablets: 5, 10 mg; Zyprexa Intramuscular: IM injection for immediate effects
Quetiapine (Seroquel)	25 mg	Sedation, weight gain; less risk for EPS due to low binding	Oral tablets: 25, 100, 200, and 300 mg; recommended for patients with Lewy body dementia or parkinsonian movement problems
Ziprasidone (Geodon)	20-80 mg	May cause Q-T interval prolongation	Oral tablets and IM injection formulation for immediate effects
Aripiprazole	10-15 mg	Novel agent with dopaminergic agonist/antagonistic effects	Oral tablets and oral solution

EPS, extrapyramidal syndrome; IM, intramuscular.

Table 17-11

Conventional Antipsychotic Agents Used for Behavioral Disturbances in Patients with Dementia

Medication	Initial Daily Dose	Properties	Dosage Forms*
Chlorpromazine (Thorazine)	10-50 mg	Low potency; medium anticholinergic effects; hypotensive and high sedating effects; low risk for EPS; associated with allergic dermatitis, photosensitivity, possible ECG changes	150 mg max dose; available as oral tablets, liquid concentrate, IM formulation for immediate administration, sustained release form, and suppository
Haloperidol (Haldol)	0.25-0.5 mg	High potency; very low anticholinergic, sedating, and orthostatic hypotensive effects; high risk for EPS	4 mg max dose; can be used in emergency; available as oral tablets, liquid concentrate, and IM formulation for immediate administration and long-acting decanoate form
Fluphenazine (Prolixin)	0.5 mg	High potency; low hypotensive and anticholinergic effects; Medium sedating effects; high risk for EPS	5 mg max dose; available as oral tablets, liquid concentrate, IM formulation for immediate administration and in long-acting decanoate form

Continued

Table 17–11

Conventional Antipsychotic Agents Used for Behavioral Disturbances in Patients with Dementia—cont'd

Medication[†]	Initial Daily Dose	Properties	Dosage Forms*
Trifluoperazine (Stelazine)	1 mg	Medium potency, medium sedative, hypotensive, and anticholinergic effects; high risk for EPS	15 mg max dose; available as tablets, liquid concentrate and immediate IM formulation
Loxapine (Loxatine)	5 mg	Medium potency; medium sedative, hypotensive, and anticholinergic effects; high risk for EPS	30 mg max dose; available as tablets, liquid concentrate, and immediate IM formulation
Perphenazine (Trilafon)	2 mg	Medium potency; low sedating, hypotensive, and anticholinergic effects; high risk for EPS	10 mg max dose; available as tablets, liquid concentrate, and immediate IM formulation

*Divided doses may be necessary to decrease adverse effects.
[†]These medications may not be readily available in the emergency department in the United States, but they are usually available worldwide.
ECG, electrocardiography; EPS, extrapyramidal syndrome; IM, intramuscular.

Table 17–12

Pharmacological Agents Used for Cognitive Decline in Alzheimer's Disease

Medication	Dosage Forms	Recommended Dosing	Titration	Possible Side Effects
Donepezil hydrochloride (Aricept)	Tablets: 5 and 10 mg	Once daily at night, before bed; can be taken with or without food	Starting dose is 5 mg daily for 4 to 6 weeks before increasing dose to 10 mg daily	Anorexia, diarrhea, vivid dreams, fatigue, insomnia, muscle cramps, nausea, vomiting, weight loss
Galantamine hydrobromide (Reminyl)	Tablets: 4, 8, and 12 mg; oral solution: 4 mg/mL	Twice daily in morning and evening with full meals	Starting dose is 4 mg twice daily; increase dose to 8 mg or 12 mg twice daily, as tolerated, after a minimum of 4 weeks of treatment at the lower dose	Anorexia, diarrhea, nausea, vomiting, weight loss
Rivastigmine tartrate (Exelon)	Capsules: 1.5, 3, 4.5, and 6 mg; oral solution: 2 mg/mL	Twice daily in divided doses in morning and evening; patient tolerance is improved if taken with full meals	Starting dose is 1.5 mg daily; most clinicians recommend increasing the dose to 3 mg twice daily after 4 weeks of treatment; thereafter, at 4-week intervals, the dose may be increased to 4.5 mg and 6 mg twice daily	Anorexia, nausea, vomiting, weight loss

Continued

Table 17–12

Pharmacological Agents Used for Cognitive Decline in Alzheimer's Disease—cont'd

Medication	Dosage Forms	Recommended Dosing	Titration	Possible Side Effects
Memantine hydrochloride (Namenda)	Tablets: 5 and 10 mg	Twice daily in divided doses; can be taken with or without food	Starting dose is 5 mg four times daily; dose increases should be in 5-mg increments after a minimum of 1 week of treatment	Agitation, constipation, dizziness, hallucinations, headache, insomnia

Adapted from Ellis JM: Cholinesterase inhibitors in the treatment of dementia. J Am Osteopath Assoc 2005;105:145-158.

administration has been associated with improvement in the cognitive deficit observed in patients with AD. Tacrine was the first such agent approved for this use, but hepatotoxicity and the four-times-daily dosing schedule have limited its use.

The newer ChE inhibitors donepezil, galantamine, and rivastigmine are better tolerated, easier to administer, and selective for neural tissue. Treatment of patients with mild to moderate AD with ChE inhibitors resulted in improvement (or maintenance) of activities of daily living (ADLs), cognition, and behavioral control. In one long-term study, use of antipsychotics was reduced from 58% to 23% in patients taking rivastigmine. Starting therapy early is important. When patients with MMSE scores of 21 to 26 were treated, significant improvement in cognition and behavior was seen. In those with scores of 10 to 20, the improvement was much less pronounced, although still significantly better than in placebo-treated patients, whose function and cognition declined.

ChE inhibitors may be effective in other forms of dementia, especially Lewy body dementia. Because a cholinergic deficiency also appears to underlie the development of behavioral and psychological symptoms of dementia, ChE inhibitors also are likely to ameliorate behavioral disturbances in AD.

Memantine Hydrochloride
Memantine is not a ChE inhibitor as are the other agents listed in Table 17-12. Memantine is an antagonist at the N-methyl-D-aspartate receptor, which is involved in the excitatory glutamatergic neurotransmitter system. Memantine can be used alone or as an adjunct to ChE inhibitors.

Although ED clinicians may be reluctant to initiate pharmacological treatment for cognitive dysfunction in patients with dementia because of their cost, studies suggest that the use of ChE inhibitors is cost-effective. One recent study in a group of veterans with AD showed that the overall cost of care for those on ChE inhibitors was completely offset by reduced hospitalization times and ED visits.

Other Pharmacological Therapies
Estrogen
The influence of estrogen on cognitive function in women has been difficult to establish. A number of studies both affirm and refute the efficacy of estrogen therapy in enhancing cognition in nondemented women. The use of estrogen in women with

AD does not appear to be effective. Thus, given the potential side effects of estrogen, its use for the prevention or treatment of dementia is not yet recommended.

Vitamin E

Antioxidants such as vitamin E, which limits free radical formation, oxidative stress, and lipid peroxidation, may have disease-modifying effects in AD and other forms of dementia. The dose of vitamin E was initially recommended as 2000 IU/day for patients with AD; however, that dose has been associated with hepatic and cardiovascular complications. The role and benefits of vitamin E at a lower dose of 800 IU/day for dementia prevention and the optimal dose for dementia treatment still remain unclear.

Nonsteroidal Anti-inflammatory Drugs (NSAIDs)

Inflammatory mediators probably contribute to progressive neurodegeneration in AD and potentiate damage after stroke. Several retrospective studies have found that patients chronically treated with NSAIDs have a lower incidence of AD than expected. However, because of the multiple adverse effects of standard NSAIDs and the potentially life-threatening toxicities of selective COX-2 inhibitors, these agents are no longer recommended for the treatment of dementia.

Ginkgo biloba

Standardized extracts of the leaves of the *Ginkgo biloba* tree have been used widely in Europe for treating both AD and vascular dementia. In vitro studies have shown that the extracts have anti-inflammatory, antioxidant, and neurotrophic properties. Due to the increased popularity of herbal therapies, family members of patients with dementia may tend to use it. However, because of the anticoagulant effects of ginkgo and the adverse side effects of insomnia, restlessness, and nausea, it is not advisable to use this agent in treating dementias. Patients taking ginkgo biloba and who are maintained on anticoagulant or aspirin therapy require regular monitoring of prothrombin time and international normalized ratio.

Antidepressants

Because depression commonly occurs in patients with all types of dementia, a trial of antidepressants is warranted in any patient with dementia. The treatment of depression is addressed in the following section of this chapter.

Treatment of Coexisting Conditions

Exacerbation of medical conditions, changes in environment, and infections are common causes of cognitive and functional decompensation in patients with dementia and may lead to delirium. Once delirium develops, patients with dementia may experience a permanent loss of cognitive function if the cause is not treated promptly.

Thus, ED clinicians evaluating patients with dementia need to institute up-front preventive measures. These may include strict avoidance of medications known to exacerbate dementia such as sedatives/hypnotics, anticholinergics, H_2 blockers, and low-dose maintenance regimens. Creating a calm environment with few or no changes in personnel, although difficult to achieve in the ED setting, nevertheless is of paramount importance, in addition to minimizing the use of lines and tethers such as Foley catheters and IV fluids.

Advance Care Planning

ED clinicians may be the first line of providers who can advise patients and their families about advance care planning. Dementia, especially AD dementia, is usually a terminal condition within 2 to 10 years of diagnosis, depending on the cause and the stage at diagnosis; therefore, it is critically important to address advance directives early in the course of AD because the patient will be unable to articulate or even comprehend important treatment decisions later.

Documentation of the patient's wishes for end-of-life care, especially regarding feeding tubes, intravenous hydration, and choice of durable power of attorney, can prevent much heartache otherwise faced by family caregivers. Most patients choose to have care directed toward maintaining comfort and quality of life rather than length of life once they become physically and cognitively dependent on others and unable to recognize loved ones and interact with their environment. To ensure fulfillment of such directives, it is critical to have a strong, well-informed proxy who will uphold the patient's wishes in the face of pressure for aggressive late intervention.

THE THIRD D = DEPRESSION

Overview

Depression, which can occur for the first time late in life, is an important cause of behavioral problems in the elderly. Unipolar depression in elderly patients often has a psychotic or delusional component, such as auditory hallucinations or somatic delusions. Effective treatment of psychotic depression often requires a combination of an antidepressant and antipsychotic.

ED Depression Pearls

The ED assessment and diagnosis of depression in geriatric patients with dementia poses a challenge because of the variability of symptom patterns, differences between self-report and observer ratings, and frequency of atypical cases. Depression causes excessive disability and suffering in patients and is associated with increased distress in caregivers. Psychosocial treatments, which often involve the caregiver, are indicated for patients with mild to moderate depression; the choice of antidepressants for treatment of more severe depression should be based on how the patient tolerates the medication. Treatment resistance is common, and serial therapy involving combinations of psychosocial and pharmacological treatment may be required.

   The ED clinician needs to be able to differentiate the presence of depression in association with dementia from the cognitive symptoms associated with depression, which may be a presentation of dementia. This presentation was formerly termed "pseudodementia"; the currently preferred term is "dementia spectrum of depression." Patients with this presentation are at risk for developing dementia later in life.

Patients with late-life depressive syndromes commonly present with somatic complaints. Typically, patients deny having a mental illness and believe that their symptoms are due to medical problems; many elderly patients were raised in an atmosphere where showing feelings was discouraged, and this adds to diagnostic difficulties. Comorbid medical conditions, the tendency of patients to somatize, cognitive deterioration, and multiple late-life medical complications further complicate the diagnostic process. Although the presenting symptoms often do not meet criteria for major depression, they may be debilitating and can lead to suicide.

Table 17-13 describes features distinguishing depression from dementia.

Risk Factors for Depression

The following factors are considered to be linked to the development of depression and can be used as a means of identifying high-risk groups:

- Physical illness, especially if painful or disabling
- Feeling lonely despite living with others
- Recent bereavement or other adverse life-event
- Hearing and visual difficulties

Table 17–13

Differentiation of Depression and Dementia

Depression	Dementia
Abrupt onset associated with expressed mood	Insidious onset associated with significant impairment in social or occupational functioning
Short duration; symptoms cause significant distress in function	Long duration; significant impairment in social or occupational functioning.
Previous psychiatric history (including undiagnosed depressive episodes)	May have psychiatric history, but majority of patients with dementia have no history of psychiatric disorders; deficits do not occur exclusively during the course of delirium
Complaints of memory loss; "I don't know" answers to questions; fluctuating cognitive loss; equal memory loss for recent and remote events	Often unaware of memory loss; near-miss answers; stable cognitive loss (although loss is progressive over time); memory loss greatest for recent events; memory impairment and at least one of these—aphasia, apraxia, agnosia
Depressed mood (if present) occurs first	Memory loss occurs first; impaired executive functioning (e.g., planning, organizing, abstracting) occurs later

Adapted from Birrer RB, Vemuri SP: Depression in later life: A diagnostic and therapeutic challenge. Am Fam Physician 2004;69:2375-2382.

- Personal or family history of depression
- Co-occurrence with dementia
- Medications
- Female gender (female-to-male ratio of about 70:30); however, older white men are at particularly high risk for completed suicide using firearms
- Psychosocial losses; may include the death of a spouse, sibling, or peer or moving from one's longtime home to assisted living, nursing home, or living with relatives
- Alcohol abuse; a second peak of alcoholism occurs in the eighth decade of life and can confound diagnosis of depression in patients of this age
- Depressed phase of bipolar disorder

Assessment and Diagnosis of Depression

Diagnosis of depression can be very difficult in the ED setting. Physical signs of aging, such as stooped posture and a lined face, may influence the perception of elderly patients by others and result in a tendency to consider a person depressed. Conversely, depressive symptoms and signs, such as complaints of pain or fatigue, may be mistakenly attributed to the process of aging or to medical disorders.

The ED is often noisy with little privacy and other emergencies may be obtrusive, making it difficult for the clinician to conduct a comprehensive assessment. Patients may have speaking, hearing, and visual difficulties or they may be too ill to be moved to an interview room or other quiet and private situation. They may be fatigued by their illness or by multiple medical evaluations, or they may be sedated and/or confused by prescribed medication.

Allowing time for the assessment is very important; more symptoms will be revealed if the clinician allows time for rapport to develop. Diurnal variation of mood may affect answers. Some elderly patients may not feel comfortable revealing depression to clinicians they do not know and may withhold information about personal matters and feelings, so that depression may only be identified upon repeated evaluation.

Clinical clues to depression in elderly patients are summarized in Box 17-4.

The medical evaluation of elderly patients with major depression requires a complete physical examination to rule out underlying medical conditions and laboratory tests, including

Box 17–4. Clinical Clues to Depression in Elderly Patients

Unexplained Somatic Complaints
Older patients with depression may present with somatic complaints for which a medical etiology cannot be found or that are disproportionate to the extent of medical illness.

Hopelessness
Hopelessness, not sadness, has been associated with suicidal ideation. Although thoughts about the end of life may be developmentally normal in older persons, suicidal thoughts are not. Statements such as "What's the use?" or "I might as well be dead" should prompt an assessment of the degree of hopelessness and coping skills.

Helplessness
Ask elderly patients about whether they feel helpless about life and about concerns they have about the future.

Memory Complaints
Memory complaints, with or without objective signs of cognitive impairment, should prompt the ED clinician to determine the presence of memory deficits related to an underlying dementia or the presence of dementia spectrum of depression formerly known as pseudodementia.

Irritability
Irritability may be an atypical presentation of depression in the elderly.

Anxiety
Worry and nervous tension (as opposed to specific anxiety syndromes such as panic disorder) are common presentations of depression in older people.

Slowed Movement
Nonverbal clues such as stooped posture and slowed movement and speech may signal depression even in the absence of complete psychomotor retardation.

Continued

Box 17–4. Clinical Clues to Depression in Elderly Patients—cont'd

Loss of Feelings of Pleasure (Anhedonia)
The inability to derive pleasure from life (anhedonia) is a core symptom of depression. Patients with depression may lose their overall zest for life and the satisfaction normally derived from everyday events. Anhedonia may be expressed as no longer enjoying time spent with grandchildren or losing a sense of closeness to God.

Lack of Interest in Personal Care
Lack of interest in personal care in an older patient, including diminished concern for personal appearance and poor adherence to medical or dietary regimens, should prompt an evaluation for depression.

ECG, urinalysis, general blood chemistry screen, CBC, and determination of thyroid-stimulating hormone, vitamin B_{12}, folate, and medication levels.

The gold standard for diagnosis of depression continues to be a complete mental status examination. In patients who present with symptoms and risk factors for late-life depression, depression rating scales can help confirm the diagnosis. The Geriatric Depression Scale—Short Form described in Box 17-5, if it is clarified by the use of simple, nonmedical language and administered in private in an unhurried manner, can identify at-risk patients who require further evaluation.

Medical Causes of Depression

The mnemonic DEPRESSION described in Table 17-14 can be used by the ED clinician to recall medical causes of depression (also see Chapters 3, 4, and 25). The following medications may cause significant depression in the elderly:
- Cardiac and antihypertensive (heart and blood pressure) drugs
  - Bethanidine, clonidine, guanethidine, hydralazine, methyldopa, propranolol, reserpine, digitalis, prazosin, procainamide, Veratrum, lidocaine, oxprenolol
- Sedatives and hypnotics
  - Barbiturates, chloral hydrate, ethanol, benzodiazepines, chlormethiazole, chlorazepate
- Steroids and hormones

Box 17–5. Geriatric Depression Scale— Short Form

1. Are you basically satisfied with your life? Yes No
2. Have you dropped many of your activities and interests? Yes No
3. Do you feel that your life is empty? Yes No
4. Do you often get bored? Yes No
5. Are you in good spirits most of the time? Yes No
6. Are you afraid that something bad is going to happen to you? Yes No
7. Do you feel happy most of the time? Yes No
8. Do you often feel helpless? Yes No
9. Do you prefer to stay at home, rather than going out and doing new things? Yes No
10. Do you feel you have more problems with memory than most? Yes No
11. Do you think it is wonderful to be alive now? Yes No
12. Do you feel pretty worthless the way you are now? Yes No
13. Do you feel full of energy? Yes No
14. Do you feel that your situation is hopeless? Yes No
15. Do you think that most people are better off than you are? Yes No

(Total the number of underlined answers. Normal = 3 ± 2; mildly depressed = 7 ± 3; very depressed = 12 ± 2.)

Score:_____

Compiled from Sheikh JI, Yesavage JA: Geriatric Depression Scale (GDS): Recent evidence and development of a shorter version. Clin Gerontologist 1986;5:165-173.

- Corticosteroids, oral contraceptives, prednisone, triamcinolone, norethisterone, danazol
- Stimulants and appetite suppressants
  - Amphetamine, fenfluramine, diethylpropion, phenmetrazine
- Psychotropic drugs
  - Butyrophenones, phenothiazines
- Neurologic agents
  - Amantadine, bromocriptine, levodopa, tetrabenazine, baclofen, carbamazepine, methsuximide, phenytoin
- Analgesics and anti-inflammatory drugs
  - Fenoprofen, ibuprofen, indomethacin, opiates, phenacetin, phenylbutazone, pentazocine, benzydamine

Table 17–14

The Mnemonic DEPRESSION Used to Identify Medical Conditions Causing Depression

Acronym	Conditions
D = Demoralizing	Dementia, drug and alcohol abuse, cerebral arteriosclerosis, cerebral infarction
E = Endocrine	Addison's disease, hypothyroidism, hyperthyroidism, hyperparathyroidism, Cushing's disease, diabetes, hypoglycemia
P = Pressuring	Hypertension, myocardial infarction, angina, stroke
R = Recurrent	Porphyria, rheumatoid arthritis, Huntington's disease
E = Electrolyte abnormalities	Hypernatremia, hypercalcemia, hypokalemia, hyperkalemia
S = Systemic	Systemic lupus erythematosus
S = Space-occupying lesions	Intracranial tumors (malignant or benign), primary or due to secondary metastasis; cancer of the pancreas, oropharynx, or colon; breast cancer, gynecologic cancer, gastric cancer; lymphoma
I = Infectious, inflammatory	Hepatitis, influenza, viral pneumonia, acquired immunodeficiency syndrome (AIDS), syphilis, temporal arteritis
O = Others	Folate and thiamine deficiencies; renal disease, pernicious anemia
N = Neurologic	Temporal lobe epilepsy, multiple sclerosis, Parkinson's disease

Compiled from Birrer RB, Vemuri SP: Depression in later life: A diagnostic and therapeutic challenge. Am Fam Physician 2004;69:2375-2382.

- Antibacterial and antifungal drugs
  - Ampicillin, sulfamethoxazole, clotrimazole, cycloserine, dapsone, ethionamide, tetracycline, griseofulvin, metronidazole, nitrofurantoin, nalidixic acid, sulfonamides, streptomycin, thiocarbanilide
- Antineoplastic drugs
  - L-Asparaginase, mithramycin, vincristine, 6-azauridine, bleomycin, trimethoprim, thiocarbanilide
- Miscellaneous drugs

- Acetazolamide, choline, cyproheptadine, disulfiram, methysergide, meclizine, pizotifen, anticholinesterases, cimetidine, diphenoxylate, lysergide, mebeverine, metoclopramide, salbutamol

Treatment of Depression

Antidepressant Treatment

Antidepressant treatment in combination with psychotherapy usually is warranted when treating nonpsychotic late-life depression. In patients with psychosis, antipsychotics and electroconvulsive therapy can help achieve remission.

When antidepressant therapy is indicated in older patients, the ED clinician needs to be aware of the physiologic changes that occur with aging, including:

- Decreased metabolic rate, especially decreased demethylation of medications
- Increased body fat-to-water ratio, which increases the volume of distribution for lipophilic psychiatric medications
- Decreased glomerular filtration rate, which may account for higher serum concentrations of kidney-excreted medications and their metabolites
- Increased brain sensitivity to medication effects

Older patients generally require prolonged titration rates and a longer course of treatment than do younger patients. Thus the recommended starting dosages are usually half of those used in younger adults. For the frail older patient, the starting dosage should probably be even lower—about one fourth the typical starting dosage in young adults. As in younger patients, the treatment goal is to achieve the maximal therapeutic effect with the lowest effective dosage while avoiding side effects.

More time may be required to achieve a therapeutic effect in older patients. Substantial improvement may not be seen until an older patient has been taking an antidepressant for 9 weeks or longer.

Selective Serotonin Reuptake Inhibitors (SSRIs)

Currently, SSRIs are the first choice for treatment of depression in elderly patients. Compared with TCAs, for the most part their side effects are better tolerated. SSRIs are less sedating than TCAs and are associated with minimal adverse effects on cognition; both qualities make these agents appropriate for elderly patients. Risk of overdose with SSRIs also is much

Table 17–15

Antidepressants Recommended for Treatment of Elderly Patients

Antidepressant Drug Class/Dosage Forms	Usual Daily Dose Range (mg)	NE Effects	MO Effects	5-HT Effects	DA Effects
TCAs					
Tertiary amines					
Amitriptyline (Elavil) IM, T	50–150	++	0	+++	0
Clomipramine (Anafranil) C	75–150	+++	0	+++++	0
Imipramine (Tofranil) C, T	50–150	++	0	+++	0
Trimipramine (Surmontil) C	50–150	++	0	++	0
Secondary amines					
Desipramine (Norpramin) T	75–150	+++++	0	0	0
Nortriptyline* (Aventyl, Pamelor) C, L	50–150	+++	0	++	0
Protriptyline (Vivactil) T	15–20	++++	0	+	0
Dibenzoxazepine derivatives					
Amoxapine (Asendin) T	50–150	++++	0	++	0
Doxepin (Sinequan, Adapin) C, L	75–150	+++	0	++	0
Tetracyclic Antidepressants					
Maprotiline (Ludiomil) T	50–150	+++++	0	0	0

Antidepressant Drug Class/Dosage Forms	Usual Daily Dose Range (mg)	NE Effects	MO Effects	5-HT Effects	DA Effects
Triazolopyridines					
Nefazodone[†] (Serzone) T	200–400	+	0	++++	0
Trazodone (Desyrel) T	75–300	+/0	0	+++++	0
Aminoketone derivatives					
Bupropion (Wellbutrin, Zyban); bupropion SR (Wellbutrin SR) T	150–300	+++	0	0	++
MAOIs					
Phenelzine (Nardil) T	15–60	+++	+++++	+++	+++
Tranylcypromine (Parnate) T	20–40	+++	+++++	+++	+++
Isocarboxide (Marplan) T	20–60	+++	+++++	+++	+++
SSRIs					
Citalopram (Celexa) L, T	20–40	0	0	+++++	0
Escitalopram (Lexapro) L, T	10–20	0	0	+++++	0
Fluoxetine daily (Prozac, Sarafem); fluoxetine weekly (Prozac) C, L, T	10–50	0	0	+++++	0
Fluvoxamine‡ (Luvox) T	100–300	0	0	+++++	0

Table 17–15

Antidepressants Recommended for Treatment of Elderly Patients—cont'd

Antidepressant Drug Class/Dosage Forms	Usual Daily Dose Range (mg)	NE Effects	MO Effects	5-HT Effects	DA Effects
Paroxetine (Paxil) L, T; paroxetine CR (Paxil CR) T	10-40	+	0	+++++	0
Sertraline (Zoloft) L, T	50-150	0	0	+++++	0/+
SNRIs					
Venlafaxine (Effexor) T; venlafaxine XR (Effexor XR) C	75-225	++	+++++	+++	+
Duloxetine (Cymbalta)	20-60	++++		++++	
α-2 A-SSA					
Mirtazapine (Remeron) T, ODT	15-45	++	0	++	0

*Efficacy of nortriptyline plasma concentrations has been reported to be associated with a therapeutic window between 50 to 150 ng/mL.
†Nefazodone has been reported to cause liver failure and is usually not prescribed except for maintenance of patient already receiving the drug who did not develop hepatic dysfunction.
‡Fluvoxamine has not been approved to treat depression in the United States; it is only approved for treatment of obsessive-compulsive disorder.
α-2 A-SSA, alpha-2 antagonist-specific serotonergic antagonist; C, capsule; DA, dopamine effects; 5-HT, 5-hydroxytryptamine (serotonin); L, liquid; NE, norepinephrine; MAOIs, monoamine oxidase inhibitors; MO, monoamine oxidase; ODT, oral disintegrating tablets; SNRIs, serotonin-norepinephrine reuptake inhibitors; SSRIs, selective serotonin reuptake inhibitors; SR, sustained release; T, tablets; TCAs, tricyclic antidepressants; XR, extended release; ++++ = high; +++ = moderate; ++ = low; + = low; + = very low; 0 = none.

lower than with TCAs. Also, unlike TCAs, SSRIs do not significantly affect cardiac conduction, which is an important quality in the older population with its relatively high incidence of heart disease.

Given the fact that most antidepressants are effective in the elderly, choice of medications should be based on their side effect profile and their potential to interact with other medications. Table 17-15 summarizes the various classes of antidepressants recommended for treatment of elderly patients, with their main neurotransmitter actions and dosages.

The ED clinician should be aware that medication half-lives may be extended 1.5- to 2-fold in elderly patients and that, due to the heterogeneity of this population, there is a wide variation in antidepressant dosages. Therefore, in some older patients effective dosages may be the same as for younger adults.

Side Effects of SSRIs

Nausea, the most common side effect of SSRIs, is usually mild and occurs in the first weeks of treatment. Dry mouth is related to noradrenergic influences on the salivary gland.

Anxiety is usually transient. TCAs and SSRIs have been reported to cause movement disorders such as extrapyramidal syndrome and tardive dyskinesia, but these side effects are much rarer with SSRIs than with TCAs.

Sedation can be a problem in older patients. Among the six SSRIs indicated for depression, paroxetine appears to be the most sedating. Paroxetine exhibits the most anticholinergic side effects; however, it does not appear to compromise cognitive functioning, as it has been observed with other antidepressants with anticholinergic action.

Sexual function can be diminished by SSRIs; the most common sexual side effects are anorgasmia and delayed orgasm. Preserving sexual function is important to many older men and women who retain their interest in sexual activity well into later life.

Abrupt discontinuation or interruption of some SSRIs with shorter half-lives, such as citalopram, escitalopram, paroxetine, and sertraline, may lead to a discontinuation/interruption syndrome with withdrawal symptoms similar to those of the flu, such as dizziness, fatigue, and nausea. In a study of both young and older adults, this syndrome followed abrupt discontinuation at rates of 14% with fluoxetine and 60% with sertraline or paroxetine.

The half-lives of medications tend to be prolonged in elderly patients because of age-related pharmacokinetic changes. SSRIs with a relatively shorter half-life, such as citalopram, sertraline, paroxetine, and escitalopram, can be eliminated fairly rapidly should adverse events arise. On the other hand, use of a longer-acting agent such as fluoxetine may be an advantage if compliance is a problem. In this case, fluoxetine's prolonged washout rate could help protect a patient from relapse, even when doses are missed.

Potential drug-drug interactions vary because individual SSRIs have different effects on the cytochrome P450 system. The ED clinician should assess various medications being taken by elderly patients and determine if such interactions will occur with an SSRI.

Electroconvulsive Therapy (ECT)

ECT is a recommended option for patients with depression and psychotic features who have not responded to antipsychotic and antidepressant medications and for patients with severe nonpsychotic depression who have not responded to adequate trials of at least two antidepressants. ECT is used most often in patients older than age 60. Patients with delusions, psychomotor retardation, early morning awakening, and a family history of depression are most likely to benefit from ECT. ECT may reverse the memory loss and confusion associated with pseudodementia.

Contraindications include recent myocardial infarction, brain tumor, cerebral aneurysm, and uncontrolled heart failure.

ECT is an effective short-term therapy but has higher relapse rates over 6 to 12 months; patients with a history of medication resistance have higher relapse rates following ECT.

Psychosocial Therapy

Various psychotherapies are recommended for elderly patients to intervene in stressful life events such as family conflicts and to help patients reestablish their lost social support network. Cognitive-behavioral therapy and interpersonal and insight-oriented psychotherapy have been shown to be effective in late-life depression. Supportive psychotherapy and problem-solving therapy in combination with social and spiritual interventions aimed at preventing isolation are also recommended.

In milder cases of depression, psychotherapy alone may be sufficient.

The ED clinician needs to be aware that the potential benefits of psychotherapy are not diminished by increasing age. Older adults may often have better treatment compliance, lower dropout rates, and more positive responses to psychotherapy than younger patients.

Although the initiation of psychotherapy usually is not feasible in the ED, clinicians should provide patients and their families with access to information and referral sources.

Other appropriate psychosocial interventions include education related to coping and adaptation, family counseling, participation in bereavement groups, involvement with a senior citizen center, and use of visiting nurse services to help with outpatient care.

THE FOURTH D = DRUGS/MEDICATIONS

Overview

Persons over the age of 65 make up almost 13% of the U.S. population, but they receive 30% of prescriptions filled. The elderly generally have more medical problems, and many of them are taking medications for more than one of these conditions. In addition, they tend to be more sensitive to medications. Even healthy older people eliminate some medications from the body more slowly than younger persons and therefore require a lower or less frequent dosage to maintain an effective level of medication.

The elderly are also more likely to take too much of a medication accidentally because they forget that they have taken a dose and take another one. The use of a 7-day pill-box, as described earlier in this brochure, can be especially helpful for an elderly person.

ED clinicians, as well as those who are close to the elderly such as friends, relatives, and caretakers, need to pay special attention to and watch for adverse physical and psychological responses to medication. Because the elderly may often take other medications beside those prescribed, such as over-the-counter (OTC) preparations and home, folk, or herbal remedies, the possibility of adverse drug interactions is high.

This section summarizes some of the adverse effects associated with psychotropic medications that can lead elderly patients to seek ED assessment and treatment (also see Chapters 3, 4, 5, and 25).

Box 17-6 lists certain medications that can cause cognitive impairment and behavioral problems.

Box 17–6. Medications That Can Cause Cognitive Impairment and Behavioral Problems

Stimulants
Caffeine
Phenylpropanolamine
Pseudoephedrine

Sedatives
Alcohol
Barbiturates
Benzodiazepines
Narcotics

Anticholinergics
Trihexyphenidyl hydrochloride
Diphenhydramine hydrochloride
Benztropine
Oxybutynin chloride
Propantheline bromide
Tricyclic antidepressants

Dopaminergics
Bromocriptine
Conventional neuroleptics
Metoclopramide
Carbidopa-levodopa
Amantadine

Miscellaneous
Digoxin
H_2 antagonists
Phenytoin
Salicylates
Steroids
Theophylline
Lidocaine

Disorders Related to Adverse Effects of Psychotropic Medications
Neuroleptic Malignant Syndrome (NMS)

NMS is an idiosyncratic reaction that is attributed to an acute blockade of dopamine. Onset is relatively sudden, from hours to days, which helps distinguish NMS from lethal catatonia.

Risk factors for NMS include:

- Male gender
- Increased environmental temperature
- High-potency antipsychotics
- Recent use of antipsychotics or recent increase in the dose of antipsychotics
- Concurrent antipsychotic and lithium treatment
- Dehydration
- Preexisting medical or neurologic illness
- Diagnosis of mood disorder

  Signs and symptoms include:
- Abnormal vital signs: Fever, labile blood pressure, increased pulse rate
- Medical signs: Diaphoresis, dysphagia
- Neurologic signs: Rigidity, altered mental state, delirium
- Laboratory findings: Increased white blood cell (WBC) count, increased creatine phosphokinase, aspartate aminotransferase (AST), and lactate dehydrogenase levels.

  Mortality has been reported as 5% to 20% and is usually the result of rhabdomyolysis (acute renal failure) or thrombosis (pulmonary emboli).

Differential Diagnosis

NMS should be differentiated from lethal catatonia, anesthesia-induced hyperthermia, and serotonin syndrome.

ED Treatment

Supportive treatment includes IV hydration, cooling blankets, and monitoring of respiratory status. Any antipsychotics and other dopaminergic blockers should be immediately discontinued. The patient may require immediate transfer to ICU.

The value of the medical therapy of NMS (dantrolene, bromocriptine, amantadine, and ECT) still remains uncertain.

Medical therapy includes IV dantrolene, given at the rate of 2-3 mg/kg/day in tid to qid doses. Side effects include hepatotoxicity, drowsiness, dizziness, weakness, and diarrhea. An alternative drug is bromocriptine, given 5 mg qid PO, which can be increased up to 40 mg/day if needed.

It is reasonable to start both these drugs at the same time. Once symptoms start to resolve the IV dantrolene can be discontinued and the oral bromocriptine can be maintained. The duration of treatment should be at least 10 days for patients who were treated with oral antipsychotics, and 2 to 3 weeks for patients who had been taking parenteral antipsychotics.

An alternative is amantadine, given orally at 100 mg bid. Other drugs that can be used include levodopa, pergolide, and benzodiazepines.

ECT is an option if the symptoms remain unresolved with ongoing pharmacotherapy.

If NMS occurs in the setting of Parkinson's disease, the treatment is basically the same except the parkinsonian medication should be reinstituted as quickly as possible. Because of the risk of NMS, drug holidays are no longer routinely recommended for Parkinson's disease.

If the antipsychotic is to be reintroduced, a waiting period of 2 weeks is recommended for oral medication, and at least 6 weeks for parenteral medication. It is prudent to use a different antipsychotic than the one that originally caused the NMS.

Lethal Catatonia

Lethal catatonia is a severe form of catatonia that may be a manifestation of psychosis or a mood disorder with psychotic features.

Early signs include increased psychomotor activities progressing to wild agitation and choreiform movements, which can alternate with rigidity, stupor, mutism, and refusal of food and fluid intake. Fever, hypotension, and diaphoresis, similar to symptoms of NMS, also may be present.

Patients may become violent and despite their rigid posture may throw heavy objects at bystanders.

Severe end stages of lethal catatonia are associated with convulsions, delirium, coma, and even death.

In contrast to NMS, lethal catatonia usually has a longer prodromal phase of days to weeks; also, abnormal laboratory values are less common than in NMS.

ED Treatment

Immediate medical supportive care includes fluids and nutrition by the IV or nasogastric route if necessary.

Short-term use of lorazepam has been helpful in treating the symptoms of immobility. However, the effects of each dose rarely last more than 1 hour.

The treatment of choice is to restart or increase the formerly prescribed antipsychotic medication.

Malignant Hyperthermia (MH)

MH, also called anesthesia-induced hyperthermia, is a hypermetabolic response to anesthesia leading to acute changes in hemodynamics and resulting in tachycardia, tachypnea, acidosis, hyperkalemia, myoglobinuria, and hyperthermia.

MH is an inherited condition triggered in some patients by anesthesia. It usually occurs during operating procedures. Therefore, this condition is rare in elderly patients in the ED setting, unless they have a history of MH.

If MH is suspected in an elderly patient with a history of a recent anesthesia exposure, immediate admission to the ICU is mandatory.

Serotonin Syndrome

Serotonin syndrome is a cluster of symptoms caused by the administration of monoamine oxidase inhibitors (MAOIs) in combination with other antidepressants such as SSRIs, bupropion, tryptophan, or TCAs. The sudden systemic build-up of serotonin can be life-threatening.

Signs and symptoms include hyperthermia, diaphoresis, excitement or confusion, hyperreflexia, hypotension, and tremor.

Complications include disseminated intravascular coagulation (DIC), rhabdomyolysis, and cardiovascular compromise.

ED Treatment

Immediate medical consultation and, if needed, ICU admission are warranted. The offending agents should be discontinued.

Vital signs should be stabilized and monitored. Dantrolene can be helpful because of its potent muscle relaxant properties. Cyproheptadine, a potent antihistamine and serotonin antagonist, can also be used

Tardive Dyskinesia (TD)

TD is a serious neurologic disorder caused by the long-term use of dopaminergic antagonist medications. Although it is usually associated with the use of antipsychotics, TD apparently was recognized before the development and use of antipsychotics.

It is most common in patients with schizophrenia, schizo-affective disorder, or bipolar disorder who have been treated with conventional antipsychotic agents for long periods, but it can occasionally occur in other patients.

TD is characterized by involuntary movements of the tongue, lips, face, trunk, and extremities.

ED Treatment

TD can be prevented by using the lowest effective dose of antipsychotics for the shortest period of time possible. Reduce or discontinue the causative agent if possible. The risk of a permanent movement disorder must be weighed against the risks of exacerbating psychosis. Also, the symptoms of TD may initially worsen when antipsychotics are discontinued.

Atypical antipsychotics may control psychosis while reducing the risk of TD.

In particular, clozapine is recommended as treatment for patients with TD who require antipsychotics. Clozapine is one of the most effective atypical neuroleptics for treatment-refractory schizophrenia. Although its use has been associated with TD, the incidence of TD with this and other atypical agents appears markedly less than that with conventional antipsychotics. Treatment with clozapine requires close hematologic monitoring to avoid fatal agranulocytosis.

Other, anecdotal treatments include vitamin E, levodopa, benzodiazepines, botulinum toxin, reserpine, tetrabenazine, and dopamine-depleting agents. Ondansetron, a selective 5-hydroxytryptamine-3 antagonist, has been effective in some cases of TD.

Discontinuation of treatment with antipsychotics may worsen or may relieve TD. A controversial strategy to treat TD is continuing and/or increasing the dose of the dopamine antagonist.

Tardive blepharospasm may respond favorably to reduction or cessation of dopamine antagonists. Consultation with an ophthalmologist is indicated to evaluate tardive blepharospasm and/or to exclude Wilson's disease with slit lamp examination.

Drug-Induced Agranulocytosis

Although drug-induced agranulocytosis is relatively rare in the elderly population, it is a potentially life-threatening condition. Very often, a history of a new medication being used or a recent change in medication is reported in elderly patients with agranulocytosis. Because the offending medication may no longer be in use, the inquiry by the ED should include a detailed history of medication intake.

Drug-induced agranulocytosis is a severe condition associated with a mortality rate of approximately 30% due to life-threatening infection. It is defined by the absence of polymorphonuclear leukocytes, relative lymphopenia, and a WBC count of 2000/mm^3 or less. Many drugs associated with agranulocytosis have been reported to the FDA under its adverse reactions reporting requirement. Many are also reported to a registry maintained by the American Medical Association. The reported drugs were used alone, in combination with another drug known to be potentially toxic, or in combination with another drug without known toxicity. Some medications associated with drug-induced agranulocytosis are described in Box 17-7.

Box 17–7. Medications Associated with Drug-Induced Agranulocytosis

Antipsychotics
Chlorpromazine
Clozapine
Prochlorperazine
Promazine
Thioridazine

Antidepressants
Desipramine
Mirtazapine

Anti-inflammatory Agents
Fenoprofen
Gold salts
Ibuprofen
Indomethacin
Phenylbutazone

Others
Carbamazepine
Chlordiazepoxide
Meprobamate
Metoclopramide

ED Treatment

Care is based on the etiology of the agranulocytosis. In most cases in which drug exposure is involved, the most important step is to discontinue the offending agent. If the identity of the causative agent is not known, stop administration of all drugs until the etiology is established.

Specific antibiotic therapy may be required to combat infections. This often involves the use of third-generation cephalosporins or equivalents.

In cases caused by heavy metals such as gold, chelation with British antilewisite (dimercaprol) may be needed.

If agranulocytosis was induced by a specific psychiatric medication (e.g., clozapine), to avoid risk of recurrence, the patient should not be retreated with the same agent.

Extrapyramidal Syndrome (EPS) Side Effects of Medications

EPS side effects include akathisia, parkinsonian side effects, and acute dystonias.

Akathisia

Akathisia is a subjective sensation of inner restlessness that often is associated with the inability to keep still, and is erroneously attributed to a worsening of psychotic agitation and an inappropriate escalation in antipsychotic dose. Acute akathisia may respond to one or more of the following:

- Dose reduction
- A change to a less potent agent or a change to an atypical agent
- The addition of an anticholinergic agent
- The addition of a benzodiazepine or beta blocker

Parkinsonian Side Effects

Parkinsonian side effects are clinically indistinguishable from symptoms of idiopathic Parkinson's disease and include tremor, rigidity, and bradykinesia after months of therapy.

Treatment consists of:

- Dose reduction or withdrawal (if possible)
- A lower-potency traditional agent or an atypical antipsychotic
- Addition of an anticholinergic such as benztropine, trihexyphenidyl, or the dopamine agonist amantadine

Acute Dystonias

Acute dystonias are characterized by sustained posturing due to involuntary muscle spasms involving the head, neck, trunk, and/or limbs. Treatment involves decreasing the dosage or withdrawal of the antipsychotic, or addition of an anticholinergic. Acute dystonic reactions are rare in the elderly.

Psychotic Disorders in Geriatric Patients

When psychotic symptoms occur in conjunction with delirium, dementia, or other medical conditions, the proper diagnosis and treatment of these conditions need to be implemented, in addition to the treatment of psychotic symptoms. Pharmacological and nonpharmacological treatments of psychosis in the elderly are mentioned in other sections of this chapter (also see Chapters 4 and 5). An overview of conditions associated with psychosis in the elderly is described in Box 17-8.

The ED clinician needs to conduct a detailed medical and psychosocial history in conjunction with the medical workup before initiation of treatment of psychosis in the elderly.

Monitoring Adverse Effects of Atypical Antipsychotics

Recent studies have indicated that patients receiving atypical antipsychotic drugs are at increased risk for developing a host of metabolic disorders, including insidious non-insulin–dependent diabetes mellitus (NIDDM) (type II), elevated lipid profiles, and hyperprolactinemia. Other side effects include increased body weight, hemodynamic changes, sleep apnea, arthritis, cardiac conduction delays, bone marrow suppression, cardiomyopathy, and seizures.

As a result, the FDA has asked the makers of atypical antipsychotics to include a warning in the label about a possible link with diabetes. Studies have shown a higher incidence of diabetes among patients with schizophrenia regardless of whether they use antipsychotics when compared with the general population, but it is not known whether these agents aggravate that risk.

Various strategies may be employed to address issues related to weight gain, such as lowering the dose, diet, exercise and adjunctive medications. These, however, are difficult interventions in most cases, and a switch to another atypical agent may

Text continues on page 374.

Box 17–8. Conditions Associated with Psychosis in the Elderly

Brief Reactive Psychosis

There is a sudden onset of psychotic symptoms with a duration of less than 1 month. The symptoms are usually precipitated by stressful or unpredictable situations. Eventually recovery occurs, with return to premorbid functional levels once the stressors are identified and managed.

Schizophreniform Disorder

This condition is similar to schizophrenia; however, symptoms have a duration of less than 6 months. Elderly patients with schizophreniform disorder present with prominent psychotic symptoms and, despite good premorbid social and occupational functioning, they may become perplexed and confused at the height of the psychotic episode. Schizophreniform disorder is rare in the elderly.

Schizoaffective Disorder

To meet the criteria for schizoaffective disorder, a major depressive episode or a manic episode occurs at the same time with symptoms that meet the criteria for diagnosis of an active phase of schizophrenia. The psychotic symptoms of delusions and hallucinations must be present for at least 2 weeks in the absence of prominent mood symptoms. The mood symptoms must coexist for a substantial period during the active and residual periods of psychotic symptoms.

In schizoaffective disorder bipolar type, a manic or a mixed episode with or without major depressive episodes occurs. In the depressed type of schizoaffective disorder, no manic episodes occur.

Induced Psychotic Disorder

Induced psychotic disorder, also called "Folie à deux," is characterized by a close relationship with a person (or persons) with an established delusion that leads to the onset of a similar delusion in that person or persons. Induced psychotic disorder appears to be similar in young and elderly patients, with the exception of an unusually strong interdependence when it occurs in the elderly.

Box 17–8. Conditions Associated with Psychosis in the Elderly—cont'd

Depression with Psychotic Features

This disorder, which is also known as psychotic depression, is more common in depressed patients whose first depressive episode occurs later in life than in patients with early episodes. Delusions are usually somatic in nature; patients often believe that they have an incurable illness or that they are receiving deserved punishment for unforgiven sins, or they have a sense of impending catastrophes affecting loved ones. The psychotic symptoms are usually mood-congruent. Mood disturbance and neurovegetative signs of depression are also present.

Bipolar Disorder

The first episode of mania in bipolar disorder usually has an earlier onset; however, mania can occur for the first time in late life. Mania in the elderly often is characterized by grandiose delusions (e.g., possessing great wealth, exceptional talents, and supernatural powers), irritability, and sexually inappropriate behaviors that are not characteristic of the individual and often surprise persons close to the individual.

Hallucinations of Widowhood

Although this condition is not described in the American Psychiatric Association's *Diagnostic and Statistical Manual of Mental Disorders, 4th Edition, Text Revision* (DSM-IV-TR), it has been reported in the elderly. These hallucinations, which occur in women with intact cognitive functioning, are usually visual in nature; however, both auditory and tactile hallucinations have been reported. Patients report seeing, speaking, and even touching the deceased spouse. The majority of these experiences occur at night. Patients generally acknowledge that the spouse looks different ("ghost-like"), and they do not believe that the deceased spouse is really present. In almost all cases, the patient describes the hallucinatory event as a positive experience.

Continued

Box 17–8. Conditions Associated with Psychosis in the Elderly—cont'd

Paranoid Personality Disorder

Although the disorder begins in early adulthood, as the person grows older, the degree of paranoia and suspiciousness can increase and may evolve into a delusional disorder. The development of late-life medical conditions may worsen the degree of paranoia. It is notable that elderly patients with underlying paranoid personality disorder rarely present to the ED for psychiatric treatment.

Psychosis Due to General Medical Conditions

Psychotic symptoms often occur in patients with delirium and with CNS tumors, including meningiomas, gliomas, and pituitary tumors. The psychotic symptoms are characterized by misinterpretations, illusions, visual hallucinations, and poorly systematized and persecutory delusions.

Substance-Induced Psychosis

Alcohol intoxication and withdrawal can induce hallucinations and paranoid delusions. Hallucinogens and stimulants such as cocaine and amphetamines can also cause psychotic symptoms. OTC and prescribed medications, as well as herbal and other alternative medicine products, can precipitate psychosis in the elderly. Because drug abuse is usually associated with younger age groups, substance-induced psychosis in the elderly may be under-diagnosed or misdiagnosed by ED clinicians.

Traumatic Brain Injury

Patients with moderate to severe head injury have a two to five times greater risk of developing psychosis than the general population. Psychosis in these patients has a distinctive profile of delusions and hallucinations. Psychosis may occur in association with posttraumatic seizures.

Psychosis of Epilepsy

In epilepsy, psychotic symptoms can occur postictally, interictally, and under conditions of forced normalization with anti-seizure medications. Because of the increasing incidence of seizures over the lifespan of a person with epilepsy, it is important to rule out an active seizure disorder in elderly psychotic patients, especially those with a history of seizures.

Box 17–8. Conditions Associated with Psychosis in the Elderly—cont'd

Visual and Auditory Deficits in Patients with Late-Onset Psychosis

Elderly patients who develop late-onset psychosis have a high rate of decreased visual and auditory acuity, and some controversy surrounds the relationship between these sensory deficits and predisposition to psychosis. Improved hearing or vision has been reported to decrease the incidence of paranoid delusions and hallucinations in the elderly. Thus a clinical assessment of vision and hearing is needed for patients with these sensory deficits who develop late-onset psychosis.

Psychosis with Dementia

Various types of dementias can present with psychotic features, including Alzheimer's disease, Pick's disease, vascular dementias, infections (neurosyphilis, Creutzfeldt-Jakob disease), and toxic etiologies (alcoholic dementia).

Schizophrenia

Although schizophrenia usually has its onset in adolescence or early adulthood, it can present for the first time in middle age or later and persist into old age. Some similarities and differences exist between the clinical presentations of early-onset schizophrenia and late-onset schizophrenia. Late-onset schizophrenia generally is similar to early-onset schizophrenia in terms of positive symptoms (delusions and hallucinations), family history, and chronicity. However, late-onset schizophrenia is two to five times more common in women than in men. Negative symptoms (social withdrawal or emotional blunting) and the presence of formal thought disorder are much rarer in patients with late-onset schizophrenia.

Compiled from Khouzam HR, Battista MA, Emes R, Ahles S: Psychoses in late life: Evaluation and management of disorders seen in primary care. Geriatrics 2005;60:26-33.

be a suitable option. In some cases, treatment with cholesterol-lowering agents may help to decrease the hyperlipidemia.

⚠ The mnemonic E-FALCONS outlined here can be used as a tool to recall the parameters used to monitor for adverse effects of atypical antipsychotics.

E = ECG (electrocardiogram) at baseline and every 6 months to monitor for reactions to clozapine and determine whether cardiac risk factors are present for ziprasidone.

F = Fasting glucose at baseline and every 3 months if weight gain is >7% body weight; & **F** = Fall risk assessment to monitor for orthostatic hypertension; measure blood pressure at baseline 1 hour after first dose, then every 3 months, or at clinician's discretion

A = AIMS (abnormal involuntary movement scale) to monitor for EPS side effects at baseline and at every follow-up appointment

L = Lipids (cholesterol/triglyceride) at baseline and every 3-4 months if weight gain >7%; otherwise every year; & **L** = LFTs (liver function tests) at baseline and yearly

C = CBC (complete blood count) and differential at baseline and every week for 6 months, and then every 2 weeks with clozapine and yearly with the other atypical antipsychotics to rule out possible undiagnosed infections (especially pulmonary and urinary tract infection); & **C** = CVAE (cardiovascular adverse events), especially in elderly patients with dementia, such as stroke (transient ischemic attacks were reported in patients with prior risks of cardiovascular diseases and in elderly patients with dementia-related psychosis)

O = Obesity (check body weight at baseline and every 3 months)

N = Noncompliance needs to be checked if new medications are added; it is especially important to monitor if the additional medications can prolong the action or can alter levels of antipsychotic medications; & **N** = NMS (neuroleptic malignant syndrome) can occur with atypical antipsychotics, especially in the elderly, who may be more vulnerable to develop this adverse effect; if signs and symptoms appear, immediate discontinuation is recommended.

S = Seizures; inquire about history of seizures and monitor every 3 months for emergence of any pre-ictal, ictal, and post-ictal phenomena.

Schizophrenia

Although rarely diagnosed for the first time in elderly persons, schizophrenia does continue its course throughout life. For elderly patients with schizophrenia, maintenance treatment with antipsychotics is often necessary. However, elderly patients with schizophrenia sometimes experience a lessening of primary symptoms, allowing management with lower doses or no medication at all.

Delusional Disorder

Delusional disorder consists of a focused delusion without other psychotic features, often occurring in the context of dementia. Although antipsychotic medications are usually prescribed for delusional disorder, they are not always beneficial.

Sleep Disturbances

Families of elderly patients can often tolerate agitation, delusions, and wandering as long as nighttime sleep remains uninterrupted. However, when behavioral disturbances occur at night, families often feel compelled to resort to institutionalization. Educating families about strategies for preventing or correcting sleep problems may help delay nursing home placement.

Many factors can contribute to poor sleep habits in elderly patients, especially those with dementia, including disrupted sleep patterns, alterations in circadian rhythm, concurrent medical problems that cause frequent urination, and daytime use of sedating medication,

Causes of Sleep Disturbances

The main causes of sleep disruption appear to be frequent napping and excessive expectation of sleep needs. Because daily sleep requirements do not increase as a person ages, no more than 7 to 8 hours are required for most persons to feel rested.

Medication-Induced Insomnia
Although many types of medications can alter rest patterns, the following are the most common culprits: antidepressants,

anti-asthma medications, anticonvulsants, antihistamines, anti-hypertensives, bronchodilators, thyroid medication, diuretics, and decongestants. Many of these pharmaceuticals are available as OTC preparations.

Antidepressants

Antidepressants can alter sleep patterns. Lithium in some patients can also alter sleep patterns. The MAOIs commonly cause insomnia and they are also known to cause restlessness if treatment is suddenly stopped, which can further compromise sleep patterns. SSRIs may increase energy levels and awareness, thus interfering with sleep if taken at bedtime. The antidepressant bupropion can also increase energy levels and should not be taken at bedtime. Stimulants can also cause insomnia.

Anti-asthma Medications

Theophylline and prednisone often make nighttime sleep difficult, especially in the beginning of treatment.

Decongestants

OTC decongestants often contain the vasodilators pseudoephedrine and phenylpropanolamine, two medications that can interfere with regular sleep patterns.

So-Called "Sleeping Pills"

OTC sleeping pills often are used to treat insomnia, but with long-term use tolerance develops, leading to worsening of insomnia. If hypnotics are used to induce sleep, they should be used as an adjunct in combination with behavioral therapy to develop better sleeping habits, and they should not be mixed with alcohol. OTC sleeping pills often include sedating antihistamines. As with prescribed sedative/hypnotics, OTC medications should not be mixed with alcohol, or used for long-term relief. Also, withdrawal from sedative agents and alcohol can cause insomnia.

Anticonvulsants

Anticonvulsants such as phenytoin and the newer anticonvulsants felbamate and lamotrigine may cause insomnia.

Other Agents/Causes

Carbon monoxide, idiosyncratic reactions to other medications, and toxin-related reactions can cause insomnia.

Medical Conditions

Medical conditions can cause chronic insomnia, including allergies, arthritis, cancer, fibromyalgia, heart disease, gastroesophageal reflux disease (GERD), hypertension, asthma, emphysema, rheumatologic conditions, Parkinson's disease, and hyperthyroidism.

Pain syndromes and discomfort are major factors leading to impaired sleep.

Nightly Leg Problems

Leg disorders that occur at night, such as restless legs syndrome and leg cramps, are of special note. They are very common and an important cause of insomnia, particularly in the elderly. These disorders may require treatment with benzodiazepines or anticonvulsants.

Psychiatric Conditions

Most psychiatric conditions can cause sleep disturbances in the elderly, especially AD and anxiety disorders such as generalized anxiety disorder (GAD), panic disorder, and post-traumatic stress disorder (PTSD). Mood disorders sometimes are difficult to differentiate from psychophysiologic insomnia because a dysphoric mood, ascribed to the effects of poor sleep, often accompanies psychophysiologic insomnia. The two conditions can often be distinguished on the basis of other "vegetative" signs such as loss of appetite or libido or the typical diurnal fluctuation (worse in the morning) of depression. Manic episodes are usually manifested by decreased need for sleep and may be misinterpreted as insomnia. Insomnia initially may be unrelated to depression but may be a major risk factor for development of depression or anxiety.

Alcohol and Illicit Drug Abuse

An estimated 10% to 15% of chronic insomnia cases result from substance abuse, especially of alcohol, cocaine, and sedatives. Although one or two alcoholic drinks at dinner, for most people, poses little danger of developing dependence in a younger age group, elderly patients may become alcohol- or drug-dependent with that small amount. Elderly patients may believe that excess alcohol promotes sleep; however, to the contrary, it tends to fragment sleep and cause wakefulness a few hours later.

Alcohol consumption also increases the risk for other sleep disorders, including sleep apnea and restless legs syndrome.

Alcohol-dependent patients will often suffer insomnia during withdrawal and, in some cases, for several years during recovery.

Effect of Environment on Sleep Patterns

Environmental lighting may play a role in sleep disturbances. Light is an important modulator of circadian rhythms, which may be disrupted in the elderly, especially patients with dementia. Increased lighting during afternoon and early evening hours may lead to improved sleeping patterns.

Treatment of Sleep Disturbances

The ED clinician should focus on initial treatment of the medical condition(s) and/or co-existing psychiatric conditions that contributed to the sleep disturbance, followed by thorough outpatient care.

Nonpharmacological Interventions

Nonpharmacological interventions are often successful and may include:

- Decreasing excessive time in bed
- Increasing exercise and aerobic fitness during the daytime but not prior to bedtime
- Eliminating clocks in the bedroom
- Using distracting or boring activities to induce sleep onset
- Curtailing caffeine intake in the evening
- Avoiding nicotine
- Avoiding alcohol
- Following a regular sleep-wake schedule
- Using the bed only for sleep and for intimate relationships but not for reading, eating, working, or watching television

Pharmacological Interventions

It is important to avoid the use of any drug with anticholinergic properties for the treatment of insomnia, especially diphenhydramine, hydroxyzine, and similar drugs. Long-acting benzodiazepine hypnotics are often used in nursing homes, where the institutional setting, nighttime light, noise, and the underlying medical problems of older patients worsen problems with sleeplessness. The chronic use of these agents, however, may produce side effects such as impaired memory and alertness, urinary incontinence, daytime sleepiness, and gait imbalance, that can make care even more difficult on a long-term basis. The short-acting benzodiazepines and the hypnotic non-benzodiazepines pose less risk for these side effects (also see Chapters 3, 4, 5, and 11).

The antidepressant trazodone, when given at a relatively low dose of 25 to 75 mg at night, may improve deep sleep, has milder anticholinergic properties, and produces a state of restfulness with minimal cognitive impairment. However, trazodone can cause dizziness and orthostatic hypotension. Medications recommended for treatment of sleep disturbances in the elderly are listed in Table 17-16.

If chronic insomnia coexists with depression or anxiety, treating these problems first may be the best approach. Antidepressants such as trazodone and mirtazapine may be effective in treating depression, anxiety, and sleep disturbances.

ED Interventions

Sleep disturbances may be the presenting symptom in the ED of medical conditions rather than of psychological or psychiatric illness. Untreated, sleep disturbances can cause significant economic hardship, morbidity, and mortality, and they may be a risk factor for development of depression or anxiety. Treatment includes both pharmacological and behavioral interventions.

The first step in reestablishing a normal sleep pattern is to establish sleep hygiene to limit daytime napping. Placing elderly patients in front of a television set almost always leads

---

Table 17–16

Optional Treatment for Sleep Disturbances in the Elderly

Medication	Average Nightly Dose
Benzodiazepines, preferably short-acting:	Can be prescribed 30 min before bedtime;
Lorazepam (Ativan)	0.5-1.5 mg
Oxazepam (Serax)	7.5-15 mg
Hypnotics:	Can be prescribed before bedtime:
Zolpidem (Ambien)	2.5 -5 mg
Zaleplon (Sonata)	2.5-5 mg
Esopiclone (Lunesta)	1-1.5 mg
Ramelteon (Rogerem)	4-8 mg 30 min before bedtime

to napping. To prevent this, caregivers should engage patients in activities that are tailored to their degree of physical activity and psychiatric stability, such as household tasks and, most important, regular physical exercise. These activities can be carried out at home.

The most difficult part of managing sleep problems is the need for continued adherence to a rigid schedule. Families and patients should be advised that periodic disruption of the schedule will likely result in a return to irregular sleep patterns.

Anxiety in the Elderly

This section is an overview of anxiety disorder in elderly patients who present to the ED. Until recently, anxiety disorders were believed to decline with age. Now it is well established that anxiety is as common in the old as in the young. Depression and anxiety may coexist in the elderly, as they do in the young, with almost half of those with major depression also meeting the criteria for anxiety and about one fourth of those with anxiety meeting criteria for major depression. As with younger persons, female gender is a risk factor for anxiety in older adults.

Anxiety in the elderly can lead to disorganized behaviors that appear psychotic. Anxiety secondary to a medical condition is the most common anxiety diagnosis in medically ill elderly patients. This form of anxiety disorder, which often occurs in the context of delirium, is best treated with low-dose antipsychotic agents (also see Chapter 5 and the section on delirium in this chapter). Generalized anxiety disorder (GAD) accounts for most primary anxiety disorders in the elderly; new-onset panic disorder is a rare occurrence in this patient population. GAD may contribute to agitation and, if recognized, can be treated with buspirone. Because of difficulty in processing new situations, fearful anticipatory anxiety is common in patients with dementia when faced and confronted with changes.

A preexisting anxiety disorder may be magnified in the elderly because of the various stressors and vulnerabilities of aging, the presence of chronic medical conditions, the association with cognitive impairment, and the occurrence of significant losses, especially the loss of a significant other.

Treatment options for specific anxiety disorders are summarized in Table 17-17.

Table 17-17

Treatment Options for Specific Anxiety Disorders

Anxiety Disorder	Medication	CBT and Other Non-Drug Therapies
GAD	Benzodiazepines, buspirone, antidepressants, particularly extended release venlafaxine (Effexor) and some TCAs; SSRIs and newer designer antidepressants show promise; antipsychotics in severe cases; agents being studied include gabapentin and other anti-seizure agents	CBT (individual or group), interpersonal therapy, stress management, biofeedback
Panic attacks	SSRIs are treatment of choice; benzodiazepines used only when necessary and short-term if possible; drugs to consider for increasing effectiveness in patients who do not respond to SSRIs alone include beta blockers, buspirone, tricyclics, anticonvulsants	Studies suggest that CBT offers the best chance for a persistent response; CBT also effective in preventing the development of panic disorder in high-risk patients and in helping patients withdraw from SSRIs
Phobias	SSRIs, beta blockers, benzodiazepines; SSRIs are treatment of choice for social anxiety	CBT, hypnosis; CBT may prevent progression of phobias to full-blown panic disorder or agoraphobia

Continued

Table 17-17

Treatment Options for Specific Anxiety Disorders—cont'd

Anxiety Disorder	Medication	CBT and Other Non-Drug Therapies
Obsessive-compulsive disorder	SSRIs are treatment of choice; clomipramine (a combined SSRI and TCA) is an alternative;however, it is rarely used in the elderly due to its adverse effects	CBT (exposure and response prevention)
PTSD	Antidepressants, particularly SSRIs; medications to improve sleep	CBT (individual or group); behavioral measures for improving sleep

CBT, Cognitive-behavioral therapy; GAD, generalized anxiety disorder; PTSD, posttraumatic stress disorder; SSRIs, selective serotonin reuptake inhibitors; TCAs, tricyclic antidepressants.

Ruling Out Conditions Resembling Anxiety

Patients with anxiety disorders are more likely to see general practitioners rather than mental health clinicians, because so often their symptoms are physical, such as muscle tension, trembling, twitching, aching, soreness, cold and clammy hands, dry mouth, sweating, nausea or diarrhea, and urinary frequency. Anxiety attacks can mimic or accompany nearly every acute disorder of the heart or lungs, including heart attacks and angina. In fact, nearly all individuals with panic disorders are convinced that their symptoms are physical and possibly life-threatening. Although no causal relationships have been established, certain medical conditions have been associated with panic disorder. They include migraines, obstructive sleep apnea, mitral valve prolapse, irritable bowel syndrome, and chronic fatigue syndrome.

Depression
Depression is very common in people with an anxiety disorder, and it is sometimes difficult to distinguish one from the other because either or both can be accompanied by anxious feelings, agitation, insomnia, and problems with concentration.

Heart Problems
Studies suggest that up to a third of patients presenting to the ED with chest pain and who have a low to moderate risk for a heart attack are actually suffering from panic attacks. It is often difficult even for specialists to distinguish between symptoms of a heart condition and a panic attack.

Asthma
Asthma attacks and panic attacks have similar symptoms and can also coexist.

Hyperthyroidism
Hyperthyroidism can cause many of the same symptoms of GAD.

Epilepsy
The symptoms of partial seizures and panic attacks often overlap.

Other Medical Conditions

Anxiety-like symptoms are seen in many other medical problems, including hypoglycemia, recurrent pulmonary emboli, and adrenal gland tumors. Women can also experience intense anxiety attacks with hot flashes during menopause.

Medication Side Effects

Many drugs, including some for high blood pressure, diabetes, and thyroid disorders, can produce symptoms of anxiety. Withdrawal from certain drugs, often those used to treat sleep disorders or anxiety, can also precipitate anxiety reactions (also see Chapters 2, 3, 4, and 11).

 ## Substance Abuse

People with anxiety disorders often drink alcohol or abuse drugs in order to conceal or ameliorate symptoms, but substance abuse and dependency can also cause anxiety. In addition, withdrawal from alcohol can produce physiologic symptoms similar to those of panic attacks. Clinicians often have difficulty determining whether alcoholism or anxiety is the primary disorder. Overuse of caffeine or abuse of amphetamines can cause symptoms resembling anxiety.

Box 17-9 outlines a proposed protocol for management of substance abuse disorders (see also Chapter 15).

Treatment

Pharmacological Interventions
Antidepressants

Antidepressants usually take 2 to 4 weeks, and sometimes up to 12 weeks, especially in the elderly, before they are fully effective. Patients may initially experience a temporary period of increased anxiety while on the medication. Consequently, about a third of patients stop taking antidepressants for anxiety disorders before completing the initial phase of therapy. A combination of a benzodiazepine and an antidepressant is sometimes used to avoid the initial anxiety symptoms and to hasten control of panic symptoms. The benzodiazepine can then be withdrawn and the antidepressant, with its negligible risk for long-term abuse, is continued.

The ED clinician initiating antidepressants for the treatment of anxiety disorders should warn patients not to be disheartened if one medication treatment fails. Another may prove to

Box 17–9. Proposed Pharmacological Interventions in the Management of Substance Abuse Disorders

Alcohol Withdrawal States

For agitation, tremors, or change in vital signs:
chlordiazepoxide, 10-25 mg PO every 4 to 6 hours if good liver function tests

For patients with liver disease: lorazepam, 0.5-2 mg PO or IM every 1-2 hours

For severe agitation: lorazepam, 2-4 mg IM every hour; or antipsychotics as prescribed below.

Cocaine and Amphetamine Intoxication

For mild agitation: diazepam, 2.5-5 mg PO or lorazepam, 1-2 mg, every 8 hours

For moderate agitation: haloperidol, 1-2 mg concentrate or 2.5 mg IM; risperidone, 0.5-1 mg concentrate; olanzapine, 2.5 mg IM; or ziprosadone, 2 mg IM

For severe agitation: haloperidol, 5 mg concentrate or 5 mg IM; risperidone, 2 mg concentrate; olanzapine, 5 mg IM; or ziprosadone, 4 mg IM

Phencyclidine Intoxication

For hyperactivity, mild agitation, tension, anxiety, excitement: diazepam, 2.5-5 mg PO; or lorazepam, 1-2 mg PO or IM (0.05 mg/kg)

For severe agitation and excitement with hallucinations, delusions. bizarre behavior: haloperidol, 2-5 mg IM every 30 to 60 minutes

IM, intramuscularly; PO, orally.
Compiled from Dubin WR, Weiss KJ: Handbook of Psychiatric Emergencies. Springhouse, PA, Springhouse Corp., 1991.

be very effective, even if it is a medication of a similar type. Medication combinations should also be considered if a single medication has not been effective. Treatment with antidepressants has been described previously in this chapter and in other chapters throughout this book.

Benzodiazepines

Benzodiazepines are effective medications for most anxiety disorders and have been the standard of treatment for years. However, their use has been associated with a high risk of dependency and abuse, and they have been supplanted in most cases by SSRIs and newer antidepressants. Benzodiazepines include alprazolam and clonazepam, which are effective for panic disorder, some phobias, and generalized anxiety disorder. Benzodiazepines in combination with SSRIs may be particularly helpful in the treatment of panic attacks, although there is no standard as yet for the safest and most effective method for administering this combination.

Other benzodiazepines, including diazepam, lorazepam, and chlordiazepoxide, are used mainly for GAD.

Benzodiazepines have many side effects. The most common are daytime drowsiness and a hung-over feeling. In rare cases, they actually cause agitation. Some respiratory problems may be exacerbated by their use. They appear to stimulate the appetite and can cause weight gain. They can interact with certain drugs, including cimetidine and antihistamines.

Benzodiazepines are potentially dangerous when used in combination with alcohol. Overdoses can be serious, although they are very rarely fatal.

The elderly are more susceptible to side effects, and they should usually start at half the dose prescribed for younger people. Benzodiazepines increase the risk of falling, and some studies have reported a higher risk for hip fracture in older people who take them, although this may occur only with certain benzodiazepines (e.g., lorazepam) or with the use of more than one. Also of concern are studies showing a high risk of automobile accidents in people who take benzodiazepines.

Benzodiazepines taken during pregnancy are associated with birth defects, and they should not be used by pregnant women or by nursing mothers.

Eventually these drugs can lose their effectiveness with continued use at the same dosage. As a result, patients may want to increase their dosage to prevent anxiety. This causes dependency, which can occur as early as several weeks after taking these agents. It should be noted, however, that patients with generalized anxiety disorder rarely become tolerant to the effects of benzodiazepines. Some evidence suggests that the risk for abuse exists only in people who are already susceptible to substance abuse.

Benzodiazepine Withdrawal and Its Treatment

Withdrawal symptoms can be very severe, even in people who rapidly discontinue benzodiazepines after taking them for only

4 weeks. There are some reports that benzodiazepine withdrawal is more difficult than withdrawal from heroin. Symptoms include sleep disturbance and anxiety, which can develop within hours or days after stopping the medication. Some patients experience stomach distress, sweating, and insomnia, which can last from 1 to 3 weeks. The longer the agents are taken and the higher the dose, the more severe these symptoms can become.

Simply tapering off gradually helps about 60% of people to withdraw. Certain medications (anti-seizure agents, antidepressants, buspirone) may be helpful.

Buspirone

Buspirone appears to be as effective as a benzodiazepine for treating GAD. It usually takes several weeks for it to be fully effective, and it is not useful against panic attacks. It does not produce any immediate euphoria or change in sensation, and thus it has a very low potential for abuse. In fact, unlike the benzodiazepines, buspirone is not addictive, even with long-term use, so it may be particularly useful for the patient whose anxiety disorder coexists with alcohol or drug abuse.

Buspirone also seems to have less pronounced side effects than benzodiazepines and no withdrawal effects, even when it is discontinued quickly. Common side effects include dizziness, drowsiness, and nausea. Buspirone should not be used with the MAOIs.

Beta Blockers

Beta blockers, including propranolol and atenolol, affect only the physiologic symptoms of anxiety and are most helpful for phobias, particularly performance anxiety. Beta blockers are less effective for other forms of anxiety.

Clonidine

Clonidine has been used to treat PTSD. Some experts believe it should be tried for anxiety disorders if other therapies fail. It can cause a marked decrease in blood and pulse pressure, which may be a severe side effect in elderly patients.

Anticonvulsants

Gabapentin and other anticonvulsants may be useful for certain anxiety disorders, such as social phobia and PTSD. They may also be helpful during withdrawal from benzodiazepines.

Antihistamines

Hydroxyzine and diphenhydramine may be used as adjunctive treatment for GAD; however, their anticholinergic and antihistaminic effects can potentially cause cognitive dysfunction in the elderly.

Prazosin

Prazosin is an alpha-adrenergic blocker which reduces blood pressure and is sometimes used in treatment of benign prostatic hyperplasia. It has shown effectiveness for alleviating nightmares and other symptoms of PTSD (see Chapter 20). However, it can cause a severe drop in blood pressure, leading to syncope in some patients, within the first few days of treatment.

Nonpharmacological Interventions

A healthy lifestyle that includes exercise, adequate rest, and good nutrition can help to reduce the impact of anxiety attacks. Rhythmic aerobic and yoga exercise programs lasting for more than 15 weeks have been found to help reduce anxiety. Strength, or resistance, training does not seem to help anxiety.

Substance Abuse Emergencies

The psychiatric emergencies associated with alcohol and drug abuse are described in Chapters 4, 14, and 15. This section underscores some of the facts that the ED clinician needs to recognize when assessing and managing alcohol and drug abuse in the elderly.

Alcohol-Related Emergencies

Several conditions related to alcohol require emergent intervention.

Alcohol Intoxication

Blood alcohol levels are only a rough guide to severity of intoxication. An older patient may be medically compromised with a blood alcohol level of 0.2. Other patients with a high tolerance may demonstrate little impairment at this level. Intoxicated patients are usually poor historians and if elderly patients have preexisting cognitive dysfunctions this will further complicate the ED clinician's task of obtaining an accurate history of alcohol use, abuse, or dependence. Patients should receive a complete physical examination to rule out any serious medical conditions.

Alcohol Overdose

Excess alcohol consumption can lead to a serious and sometimes fatal overdose syndrome especially in medically compromised elderly patients. Blood alcohol levels as low as 0.25 have been associated with death. Signs suggestive of alcohol overdose include low pulse rate, decreased respiratory rate, and low blood pressure. These signs may precede circulatory collapse and death. Evaluation should, of course, include a complete physical examination. Drug screens are often necessary to assess for other contributions to cardiopulmonary and neurologic compromise. Careful monitoring of arterial blood gases, oxygen saturation, and vital signs is necessary. These patients may need ventilatory and respiratory support.

Alcohol Withdrawal

The evaluation and management of alcohol withdrawal, including prevention of DT and treatment of Wernicke's encephalopathy and Korsakoff's psychosis are discussed in Chapters 3, 4, 5, 14, and 25.

Drug Intoxication and Withdrawal Syndromes

Drug intoxication and withdrawal syndromes may occur with a psychiatric disorder or as a primary presenting complaint. Phencyclidine (PCP) and cocaine are the substances that most commonly lead to violent behavior. PCP users can present with almost any psychiatric symptom (see also Chapter 15).

Patients intoxicated with PCP should be placed under observation in a secure ED location away from stimulation; talking down is not recommended. Physical restraints or sedation may be necessary for violent patients. Lorazepam, 2 to 4 mg PO, or diazepam,10 to 20 mg PO, is recommended to treat agitation.

Patients who abuse cocaine and also use MAOIs or other psychostimulants are at risk for hypertensive crisis. Haloperidol has been used to manage paranoid psychosis or schizophrenia relapse secondary to cocaine use.

Symptoms of withdrawal from barbiturates, other sedatives, hypnotics (including benzodiazepines), and alcohol are similar clinically (see also Chapter 14). When symptoms are severe, treatment in a hospital is safest and is mandatory if the patient is febrile (>38.3° C [>101° F]), cannot hold down fluids, or has a severe underlying physical disorder. Alcohol withdrawal can be life-threatening. Seizures can occur. Delirium tremens, a withdrawal syndrome that starts within 7 days of withdrawal (usually within 24 to 72 hours), is a medical emergency and should be treated in an ICU.

Overdose of prescribed psychoactive drugs can also cause intoxication. If the patient has recently taken a toxic dose and is awake, treatment consists of inducing emesis followed by administration of activated charcoal. Overdose with tricyclic antidepressants or carbamazepine requires cardiac monitoring. Overdose with barbiturates or benzodiazepines and alcohol may cause respiratory arrest. Acetaminophen overdose requires monitoring of blood levels, and if blood levels of acetaminophen indicate probable liver damage, acetylcysteine must be given according to protocol.

Bipolar Disorder in Late Life

The first episode of mania in bipolar disorder usually has an early onset; however, mania, as well as bipolar disorder itself, can occur for the first time in late life. Both manic and depressed episodes may be accompanied by psychotic symptoms.

Little is known about mania in late life or about its eventual outcome. Elderly patients with late-onset mania may have concurrent neurologic disorders, which will require neurologic evaluation of the illness. Manic symptoms are estimated to occur at some time during the illness in fewer than 10% of patients with AD. Also, onset of mania in late life is related to an increased frequency of medical disorders and drug treatment and may occur with various medical conditions (described later in this section).

 Recent epidemiological data have documented an increased incidence of sexually transmitted diseases (STDs) in elderly patients with mania.

Clinical Presentation

Similar to middle-aged and younger adults, older patients who develop mania have delusions of possessing great wealth, exceptional talents, and supernatural powers. Mania in the elderly often is characterized by grandiose delusions, irritability, and sexually inappropriate behaviors that are not normally characteristic of the patients, often surprising those closest to the patients and resulting in their presentation to the ED for assessment or treatment (see Chapter 8 for evaluation and treatment of mania).

A careful review of the patient's psychiatric history is crucial in making an accurate diagnosis of late-life bipolar disorder, which may be characterized by:

- Recent recurrent episodes of mania and or depression which have not been previously diagnosed
- A history of similar episodes and a family history of bipolar disorder
- Overlap of symptoms of mania, schizophrenia, and agitated depression has been ruled out

Although psychotic symptoms often suggest schizophrenia, patients with schizophrenia usually have a long history of recurrent psychotic symptoms, including paranoia, auditory and visual hallucinations, and ideas of reference.

In agitated depression, symptoms of irritability, decreased sleep, restlessness, and anxiety may be present. However, impulsive behavior and grandiose thoughts characteristic of bipolar disorder are usually absent in depression.

Although most patients with bipolar disorder experience symptoms of depression or mania, some report a combination of these symptoms. Patients in a "mixed state" may verbalize severe depressive symptoms such as suicidality and also may exhibit pressured speech, irritable mood, and impulsive behavior.

Assessment and Diagnosis

Evaluating patients with suspected mania requires a thorough physical examination; laboratory tests, including a urine drug screen for substance abuse; a detailed assessment of presenting symptoms; and collateral information from family or caregivers.

Diagnosing mania in the elderly can be complicated by the coexistence of current medical illnesses, medications, or alcohol and drug abuse.

Mania Due to General Medical Conditions

General medical conditions associated with mania are summarized in Table 17-18. These should be suspected in elderly patients with new-onset mania, especially in the absence of a personal and family history of mood disorders. The presenting

Table 17–18

Medical Conditions Associated with Mania

General Medical Condition	Diagnosis
Cerebrovascular accidents, strokes	Left-sided cerebral lesions are more often associated with depressive episodes; right-sided lesions are more often associated with mania
Neurologic disorders	Temporal lobe seizures, traumatic brain injuries, multiple sclerosis
Endocrine disorders	Hyperthyroidism, hypothyroidism, pheochromocytoma
Systemic diseases	Lupus erythematosus
Tumors	Primary neoplasms, gliomas, meningiomas; metastasis

symptoms of mania associated with medical conditions are the same as the manic symptoms of preexisting bipolar disorder. The ED clinician should evaluate the history of any psychiatric disorders before assuming that the mania was precipitated by a specific medical condition.

ED Interventions
The primary ED intervention in mania due to general medical conditions is to identify and treat the underlying medical disorder; when this is accomplished, the mania symptoms usually resolve.

Mania due to medical conditions such as HIV, syphilis, and/or structural brain lesions requires pharmacological treatment with antimanic agents.

Medication- and Substance-Induced Mania
Older adults are more likely than younger adults to have one or more chronic illnesses and to be on a combination of medications. The most common offending medications include levodopa, phenylephrine, sympathomimetics (i.e., in bronchodilators), steroids, and adrenocorticotropic hormone. And although illicit drug use may be less common in the elderly, cocaine and amphetamine intoxication can precipitate mania in the elderly.

Antidepressants may precipitate a manic episode in vulnerable individuals.

Treatment

Bipolar disorder is a complicated illness and difficult to treat. Severe cases of mania may necessitate admission to a psychiatric hospital, particularly when patients are found to be dangerous to self or others.

Goals of treatment are acute stabilization, symptom attenuation, and restoration of functioning.

See Chapter 8 for discussion of the pharmacological treatment of mania. Various medications for the treatment of mania are summarized in Table 17-19.

Elderly patients, who have slower metabolism and clearance rates, are generally more sensitive to medications; accordingly, treatment guidelines should always specify lower starting doses and slower titration rates for elderly patients.

Concomitant use of antipsychotics or other mood stabilizers is often required to control acute behavioral symptoms.

In addition to lithium and divalproex sodium (DVP), the FDA has approved all the atypical antipsychotics, except clozapine, for treating acute mania. All of these medications appear to have similar efficacy; choice of medication, then, is based on tolerability and side-effect profile. Lithium has FDA approval for acute, as well as maintenance therapy; however, its tolerability in the elderly is questionable due to the decrease in the glomerular filtration rate. The ED clinician should be aware that limited data are available regarding the safety and efficacy of mood stabilizers such as lithium and DVP in the elderly.

In adults, lithium has a narrow therapeutic index (0.8-1.2 mEq/dL); and in the elderly these levels may be neurotoxic. Accordingly, the recommended lithium blood level in the elderly is lower (0.4-0.7 mEq/dL) than that recommended in younger adults. It is important to note that lithium blood levels are affected by concomitant medications affecting renal filtration, such as NSAIDs and antihypertensives.

Medications such as thiazides, spironolactone, and angiotensin-converting enzyme inhibitors increase lithium levels, whereas acetazolamide, aminophylline, and caffeine decrease lithium levels. Moreover, lithium clearance is reduced in patients with congestive heart failure, renal dysfunction, and hypertension. Although subtherapeutic lithium levels increase risk of relapse, high lithium levels can lead to toxicity.

Symptoms of acute lithium toxicity include nausea, vomiting, diarrhea, renal failure, ataxia, tremor, confusion, delirium,

Table 17–19

Medications Used for the Treatment of Mania in the Elderly

Medication/Daily Dosage	Lab Tests	Specific Information	Side Effects
Lithium; 300-450 mg	CBC, electrolytes, kidney function tests, ECG, TSH	Blood level 0.4-0.8 mEq/L 5 days following treatment initiation or dose change; lithium toxic range close to therapeutic dose	Ataxia, tremor, cerebellar dysfunction, cognitive impairment; renal impairment, polyuria, polydipsia, weight gain; worsening of skin conditions, especially psoriasis
Divalproex sodium; 125-250 mg	CBC, LFTs	Blood level 50-100 mg/L 3 days following treatment initiation or dose change	GI upset, nausea, weight gain; ataxia, somnolence; thrombocytopenia, hepatic failure, pancreatitis; hair thinning
Carbamazepine, oxycarbamazepine; 150-400 mg	CBC, LFTs, ECG	Blood level 4-12 µg/L 3 days following treatment initiation or dose change	Lightheadedness, drowsiness, dizziness, ataxia; cognitive dysfunction; blood dyscrasias
Lamotrigine; 12.5-25 mg for 1 week, increase every 1-2 weeks	None needed		Headache, nausea, skin rash; may develop Stevens-Johnson syndrome

Medication/Daily Dosage	Lab Tests	Specific Information	Side Effects
Risperidone; 0.5-1 mg	HbA1c, fasting glucose, lipid profile	May have therapeutic window between 4 and 6 mg; available as rapidly disintegrating tablets, liquid concentrate, and IM long-acting formulation	EPS, hyperprolactinemia, orthostatic hypotension
Olanzapine; 2.5-5 mg	HbA1c, fasting glucose, lipid profile	Available as rapidly disintegrating tablets and immediate IM formulation	EPS, sedation, weight gain, type II diabetes, orthostatic hypotension
Ziprasidone; 20-40 mg	HbA1c, fasting glucose, lipid profile, ECG	Available as immediate IM formulation	Akathisia; may cause QT interval prolongation
Quetiapine; 25-50 mg	HbA1c, fasting glucose, lipid profile	Preferred agent in the elderly	EPS, sedation, weight gain; type II diabetes; orthostatic hypotension
Aripiprazole; 7.5 mg	HbA1c, fasting glucose	May improve cognitive functioning	Sedation, postural hypotension

CBC, complete blood count; ECG, electrocardiogram; EPS, extrapyramidal syndrome; GI, gastrointestinal; HbA1c, hemoglobin A1c; IM, intramuscular; LFTs, liver function tests; TSH, thyroid-stimulating hormone.

hallucinations, and coma. Accordingly, use caution when prescribing lithium for the elderly; patient and family education and monitoring for potential toxicity are essential.

Anticonvulsants have assumed an increasing role in treating bipolar disorder. It is important to note, however, that not all anticonvulsants are antimanic. Although carbamazepine (CBZ) and DVP are frequently used, only DVP and lamotrigine (Lamictal) have FDA approval specifically for the treatment of bipolar disorder. DVP has been particularly useful in rapid cycling mania and mania secondary to neurologic conditions.

Although no therapeutic blood level has been determined in the elderly, studies of DVP suggest that a lower therapeutic level of 50 mg/L and an upper therapeutic level of 90 mg/L are safe and effective in elderly patients.

Lamotrigine was recently approved for maintenance treatment of bipolar disorder; however, it is not an acute antimanic medication. There have been very few reports on the use of lamotrigine in the elderly, and no therapeutic dose has been determined; therefore, patients should always be started at 25 mg or less. Stevens-Johnson syndrome has been associated with rapid increase in lamotrigine dosage.

The metabolism of CBZ is decreased in the elderly; accordingly, slow titration is recommended. Although no therapeutic range has been determined for CBZ in the treatment of mania, initial doses of 100 mg/day or bid are recommended and can be progressively increased as needed. Oxcarbazepine has a similar structure to CBZ with possibly better tolerability. However, hyponatremia and syndrome of inappropriate antidiuretic hormone (SIADH) have been reported in elderly patients.

Conventional or typical antipsychotics such as haloperidol have been widely used over the last few decades for psychosis and mania; however, the risk for EPS symptoms and tardive dyskinesia limits their use. The new generation of atypical antipsychotics (e.g., ziprasidone, olanzapine, quetiapine, risperidone, aripiprazole) carries less risk for EPS symptoms and tardive dyskinesia.

 ED clinicians need to know that effective collaboration with families, caregivers, and primary care providers remains key in ensuring provision of optimal care to elderly patients who present with manic symptoms late in life.

Summary

Elderly patients with psychiatric emergencies may be suffering from several underlying medical and psychiatric conditions. The ED clinician must conduct a comprehensive assessment in order to identify reversible conditions. Many clinicians as well as family members significantly underestimate the extent to which elderly patients will respond to treatments. The prognosis for recovery is equal in young and old patients, although remission may take longer to achieve in older patients.

In patients with reversible dementia, depression, bipolar disorder, anxiety, sleep disturbances, or psychotic disorders, good recovery rates are possible. In patients with irreversible dementia, although recovery rates are markedly reduced, the ED clinician can have an important impact by recommending appropriate psychosocial and family interventions. In patients with delirium and drug-induced psychiatric disorders, all available efforts should be made to reverse the underlying causes and offending agents. Close follow-up and review of side effects are important when prescribing medications.

 The ED clinician needs to practice and implement the belief that "growing old does not translate to growing sick."

Further Reading

Alagiakrishnan K, Wiens CA: An approach to drug-induced delirium in the elderly. Postgrad Med J 2004;80:388-393.

Almeida OP, Fenner S: Bipolar disorder: Similarities and differences between patients with illness onset before and after 65 years of age. Int Psychogeriatr 2002;14:311-322.

American Psychiatric Association. Practice guideline for the treatment of patients with delirium. Am J Psychiatry 1999;156(Suppl):1-20.

American Psychiatric Association: Diagnostic and Statistical Manual of Mental Disorders, 4th ed, Text Revision. Washington, DC, American Psychiatric Association, 2000, pp 135-180.

Birrer RB, Vemuri SP: Depression in later life: A diagnostic and therapeutic challenge. Am Fam Physician 2004;69:2375-2382.

Dubin WR, Weiss KJ: Handbook of Psychiatric Emergencies. Springhouse, PA, Springhouse Corp, 1991.

Ellis JM: Cholinesterase inhibitors in the treatment of dementia. J Am Osteopath Assoc 2005;105:145-158.

Fago JP: Dementia: Causes, evaluation, and management. Hosp Pract 2001;36:59-66, 69.

FDA Public Health Advisory: Deaths with antipsychotics in elderly patients with behavioral disturbances. Rockville, MD, US Food and Drug Administration, Center for Drug Evaluation and Research. April 11, 2005. At: http://www.fda.gov/cder/drug/advisory/antipsychotics.htm. Accessed September 1, 2005.

Folstein MF, Folstein SE, McHugh PR: "Mini-mental state." A practical method for grading the cognitive state of patients for the clinician. J Psychiatr Res 1975;12:189-198.

Gill T, Khouzam HR, Tan DT: E-FALCONS: A mnemonic for monitoring the prescribing of atypical antipsychotics. Geriatrics 2004;59:41-45.

Goodroad BK: HIV and AIDS in people older than 50. A continuing concern. J Gerontol Nurs 2003;29:18-24.

Khouzam HR, Emery PE, Reaves B: Secondary mania in late life. J Am Geriatr Soc 1994;42:85-87.

Khouzam HR, Gazula K: Clinical experience with olanzapine in the course of postoperative delirium associated with psychosis in geriatric patients: A report of three cases. Int J Psychiatry Clin Pract 2001;5:63-66.

Khouzam HR, Gill T, Tan D: When "agitation spells a medical problem." Curr Psychiatry 2005;4:87-88.

Khouzam HR, Kissmeyer PM: Physostigmine temporarily and dramatically reversing acute mania. Gen Hosp Psychiatry 1996;18:203-204.

Lynskey MT, Day C, Hall W: Alcohol and other drug use disorders among older-aged people. Drug Alcohol Rev 2003;22:125-133.

Pfeiffer E: A short portable mental status questionnaire for the assessment of organic brain deficit in elderly patients. J Am Geriatr Soc 1975;23:433-441.

Pfeffer RI, Kurosaki TT, Harrah CH Jr, et al: Measurement of functional activities of older adults in the community. J Gerontol 1982;37:323-329.

Rabins PV: Cognition. In Evans JG, Williams TF, Beattie BL, et al (eds): Oxford Textbook of Geriatric Medicine,

2nd ed. Oxford University Press, Oxford and New York, 2000, pp 917-921.

Segatore M, Adams D: Managing delirium and agitation in elderly hospitalized orthopaedic patients: Part 1— Theoretical aspects. Orthop Nurs 2001;20:31-45.

Sheikh JI, Yesavage JA: Geriatric Depression Scale (GDS): Recent evidence and development of a shorter version. Clin Gerontol 1986;5:165-173.

Sink KM, Holden KF, Yaffe K: Pharmacological treatment of neuropsychiatric symptoms of dementia. A review of the evidence. JAMA 2005;293:596-608.

Snowdon DA, Greiner LH, Mortimer JA, et al: Brain infarction and the clinical expression of Alzheimer disease: The Nun Study. JAMA 1997; 277:813-817.

Sutor B, Rummans TA, Smith GE: Assessment and management of behavioral disturbances in nursing home patients with dementia. Mayo Clin Proc 2001;76:540-550.

Volicer L: Dementia and personality. In Mahoney L, Volicer L, Hurley AC (eds): Baltimore, Health Professions Press, 2000, pp 11-28.

Yesavage JA, Brink TL, Rose TL, et al: Development and validation of a geriatric depression screening scale: A preliminary report. J Psychiatr Res 1983;17:37-49.

Additional Resources

The American Psychiatric Association: Practice Guideline for the Treatment of Patients with Delirium. Copies may be obtained from the American Psychiatric Press Inc, 1400 K St NW, Washington, DC 20005. Orders can also be placed by telephone (800-368-5777) or online.

POSTSCRIPT

In loving memory of my father Raoul, who passed at age 65; my mother Jeannette, who passed at age 86; and my father-in-law Ernest "Roy" Dickerson, who passed at age 92:

"Grow old along with me! The best is yet to be . . ."
                    Robert Browning—Rabbi ben Ezra

C H A P T E R 1 8

Child and Adolescent Psychiatric Emergencies

Tirath S. Gill, MD

KEY POINTS

- It is important to gather collateral data from multiple sources when evaluating a child or adolescent presenting to the emergency department (ED).
- Medical causes for psychiatric disturbances should be sought, as in the case of an adult with psychiatric symptoms.
- Collaboration with social workers and with other agencies is crucial when making plans for disposition and follow-up.
- ED clinicians may assume the role of primary advocate for children that are being abused or susceptible to harm in their environment and should take measures to promote the physical and emotional well-being of these children.

Overview

Emergencies in children and adolescents evoke our deepest emotions. Our collective instinct for survival compels us to protect and nurture the young. When dysfunctional behaviors present in children and adolescents, our personal emotions can get in the way of making rational decisions.

An understanding of some of the common psychiatric problems seen in children and adolescents helps the ED clinician deliver the best possible care. Acute depression, suicidal and self destructive behaviors, and conduct problems are some of the usual reasons that bring children and adolescents to the ED. These and other common presenting emergencies are shown in Box 18-1.

Box 18–1. Problems Presenting as Pediatric Psychiatric Emergencies

Depressive disorders
Substance abuse disorders
Adjustment disorders
Bipolar disorder
Attention deficit hyperactivity disorder
Conduct disorder
Psychotic disorders
Anxiety disorders
Eating disorders

General Guidelines for Interviewing Children

ED clinicians should be respectful of children's anxiety about talking with a person they do not know and their discomfort in the strange environment of the ED; clinicians should also be aware of their own emotional issues that may influence consultation. Children are perceptive about others' genuineness, and clinicians should speak in a kind and a forthright manner.

State who you are and that your purpose is to try to help the child in whatever way possible. Avoid words or language that is above the comprehension level of the age group that you are dealing with. Simple sentences and questions are better than complex ones. Children who are verbally expressive should be allowed to tell their stories without interruption.

Be careful to avoid judgmental statements and premature interruptions due to your own anxiety. Acknowledge the level of distress of the child and allow the interview to proceed at the child's own pace, using gentle facilitation interview techniques. There may be periods of silence, and you should be comfortable with these. Gentle open-ended questioning and specific probing for further information may be pursued if the child is willing and cooperative.

Children sometimes express their themes through play and fantasy. One may provide a variety of toys and dolls, crayons and paper and observe the emotional themes aroused by the children's play with these materials. It is sometimes revealing to ask about favorite activities and TV programs, and what they would wish for if they could have three wishes.

Initial Clinical Presentation

The child may be tearful, angry, and irritable in affect. Eye contact may be decreased. Mood may be depressed, elated, mixed, or fearful and anxious. The child may exhibit self-soothing behaviors such as rocking, curling into a fetal position, sucking the thumb, and other repetitive motor behaviors. The psychotic child may be mouthing and responding to hallucinations. The child with bipolar disorder may be loud and intrusive and exhibit mixed features of the disorder. The intoxicated child may show signs of alcohol intoxication. Intoxication with other substances such as cannabis, psychedelics, or stimulants such as rave drugs may be noted. This can confound the clinical picture and make it more difficult to assess for other comorbid psychiatric pathology. The child with attention deficit hyperactivity disorder (ADHD) may be easily distracted, inattentive, or engaged in increased motor activity such as climbing on furniture.

Specific Problems and Their Management

The Suicidal Child

Epidemiology

The incidence of suicide in the prepubertal population is generally lower than that in the general population and is estimated as 0.5% to 0.9%. After puberty, from age 14 to young adulthood, the risk of suicidal behavior may be higher than the average for the general population, with an incidence of 12 to 14 per 100,000 population.

A marked rise in suicidal behavior was reported from 1980 to 1992; a decline in these rates has been reported for the years 1992 to present. These numbers may indicate a change in reporting methods and/or in insurance funding for inpatient child care, as well as various other tangential forces in our society. Nevertheless, the idea of potential suicide by children and adolescents should always be taken seriously.

Clinical Presentation

The suicidal child may present with the features of a clinical depression, psychosis, or emotional turmoil related to some situational or relationship crisis. The most common causes of suicidal behaviors are depressive, substance abuse, and adjustment disorders (Box 18-2). Bipolar disorder may present for the first time as a severe episode of depression, and a history of suicide attempts in blood relatives may place these individuals at higher risk for suicidal behaviors. The departure of a parent due to death, divorce, or other causes can raise intense issues of abandonment, self-worth, and purpose in the vulnerable child. Breakups with a boyfriend or girlfriend in the innocent intensity of youth can lead to serious self-harm and should not be taken lightly.

On occasion, a gradual withdrawal and decline in functioning may be a harbinger of psychosis. The acute psychotic break when it finally happens can leave the child bewildered and perplexed and call into question his or her very identity and relationship to the world. During such periods of global anxiety and disorganization, suicide risk is increased.

 Conflicts with parents, increasing school work, learning disabilities, and substance or alcohol abuse tend to have a compounding effect on the child's psychological well-being.

Physical Examination

A chaperone should always be present when a child is being examined. It is important to look for any alteration of mental status, and any physical signs of injury such as bruising or marks on the neck from hanging attempts, or cuts on the torso, arms,

---

Box 18–2. Factors Associated with Increased Risk of Suicide in Children

Physical abuse
Emotional neglect
Return to abusive environment
Insomnia
Access to firearms
Substance and alcohol abuse
Male gender
Caucasian race
Recent losses
Prior suicide attempts
Cold and distant parents
Lethality of the suicide attempt—serious or a cry for help
Family history of successful suicides

or legs. In patients with failed suicide attempts by hanging, radiologic or other imaging tests may be necessary to rule out spinal injury. A sobering listing of the modes of suicide in children is given in Box 18-3. If suspicious injuries or bruises are noted that indicate physical abuse, documentation with photographs or videotaping should be undertaken to aid in prosecution of the perpetrators of such crimes. A picture in these situations is truly worth a thousand words.

Laboratory Studies

The basic laboratory workup includes a urine drug screen, complete blood count (CBC), chemistry panel, and specific toxicology screens if overdose is suspected. Acetaminophen, aspirin, opiates, and other medications being taken by adults in the household are commonly involved in overdoses. There is often a false perception in the minds of children and many lay persons about the relative safety of acetaminophen, and accidental deaths have occurred when the victim was not actually attempting suicide but was making a gesture for help. Hence, early and sequential monitoring of acetaminophen, salicylate, and other drug levels should be considered, as well as electrocardiography (ECG). A safety bracelet, necklace, or anklet may furnish useful medical data.

A pregnancy test should be done in females of child-bearing age. Further testing, as indicated by the physical examination or the medication history, should be ordered by the clinician. For patients on anticonvulsant medications, anticonvulsant levels should be ascertained. When a family history of intermittent porphyria is present, urine levels of porphobilinogen and other byproducts of porphyrin metabolism can be checked. If this

---

Box 18–3. Common Means of Attempted Self-Harm in Children

Cutting/stabbing
Hanging/suffocation
Firearms
Gas asphyxiation
Overdosing on prescribed drugs
Overdosing on alcohol or street drugs
Other risk-taking behaviors

test is positive, it may help in explaining a diverse array of physical and psychiatric symptoms.

Disposition

High-risk adolescents such as those with a prior history of suicide attempts, an unstable home situation, abuse at home, psychotic symptoms, or access to firearms and other lethal means are at significantly increased risk for suicide and should be hospitalized. For acute agitation and anxiety, medicating with a short-acting benzodiazepine is often helpful. The ED clinician should confer with an ED physician or pediatrician before the patient is transferred to a psychiatric unit.

There is some evidence that antidepressants may help the child with severe depressive syndromes. However, there may be an increased risk of suicidal ideation and behaviors during the first few weeks of treatment with selective serotonin reuptake inhibitors (SSRIs) and possibly with other antidepressants. Therefore, it is prudent that children receiving outpatient treatment for depression are seen every week or more frequently. Hospitalization permits even closer monitoring when outpatient safety cannot be ensured.

Upon discharge, the first few days and weeks are high-risk periods, and close monitoring by telephone calls and office visits is advisable. Psychotherapy and family therapy can lead to long-term benefits and reduce the risk of repeated suicide attempts. Such therapy therefore should be a key consideration in discharge planning.

 Hospitalization and the posthospitalization period are high-risk periods for repeated suicide attempts. Approximately 1% of depressed patients attempt further self-harm while in the hospital and succeed at killing themselves.

The Agitated and Violent Child

A violent child or adolescent can cause significant harm to the clinician, and proper precautions are indicated. Patients with the diagnosis of conduct disorder, mental retardation, mania, psychosis, or brain injury, and with a history of violence and substance abuse, have a high risk for perpetrating violence in the future. Acute emotional turmoil in the frustrated child due to any cause can provoke a violent lashing out. Obviously, this risk is increased if the clinical interaction is lacking in sensitivity or respect for the child.

The ED clinician should note any gross signs of medical problems or intoxication. If self-injurious acts have occurred, proper attention should be paid to the medical issues such as suturing of lacerations, blood transfusions, if necessary, and charcoal and lavage as indicated. If ingestion of a toxin has occurred, the poison control center should be contacted for specific guidelines. Follow laboratory guidelines for the medical workup as listed previously for the suicidal child.

The Child with Psychosis

The psychotic child may have a history of growing social isolation and dysfunction, paranoia, and bizarre statements and behaviors. Often an associated decline in social and school functioning is revealed when the family is questioned about the child's recent behavior. As with adult psychotic patients, there is often neglect in self-care, and the child may have a strong body odor.

Agitation, when it occurs, may be related to acute paranoia associated with active hallucinations that are demeaning or threatening. Psychotic children may be observed talking to themselves and may appear deeply perplexed, with a tense, hypervigilant expression. At times, these children may exhibit catatonic features such as waxy flexibility and assumption of odd postures for prolonged periods of time.

Emergency Interventions

Treatment with an antipsychotic such as haloperidol, 2 to 5 mg, in combination with diphenhydramine, 25 to 50 mg by oral or parenteral route, can be helpful. Sometimes lorazepam, 0.5 to 1 mg, by the oral or parenteral route is added to the above regimen for control of severe anxiety or agitation. The dose may be repeated in 30 to 45 minutes if needed to control the agitation. Anticholinergic medications are recommended to be given in combination with doses of haloperidol greater than 5 mg to prevent the emergence of acute dystonia. The acute dystonic reaction is very frightening for the patient and can cause problems with drug compliance in the future. Oral preparations of atypical antipsychotics such as risperidone or olanzapine in rapid-dissolving form or concentrate are sometimes useful.

The Child with Substance and Alcohol Intoxication

Stimulants such as phencyclidine (PCP) may cause nystagmus, elevation of vital signs, and features of adrenergic arousal and paranoia. Use of antipsychotics and benzodiazepines may be useful, as recommended in the preceding section. Consideration should be given to the use of benzodiazepines such as lorazepam, 1 to 2 mg, by the oral or intramuscular route. Antipsychotic agents should be avoided because they may cause worsening of the muscular rigidity seen in PCP intoxication.

The alcohol blood level should be determined if there is an odor of alcohol on the breath. Levels above 400 mg/dL can be lethal and may require monitoring in an intensive care unit (ICU) with support of respiratory function. Serial assessments of alcohol level may be needed if the intoxication is recent, because the blood alcohol level will be increasing. Benzodiazepines should not be given to alcohol-intoxicated patients, in order to avoid deepening of the sedation and causing respiratory arrest.

The Child with Conduct Disorder

The differential diagnosis of conduct disorder can hinge on a history of fire setting, cruelty to animals, or criminal activity before age 18.

The ED clinician should proceed with caution when interviewing adolescents with conduct disorder because they pose a high risk for assaulting staff and others. It is useful to ask about any recent substance use and ongoing drug use habits. Some children with conduct disorder may appear boastful and reveal this information willingly, whereas others may be more guarded. Mood disorders often confound the picture of conduct disorder, as some children may act out their depression in an antisocial manner.

It is important to remember that conduct problems are not synonymous with conduct disorder, and that not all children with conduct disorder mature into sociopaths. A significant number of children with conduct problems are responding in a dysfunctional manner to depression or stressors in the environment. A punitive stance is not helpful and may retraumatize some children. When evaluating children with the pure conduct disorder, it is useful to set firm limits while offering choices that are mutually acceptable. However, ED clinicians must guard against strong countertransference in themselves and in others caring for such children.

Treatment Guidelines for the Aggressive Child

Verbal de-escalation should be attempted if possible when approaching the aggressive child. If verbal de-escalation is not possible, restraint and medication with a sedating agent may be necessary before the interview can proceed. One may use haloperidol (5 mg) or lorazepam (1 to 2 mg), by mouth or by intramuscular injection. It may be useful to also give diphenhydramine (50 mg) by mouth or intramuscular injection to prevent the emergence of acute dystonia or other extrapyramidal symptoms.

Any weapons should be removed, with the help of the police. Disposition may require referral to a juvenile detention center, where psychiatric follow-up can often be provided if other acute syndromes are ruled out. Nature programs, in which youths learn to rely on each other and work as a team, are sometimes successful.

The Child with Adjustment Disorder with Disturbance of Conduct and Emotions

A careful history of children with adjustment disorder may reveal acute stressors during the previous 3 months. The onset of the disturbance in mood, conduct, and functioning often bears a chronological relationship to the event. Supportive therapy, short-term use of benzodiazepines to help with overwhelming anxiety or insomnia, and close psychiatric follow-up are often successful in an outpatient setting. Hospitalization is warranted, however, if there is a suicide risk and when social supports are lacking.

The Child with Mania

The manic child or adolescent may present to the ED because of changes in behavior that are a marked departure from previous patterns of functioning. Such behaviors may include excessive talking and joking, increased impulsivity, and insomnia. Loud, boisterous behaviors may be noted during the interview, and the history often reveals risk-taking behaviors such as drug use, "joy rides," and promiscuity. There may be a family history of bipolar disorder, major depression, or a psychotic disorder. Substance abuse can confound the clinical picture. Any pediatric patient manifesting manic symptoms should be hospitalized for diagnostic workup and further observation.

The Child with Depressed Mood

Children suffering from depression may present with a sad, constricted, and angry affect. They may have been noted by the family to be tearful and isolated and may show a decline in school grades and lack of participation in enjoyable activities. These children usually are retiring and unmotivated but rational. This is in contrast to the bizarre affect and thought content of the psychotic patient or the labile and grandiose posturing of the manic child. If vegetative symptoms are noted along with a strong family history of depression, the symptoms of depression should be taken with great seriousness.

Untreated depression can result in a lifetime of underachievement, frustration, and quiet desperation, and it has a profound effect on the development of healthy self-esteem and competency. Untreated depression can also lead to suicidal behaviors.

Psychotherapy can be beneficial. Medications that have been effective for treating depression in family members should be given consideration when formulating a treatment plan. Caveats for monitoring for suicidal ideation should be kept in mind.

The Child with Autistic Disorder

Autistic children rarely present as emergencies unless disruptive behaviors unique to their condition cause problems for others in the home or placement facility. These behaviors may include sudden bursts of anger and aggression. In some cases, caregivers are strained and stressed due to the difficult behaviors of these children, which often are marked by stereotypic, obsessive fixations and rituals. One or both parents may possess these obsessive traits, causing some difficulties. Education of the parents, who may be intelligent and insightful, about these issues may be very productive.

Some of the symptoms associated with autism and secondary depression may be responsive to serotoninergic medications. Autistic patients may display aggression due to a specific situation such as pain or an unrecognized medical problem that is causing physical distress. A thorough physical examination and medical workup are recommended to rule these out. Use of atypical and typical antipsychotics has shown some effectiveness in limiting disruptive and aggressive behaviors.

Some success has been reported in treating the ADHD component associated with autism with stimulants such as methylphenidate (Ritalin). Once the symptoms have stabilized, the autistic patients must return to the primary psychiatrist or caregiver with the discharge summary and a record of any observations and responses to medications that were useful. This provides continuity of care and promotes stability for these patients, who are often unable to communicate with their treatment providers because of the nature of autism.

The Child with Attention Deficit Hyperactivity Disorder (ADHD)

The signs and symptoms of ADHD are protean and usually begin before 7 years of age. Clinical features include marked impulsivity and difficulty sitting still or sustaining attention. Other disruptive behaviors include distracting other children while they are trying to work. ADHD may be combined type with impulsivity and inattention, impulsive type, or predominantly inattentive type.

The symptoms of ADHD are often confused with those of bipolar disorder, and it is important to make an accurate diagnosis. The differentiating features include the presence in the bipolar manic child of insomnia, grandiose and elevated mood, and increased pressured speech. These and other differentiating features are enumerated in Table 18-1.

Proper diagnosis and treatment can make a dramatic difference in the home and school setting. Treatment usually includes the use of stimulants such as methylphenidate or dextroamphetamine. The use of atomoxetine (Straterra) and pemoline (Cylert) is complicated by the risk of significant side effects, including severe hepatotoxicity. Tricyclic antidepressants (TCAs) have been noted to have some benefit, along with clonidine, but there have been reports of sudden death with these agents, and their routine use is not recommended. Stimulant medications such as methylphenidate are remarkably safe, and the risks of addiction or stunting of growth are slight. However, this may be a concern for the parents, and provision of education and drug holidays, if feasible, should be considered.

Table 18–1

Differentiating ADHD and Bipolar Disorder

Symptom Pattern	ADHD	Bipolar Disorder
Sleep	Normal	Decreased
Speech	Normal in output	May be increased, pressured
Mood	Tends to be euthymic	Tends to be elevated or mixed
Level of dysfunction	Chronic pattern of dysfunction	Often later onset with waxing and waning of symptoms
Treatment response	Improved by stimulant medications	Exacerbated by stimulant medications
Family history	Family history of ADHD	Family history of bipolar disorder or other major psychiatric disorders

ADHD, attention deficit hyperactivity disorder.

The Abused and Neglected Child

The sexually abused child is discussed in a separate section (see also Chapter 19).

Clinical Presentation

Abused and neglected children often are brought to the ED by social service agencies. The physical examination may indicate bruising in various stages, and imaging studies may reveal spiral fractures, fractures in various stages of healing, or subdural hematomas. Fractures of the ribs in various stages of healing may be noted in a child who has been violently shaken on more than one occasion. The child may have a vacant and forlorn look of helplessness and may withdraw from touch of the examiner. See Figure 18-1 for some clinical features noted in the physically and emotionally abused child.

Injuries in any part of the body should be noted during a careful examination. The mental status may indicate a child who is difficult to engage or is overly friendly and ingratiating with remarkable lack of stranger anxiety. There may be features of depression, anxiety states, and avoidance and startle phenomena related to acute stress disorder or posttraumatic stress disorder (PTSD). Signs of malnutrition and improper medical

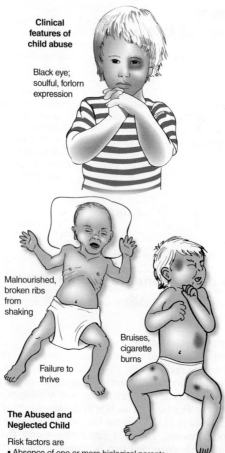

Clinical features of child abuse

Black eye; soulful, forlorn expression

Malnourished, broken ribs from shaking

Failure to thrive

Bruises, cigarette burns

The Abused and Neglected Child

Risk factors are
- Absence of one or more biological parents
- Alcoholism or drug abuse in parent or caretaker
- Personality disorder in parent or caretaker
- Parents who were abused themselves
- Deformity or physical illness in child
- Sibling order, higher risk for first and last born
- Financial and social deprivation of family

FIGURE 18–1

The abused and neglected child.

care such as missed immunizations should also be noted. Although the intent of child protective services is to try to preserve the family unit, some families are truly toxic and placing the child in a different setting (in a foster home or with adoptive parents) may be the best option.

Laboratory Studies

Routine laboratory tests and any specific tests, as indicated for sexually transmitted diseases or pregnancy, should be carried out. Photographs of bruises and injuries related to neglect should be taken to support legal advocacy for protection of the child. Imaging studies can support evidence of repeated trauma such as unique fractures in various stages of healing in the absence of genetic osteoporotic disease. These efforts will serve to protect the child from future harm.

Disposition

Abuse must be reported to the appropriate authorities. Physicians and other licensed professionals such as nurses, social workers, and psychologists are expected to be the eyes and ears of the state to fulfill its obligation to protect all its citizens. The reporting can be anonymous. It is often unsafe and unethical to return an abused child to the abusive environment, and psychiatric hospitalization is often required until appropriate placement in foster care or an alternative living situation can be arranged.

Treatment Issues of the Abused Child

The abused child may be overly inhibited or unusually seductive, social, and friendly with strangers. The ED clinician should monitor for ongoing neglect or further exploitation caused by such behaviors. Malnutrition and acute injuries and their treatment should be reviewed with a medical colleague in the ER or hospital.

Trust is a scarce resource for the abused child and is only replenished by genuine love of a loving foster family and an empathetic clinician willing to build bridges over a period of time. Issues related to chronic anxiety, nightmares, flashbacks, feelings of inadequacy, and depression and somatic complaints may persist for a long time and will need long-term, ongoing attention, support, and treatment. The potential rewards of restoring the health of an abused child are emotionally and spiritually great for the clinician and make a career in the mental health field worthwhile. Some victims of abuse later emerge as survivors and leaders. They can rise from their past and lead lives of great courage, fortitude, and strength. Such individuals abound and become beacons of inspiration for others. Individual traits, strengthened by a person who believed in them, such as a teacher, clinician, or an uncle or aunt, often are cited by the survivors as having made the difference. Depending on timely intervention, abused children can go on to lead exemplary lives or crumble under the weight of depression, drug abuse, and other means of self-destruction. The ED clinician can be a force for the former outcome. See also Chapter 19.

The Sexually Abused Child

Clinical Presentation

Sexually abused children may be acutely anxious and frightened and ashamed of the incident. They may tend to blame themselves for the incident and often are afraid of possible reprisals by the abuser, who may have appeared omnipotent to such children. Sexual abuse and rape can occur in male as well as female children, and the consequences are equally devastating. Nightmares may be reported, as well as insomnia and appetite problems. Self-injurious behaviors and suicidal ideations may be noted. Features of PTSD and clinical depression maybe present.

Physical Examination

A forensic examination by a pediatrician (preferably a female clinician) is recommended, in the presence of a chaperone (preferably someone the child trusts).

There is a special protocol for examining the sexually abused child or victim of rape, and this should be followed in accordance with hospital policies. The main purpose of the forensic examination is to collect uncontaminated specimens that may help with DNA matching of the perpetrator; treat any injuries caused by the assault; and supply prophylactic contraceptive medications if indicated. If the perpetrator's human immuno-deficiency virus (HIV) or hepatitis status is not known, testing for these infections should be done at baseline and after the routine incubation period for the infective agent. Prophylactic treatment for gonorrhea and syphilis can be provided. If the perpetrator is known to be HIV-positive, prophylactic antiviral regimens may offer some protection.

These recommendations are in transition because of the large number of new antiretroviral agents available; consultation with infectious disease or internal medicine specialists may be necessary. A pregnancy test in female patients at baseline and about 2 to 3 weeks later is recommended to rule out pregnancy resulting from the rape and abuse.

Treatment

The use of anxiolytics such as lorazepam may help with acute symptoms of anxiety. Individual psychotherapy to process the trauma will help to limit long-term complications. If the patient is suicidal, hospitalization is warranted. During the acute period of initial crisis, there tends to be significant emotional turmoil. Supportive therapy along with comfort care and provision of a secure setting can be helpful. Later, the victim should be offered support and assistance in the process of giving testimony about the crime, because this often worsens flashbacks and any PTSD symptoms related to the event.

Eating Disorders

Eating disorders seen in children, especially adolescents, include anorexia nervosa and bulimia. Anorexia nervosa is a psychiatric disorder characterized by refusal to maintain normal body weight, usually by voluntary starvation. Bulimia, also called bulimia nervosa, is a psychiatric disorder characterized by binge eating followed by inappropriate methods of weight control, such as vomiting and excessive use of laxatives (purging). Often symptoms of both disorders, combined with depressive symptoms, are seen in patients with eating disorders. Bulimia tends to occur more commonly in adolescent girls.

Anorexia

Clinical Presentation

Anorexic patients usually have a distorted body image and think they are fat. Depressed patients have associated features of loss of interest and tearfulness, in contrast to anorexic patients, who may appear energetic, normal, engaged in physical exercise, and amused by the clinician's concern.

 Anorexic patients have a dangerous lack of insight into the high risk of dying from their condition. Some studies report a 20% long-term mortality risk in this patient population.

Physical Examination

The physical examination usually shows that the patient is severely underweight and, in some cases, literally "skin and bones." These patients may continue to surprisingly feel "fat." There may be absence of menses, lanugo hair, and loosening of teeth and other features of starvation.

Laboratory Studies

These studies often show electrolyte imbalances such as hypokalemia, hyponatremia, and hypochloremia and elevated serum amylase and bicarbonate levels. ECG may show T-wave abnormalities related to the hypokalemic state. Elevated luteinizing hormone and follicle-stimulating hormone levels may be related to the starvation-induced cessation of menses and the shutdown of gonadal function. It is useful to obtain a CBC, chemistry profile, urinalysis, and urine drug screen.

Treatment and Intervention

Anorexia nervosa is one of the most dangerous conditions in childhood and adolescence, with a considerable risk of death and long-term morbidity. Hospitalization is indicated in acute cases when starvation and cardiac complications are noted. Amenorrhea in the anorexic adolescent is usually associated with starvation, but a pregnancy test should also be done. When the patient is hospitalized, close supervision is often required, with a one-to-one sitter present during mealtimes, because anorexic patients are adept at hiding their food or giving it to others.

The goal of treatment is to allow a gradual return to normal body weight. The ED clinician and other caregivers should not be distracted by the psychodynamic nuances of the case, no matter how significant they seem. Treatment in the ED setting should be focused on correcting electrolyte abnormalities and stabilizing physiologic function.

The use of antidepressants such as fluoxetine and other serotonergic agents at the upper end of normal dosage ranges has shown some efficacy in treating eating disorders. Patience on the part of the clinician may be necessary, as eating disorders are often recalcitrant and require a multimodal approach over a lengthy period of time. Consultation with an internal medicine specialist is recommended because too rapid correction of abnormalities such as a low sodium level can have adverse physiologic consequences. Cardiac function needs to be monitored as well because heart failure has occurred in starved individuals when they are suddenly placed on regular high-calorie diets.

Bulimia

Clinical Presentation
Bulimic patients may present to the ED with telltale abrasions on the back of the knuckles of the hand used to induce vomiting, corrosion and chipping of tooth enamel, swollen eyes, with petechial hemorrhages over the conjunctiva, and puffiness of the cheeks. Such patients tend to be mildly obese and may not be malnourished.

Laboratory Studies
These studies may indicate features of electrolyte imbalances and dehydration. Hypomagnesemia and hyperamylasemia may be unique laboratory findings in the bulimic patient.

Treatment and Intervention
Dietary consultation, psychotherapy, and SSRI medication are helpful. The use of bupropion and other agents that lower seizure threshold is contraindicated because of the risk for precipitation of seizures. Referral for long-term therapy with a clinician skilled in dealing with eating disorders is recommended. Bulimic patients tend to have a better prognosis than anorexic patients but may be at risk for the development of borderline personality disorder. Relationships of bulimic patients are often marred by an inability to handle interpersonal stress. Crises related to issues of abandonment and loneliness may recur during adulthood. With increasing age, however, some patients do tend to gain maturity and insight and consequently exert some control over their lives.

Recognition in childhood of these problems when patients first present to the ED may provide a golden opportunity for early intervention and referral to specialists, who can facilitate normal development and prevent heartache down the line by teaching adequate coping strategies early in these patients' lives.

Further Reading

Aharonvich E, Liu X, Samet S, et al: Postdischarge cannabis use and its relationship to cocaine, alcohol, and heroin use: A prospective study. Am J Psychiatry 2005;162:1507-1514.

Asherson P, Kuntsi J, Taylor E: Unravelling the complexity of attention-deficit hyperactivity disorder: A behavioural genomic approach. Br J Psychiatry 2005;187:103-105.

Beardslee WR, Gladstone TR, Wright EJ, Cooper AB: A family-based approach to prevention of depressive symptoms in children at risk: Evidence of parental and child change. Pediatrics 2003;112:e119-131.

Beautrais AL: Risk factors for suicide and attempted suicide among young people Aust N Z J Psychiatry 2000;34:420-436.

Brent DA, Oquendo M, Birmaher B, et al: Familial pathways to early-onset suicide attempt: Risk for suicidal behavior in offspring of mood-disordered suicide attempters. Arch Gen Psychiatry 2002;59:801-807.

Dulcan M, Martini DR: Concise Guide to Child and Adolescent Psychiatry, 2nd ed. Washington, DC, American Psychiatric Press, 1999.

Findling RL, McNamara NK, Youngstrom EA, et al: Double-blind 18-month trial of lithium versus divalproex maintenance treatment in pediatric bipolar disorder. J Am Acad Child Adolesc Psychiatry 2005;44:409-417.

Kessing LV, Sondergard L, Kvist K, Andersen PK: Suicide risk in patients treated with lithium. Arch Gen Psychiatry 2005;62:860-866.

Kowatch RA, DelBello PM: Pharmacotherapy of children and adolescents with bipolar disorder. Psychiatr Clin N Am 2005;28:385-397.

Pelkonen M, Marttunen M: Child and adolescent suicide: Epidemiology, risk factors and approaches to prevention. Paediatr Drugs 2003;5:243-265.

Roche AM, Giner L, Zalsman G: Suicide in early childhood: A brief review. Int J Adolesc Med Health 2005;17(3):221-224.

Suss A, Homel P, Wilson TE, Shah B: Risk factors for nonfatal suicide behaviors among inner-city adolescents. Pediatr Emerg Care 2004;20:426-429.

CHAPTER 19

Victims of Domestic Abuse and Rape

Hani R. Khouzam, MD, MPH, FAPA

KEY POINTS

- The general principles of emergency intervention for children, partners and elderly patients who are victims of abuse require a series of assessment and diagnostic steps.
- When emergency department (ED) clinicians suspect domestic abuse, their interventions should include establishing a diagnosis, documenting findings, addressing safety issues, reporting to appropriate social and law enforcement agencies, and recommending treatment and follow-up care.
- Awareness of the symptoms and signs of abuse and a high index of suspicion are needed when assessing and assisting victims of abuse.
- The victims of rape require special medical evaluation and psychological interventions.
- ED clinicians must be alert to the possibility of abuse within the family and home. They need to assure privacy and separation of the suspected abused and abuser during the initial interview and ongoing evaluations.

Definition

⚠ **Domestic Abuse.** Domestic abuse is a type of physical, emotional, sexual, or other violence that takes place between people who are related (e.g., family members), who are romantically involved (e.g., living together), or who have some other significant relationship (e.g., caregiver of an elderly person).

Overview

Domestic abuse can be manifested by emotional intimidation, nonconsensual sexual behavior, or physical injury exercised by a competent adult or adolescent to maintain coercive behavior in an intimate relationship. It includes physical, sexual, and emotional abuse of children, the elderly, and spouses, and may progress to rape. Although the legal definition of domestic abuse varies by state, it usually includes:

- Attempts at physical harm
- Acts causing fear of harm
- Nonconsensual sex
- Physical abuse
- Sexual abuse
- Social isolation
- Intimidation and threats
- Verbal and emotional abuse
- Economic abuse

Domestic abuse crosses all boundaries of age, race, social class, educational level, and economic background and is an important aspect of public health and safety. Being alert to abuse and its risk factors and providing vigorous intervention are important goals for ED clinicians. Steps that should be followed when reporting abuse are listed in Box 19-1.

This chapter addresses domestic violence in the context of domestic abuse of children, partners, and the elderly. This chapter also reviews emergency psychiatric interventions in relation to the rape victim.

Epidemiology

In the United States, nearly 5.3 million incidents of domestic violence occur each year among women ages 18 and older, and 3.2 million occur among men. Most assaults consist of pushing, grabbing, shoving, slapping, and hitting. According to the Centers for Disease Control and Prevention (CDC), approximately 1.5 million women and 834,700 men in the United States are physically or sexually assaulted by an intimate partner each year.

The World Health Organization (WHO) also found that "one of the most common forms of violence against women is that performed by a husband or male partner." Every year in the United States about 47 assaults occur per 1000 women and 32 assaults per 1000 men. Nearly 2 million injuries and 1300 deaths nationwide occur every year as a result of domestic violence.

One study found that 44% of women murdered by their intimate partner had visited an ED within 2 years of the homicide.

Box 19–1. Steps to Follow When Reporting Abuse

Child Abuse
- Document findings carefully; include photographs
- Contact child protective services
- Hospitalize victim if removal from the home seems indicated

Partner Abuse
- Document findings carefully; include photographs
- Assist in formulation of exit plan
- Provide resource phone numbers (e.g., shelters, spouse abuse centers, crisis hotline)
- Contact adult protective services and other agencies according to state law
- Suggest obtaining emergency protective order from courts, if indicated

Elder Abuse
- Document findings carefully; include photographs
- Contact adult protective services, if indicated
- If injuries are serious, hospitalize patient for protection until situation can be investigated

Adapted from: Steiner RP, Vansickle K, Lippmann SB: Domestic violence: Do you know when and how to intervene? Postgrad Med 1996;100:103-106, 111-114, 116.

Of these women, 93% had at least one injury visit. Women who are separated from abusive partners often remain at risk of violence. During their lifetime, 29% of women and 22% of men will experience physical, sexual, or psychological abuse. Between 4% and 8% of pregnant women are abused at least once during their pregnancy. Approximately 12 million women are raped at least once during their lifetime. Moreover, when women are victimized by male partners they are more likely to be repeatedly attacked, raped, injured, or eventually killed than are women who are assaulted by other perpetrators. In the United States, 75,000 rapes of females are reported each year; estimates of unreported rape range from 2 to 10 times that number. About 90% of rapists attack persons of the same race; 50% are known to their victims and are often members of the extended family.

Research shows that approximately 900,000 parents are beaten or abused by their children each year. The National Elder Abuse Incidence study found that approximately 115,110 elderly persons were abused or neglected in a 1-year period.

Approximately 2 million children in the United States are seriously abused by their parents, guardians, or others each year, and more than 1000 children die as a result of their injuries. In the United States, approximately 20 percent of children will be sexually abused in some way, usually by someone they know, before they become adults. More than 3 million reports are made to U.S. child protective authorities each year. Every year, nearly 1.4 million children (approximately 3% of the population <18 years of age) are victimized in some manner. Of this population, 160,000 suffer from serious or life-threatening injuries. Approximately 1200 children die each year from abusive injuries or neglect. Many of these seriously injured or murdered children had presented previously to the ED for initial care.

The U.S. total annual direct health care cost of domestic violence is estimated to be 3 to 5 billion dollars. The indirect costs of lost productivity associated with injuries and premature death and the cost of judicial proceedings or incarceration of offenders are estimated to be 1.8 billion dollars annually.

Child Abuse

Physical abuse of children is a complex phenomenon resulting from a combination of individual, family, and social factors. In some cases, physical abuse has been triggered by caregivers interacting with children who have physical, mental, temperamental, or behavioral problems. Several factors have been identified as possible causes of the physical abuse of children, including:

- Socioeconomic stressors
- Poverty
- Unemployment
- Excessive mobility
- Social isolation
- Attachment problems
- Punitive child-rearing styles
- Parent stressors
- Low self-esteem

- Abuser history of child abuse
- Depression
- Substance abuse
- Personality disorders
- Unrealistic expectations of the child
- Triggering situations
- Argument/family conflict
- Acute environmental problems

There are three categories of child abuse: neglect, physical abuse, and sexual abuse.

Neglect. Neglect occurs when basic needs of living are not met, including adequate nutrition, proper clothing, suitable and safe living conditions, emotional nurturing, age-appropriate education, and medical and dental care.

Physical Abuse. Risk factors for physical abuse include parental ignorance in relation to the child's developmental abilities combined with parental immaturity; violence in the home; and high levels of family psychosocial stressors. Premature birth or the presence of disabilities has been thought to lead to increased risk for physical trauma; however, recent studies question these findings. Children of teenage mothers have a relatively high risk for all forms of physical abuse.

Sexual Abuse. Sexual abuse or molestation may include contact with genitalia, anus, or mouth or may be in the form of exhibitionism, voyeurism, or pornography. The perpetrator usually is known to the child. Although incest is the most common form of child sexual abuse, it is usually missed or unrecognized by clinicians. Incest usually occurs between the biological father or stepfather and daughter or stepdaughter, but it can occur between father and son as well as mother and son. There is now an evolving definition of incest that takes into consideration the betrayal of trust and the power imbalance in these one-sided relationships. One such definition is "the imposition of sexually inappropriate acts, or acts with sexual overtones by one or more persons who derive authority through ongoing emotional bonding with that child." This definition expands the traditional definition of incest to include sexual abuse by anyone who has authority or power over the child. This definition of incest includes as perpetrators immediate/extended family members, babysitters, teachers, scout masters, and so forth.

Often more than one type of abuse occurs at the same time. Neglect is most commonly reported, followed by physical abuse, and then by sexual abuse. When a detailed history is not obtained due to the hectic nature of the ED, as many as one third of child abuse cases may go undetected or unreported. The categories and clinical indicators of child abuse are summarized in Box 19-2.

ED Assessment

ED clinicians may be the first line of direct contact with victims and family members at a time when early and successful intervention is possible. Therefore, it is the clinician's responsibility, when possible, to identify victims and families at risk

---

Box 19–2. Categories and Clinical Indicators of Child Abuse

Neglect
- History of untreated medical conditions, inadequate immunization
- Absence of necessary health aids (glasses, hearing aids)
- Malnutrition
- Developmental delays
- Poor hygiene, rampant dental caries

Physical Abuse
- Infants with head injuries or central nervous system (CNS) symptoms indicating shaking may present with nonspecific symptoms of lethargy, irritability, persistent unexplained vomiting, difficulty breathing, and convulsions
- Symptoms of abdominal trauma secondary to perforation, obstruction, or bleeding may include vomiting, pain, tenderness, and even shock and sepsis
- Injuries in various stages of healing in multiple sites such as the trunk, upper arms, upper legs, neck and face, and perineal area with an obvious pattern, such as from a hand; these locations of injuries are typically well protected in accidental injuries such as falls
- Bruises or welts resembling shape of article used to inflict injury
- Burns with cigarette, immersion or patterned
- Lacerations due to rope or burns associated with facial injuries
- Fractures of bones, ribs, and skull

Box 19–2. Categories and Clinical Indicators of Child Abuse—cont'd

Chemical Abuse
- Symptoms of suffocation
- Factitious disorder (Munchausen syndrome) by proxy (i.e., caregiver purposefully induces illness in a child)

Sexual Abuse
- Abrasions or bruises of labia, penis, anus, or inner thighs
- Distortion of hymen
- Abnormal anorectal tone
- Sexually transmissible disease; pregnancy
- Chronic abdominal or anal pain
- Recurrent urinary tract infections

Behavioral Findings for Any Type of Abuse
- Depression or suicidal tendencies
- Anxiety, enuresis, sleep disturbances, excessive masturbation
- Poor interpersonal relations
- Aggressive behavior
- Poor school performance
- Role reversal (e.g., child assumes the role of caregiver)

Compiled from the American Medical Association: Diagnostic and Treatment Guidelines on Child Physical Abuse and Neglect. Chicago, American Medical Association, 1992; and the American Medical Association: Diagnostic and Treatment Guidelines on Child Sexual Abuse. Chicago, American Medical Association, 1992.

of domestic violence. The prompt recognition of victims of abuse combined with the clinician's familiarity with reporting procedures presents an opportunity for appropriate referrals to community resources and close follow-up to ensure comprehensive management.

Following are some important concepts to keep in mind when conducting the initial assessment of a child suspected of being abused (see also Chapter 18).

Interview the child and the suspected abuser and/or caregiver separately.

Approach the child with respect and in a nonthreatening manner. Keep questions open-ended and nonjudgmental, using language that is simple and easily understood. Communicate with the child at a developmentally appropriate level, using the child's own words and terms.

Inquire not only about physical abuse but also about sexual abuse, domestic violence, and witnessed abuse.

When interviewing the suspected abuser and/or the caregiver, inquire not only about physical abuse but also about sexual abuse, domestic violence, and witnessed abuse. Ask about the observed injury and other signs such as bruises, poor nutrition, and soiled clothing. The physically abused child typically presents with an obvious injury. It is not uncommon, however, for the abused child to present with symptoms of occult injuries. Be aware of the fact that life-threatening abdominal trauma and head trauma may present without visible external signs or history to suggest such an injury.

Listen carefully to the caregiver's explanation of the injury and note any discrepancies with the child's version.

Signs of abuse include the following:
- Unexplained or poorly explained injuries
- Injury blamed on a sibling
- Explanations change over time
- Wounds or injuries incompatible with the stated history
- Significant delay in seeking treatment

Physical Examination

The abused child may present in extremis from circulatory or central nervous system (CNS) compromise without any history of trauma.

A high index of suspicion for occult head, chest, and abdominal trauma and a physiologic approach to resuscitation are important. Examine knees, shins, forearms, forehead and chin, and bony prominences such as elbows, hips, and spine for bruises.

Shock in these children is usually due to occult blood loss but may be due to dehydration, toxins, CNS dysfunction, external loss from lacerations or burns, or infection, such as a ruptured small bowel with resulting peritonitis.

The Shaken Baby Syndrome

The shaken baby syndrome, or shaken impact syndrome, is a well-recognized type of child abuse in which injury and even death is caused by violent shaking of a young infant, often followed by an impact to the head from being thrown onto a fixed surface. These actions result in a constellation of physical examination findings including the following:

- Retinal hemorrhages
- Intracranial trauma, particularly subdural hemorrhage
- Diffuse axonal injury
- Secondary cerebral edema
- Fractures of the posterior and anterolateral ribs or metaphyses of long bones (e.g., tibia, humerus)

ED Treatment

The treatment of the physically abused child should be the same as the treatment of the accidentally injured child, except that forensic data collection and analysis are of particular and pressing importance. The initial assessment and treatment should proceed according to established guidelines, such as those contained in the *Advanced Trauma Life Support Course for Physicians* or in the *Textbook of Advanced Pediatric Life Support*. Priorities include recognition of airway, breathing, and circulatory problems, instituting airway and ventilator management, and establishing vascular access for fluid resuscitation and medication administration.

Once these children are medically treated and their condition is stabilized, ED clinicians are mandated in all states to notify local child protective services. Clinical data about suspected abuse must be precise and detailed. Photographs of injuries may be included for supportive evidence. The importance of prompt and accurate reporting cannot be overstated. Clinician-patient confidentiality in such cases is exempted, and legal protection regarding good-faith reporting errors is in effect. Consultation with appropriate investigative authorities and careful forensic assessment must be carried out. Prematurely released information about the mechanism of a possible criminal act could impede later law enforcement interrogation as well as cause unnecessary family distress in cases where the etiology is not abuse.

Immediate removal from the home of the caregiver, with intervention by police, lawyers, and social services, may be necessary.

Abused children may need hospitalization if safety cannot otherwise be guaranteed; also hospitalization may offer time to rule out difficult diagnostic conditions and to initiate therapeutic interventions.

Most seriously injured children are best monitored in an intensive care setting. Depending on the complexity of services needed, the ED clinician should consider transferring the child to a specialized pediatric center.

Psychiatric Assessment

Child abuse and neglect frequently occur in concert with other forms of family violence, including spousal abuse and violence between siblings; abused children are at high risk for exposure to violence against their mothers. Such history of violence should be actively sought and aggressively treated in collaboration with community-based domestic violence programs.

Symptoms of psychiatric problems experienced by children who have been physically abused may include:
- Poor self-image
- Sexual acting out
- Seductiveness
- Unusual interest in or avoidance of all things of a sexual nature
- Inability to trust or love others
- Aggressive, disruptive, and sometimes illegal behavior
- Anger and rage
- Self-destructive or self-abusive behavior; suicidal thoughts
- Passive, withdrawn, or clingy behavior
- Fear of entering into new relationships or activities
- Anxiety
- School problems or failure
- Feelings of sadness or other symptoms of depression; withdrawal from friends or family
- Delinquency/conduct problems
- Drug and alcohol abuse
- Sleep problems or nightmares; flashbacks

Posttraumatic Stress Disorder (PTSD)

Normally the reactions of children and adolescents to stress are brief, and they recover without further problems. However, a child or adolescent who experiences a catastrophic event or is repeatedly physically and/or sexually abused may develop ongoing difficulties, leading to the development of PTSD (also see Chapters 20 and 21). The stressful or traumatic event may be a situation in which someone's life has been threatened or a severe injury has occurred, or a child may be the victim or a witness of physical or sexual abuse. A child's risk of developing PTSD is related to the seriousness of the trauma, whether the trauma is repeated, the child's proximity to the trauma, and his/her relationship to the victim(s). Following the traumatic event, children may initially show agitated or confused behavior, including intense fear, helplessness, anger, sadness, horror. or denial. Children who experience repeated trauma may develop a kind of emotional numbing to deaden or block the pain and trauma, leading to dissociation. Children with PTSD avoid situations or places that remind them of the traumatic event. They may also become depressed, withdrawn, and detached from their feelings.

Children with new onset of PTSD may show the following symptoms:

- Worry about dying at an early age
- Loss of interest in activities
- Physical symptoms such as headaches and stomachaches
- Sudden and extreme emotional reactions
- Problems falling or staying asleep
- Problems concentrating
- Age-inappropriate behavior, such as clingy behavior, whining, thumb-sucking

Children with preexisting PTSD who re-experience previous traumatic events may:

- Have frequent memories of the event or (in young children) playing in which some or all of the trauma is repeated over and over again
- Have upsetting and frightening dreams
- Act or feel like the experience is happening again
- Develop repeated physical or emotional symptoms when reminded of the traumatic event

Psychiatric Intervention

The ED clinician should conduct a comprehensive evaluation and initiate or refer for treatment abused children to minimize the long-term consequences of abuse.

Sexually abused children and their families need immediate professional evaluation and treatment. Psychiatrists can help abused children regain a sense of self-esteem, cope with feelings of guilt about the abuse, and begin the process of overcoming the trauma. Such treatment can help reduce the risk that the child will develop serious problems as an adult. Through treatment, the abused child begins to regain a sense of self-confidence and trust.

The family can also be helped to learn new ways of support and communicating with one another. Parents may benefit from support, parent training, and anger management.

The best approach is prevention of the trauma. Once the trauma has occurred, however, early intervention is essential. Support from parents, school, and peers is important. Emphasis needs to be placed upon establishing a feeling of safety. Psychotherapy (individual, group, or family) which allows the child to speak, draw, play, or write about the traumatic event is helpful. Behavior modification techniques and cognitive therapy may help. Medication may also be useful to deal with agitation, anxiety, or depression.

Further Outpatient Care

Parents should be educated about appropriate discipline techniques; the use of physical discipline should be discouraged, particularly in high-risk families. Parents should be made aware of the profound and long-lasting adverse effects of domestic violence on children's development.

In addition to medical follow-up needs (e.g., orthopedic, surgical, neurologic), these children often need ongoing protective and psychiatric follow-up care.

Partner Abuse

 The medical literature defines partner abuse in different ways. In this section, partner abuse refers to the victimization of a person with whom the abuser has or has had an intimate, romantic, or spousal relationship. Partner abuse encompasses violence against both men and women and includes violence in gay and lesbian relationships.

Partner abuse, which can occur alone or in combination, sporadically, or continually, includes physical violence, psychological abuse, and nonconsensual sexual behavior. Each incident builds upon previous episodes, thus setting the stage for future violence.

Forms of physical violence include assault with weapons, pushing, shoving, slapping, punching, choking, kicking, holding, and binding. Two forms of physical violence have been posited: (1) occasional outbursts of bidirectional violence, as in mutual combat, and (2) frank terrorism, the "patriarchal" form of which has been the most researched.

Psychological abuse includes threats of physical harm, intimidation, coercion, degradation and humiliation, false accusations, and ridicule. Stalking may occur during a relationship or after a relationship has ended. Of women who are stalked by an intimate partner, 81% are also physically assaulted. A new development is *cyberstalking*, psychological abuse in the form of threats made through the Internet. Stalking of a man by a woman may also occur and needs to be seriously assessed.

Rape is an extreme form of sexual abuse in which nonconsensual sexual acts are inflicted on the victim, who is often unprotected against pregnancy or disease.

Partner abuse may be associated with physical or social isolation, such as preventing communication with friends or relatives, abandonment in dangerous places, refusing to help a sick or injured partner, and prohibiting access to money or other basic necessities. Women are six times more likely than men to experience violence committed by an intimate partner. Risk factors for women include low socioeconomic status, age 17 to 28 years, pregnancy, chemical dependency of either partner, and being single, separated, or divorced. White women are more likely to be assaulted by spouses or ex-spouses, whereas black women are more likely to be victims of lovers.

Partner abuse is not a new entity; it spans history and cultures. The common law of England permitted a man to beat his wife, provided the diameter of the stick used was not wider than the diameter of his thumb—hence the term "rule of thumb."

Phases of Abuse

Most partner abuse is characterized by a battering cycle with three phases: phase I, tension building; phase II, acute abuse; and phase III, the "honeymoon phase." The cycle can happen hundreds of times in an abusive relationship. The duration of each phase varies between and within each cycle; the total cycle may be completed in a few hours or in as long as a year.

Phase I—Tension Building
In phase I, tension begins to rise and builds to the point of violence. The abuser becomes edgy and more prone to react negatively to frustrations and ceases to respond to any controls. The abuser may use alcohol as an excuse for abuse. The victim

accepts the coming violence as inevitable or may seek help to prevent the violence.

Children affected by this stage may modify their behavior to avoid anger; manipulate either parent to their own benefit; assume the parental role; use drugs or alcohol for relief; or run away as a method of escape

Phase II—Acute Abuse

This is the shortest phase. Abusers regain "control" of themselves only after the victim has "learned a lesson." The victim responds to the pain and terror by becoming emotionally detached; fighting back usually increases the violence. The police are frequently called in during this phase.

Children affected by this stage may get hurt trying to intervene; hide and be frantic; and display acting-out behavior and/or become "clingy" or withdrawn.

Phase III—the Honeymoon Phase

In this phase the abuser behaves in a contrite, loving manner while denying the extent of pain and fear the victim experienced. The victim is blamed for the abuser's past anger.

Children affected by this stage may cease to believe in or trust both the victim and the abuser.

Without intervention, this cycle of abuse usually becomes more frequent and more violent. The loving and contrite honeymoon phase gets shorter and eventually drops out entirely, and the couple moves once again into the tension-building phase.

ED Assessment

 The following guidelines are useful for the ED clinician when evaluating an abuse victim. Please also refer to Chapter 20, Figure 20-1.

The abuser often accompanies the victim and may insist on answering questions for the victim. Thus it is important to take the history in private.

Inform the victim of any limits to confidentiality imposed by mandatory reporting requirements for domestic violence and abuse. If translation is needed, friends and family members are excluded from acting as translators.

Ask direct questions, such as "Were you punched (kicked, knocked down, etc.)?" Do not ask general questions, such as

"Were you a victim of domestic violence?" This is critical because the abused victim may not interpret what occurs as domestic violence.

Phrase questions addressed to the family in an open-ended manner, because the abuser may be among those queried.

Use nonjudgmental language when questioning an abuser who has been injured.

Abusers often blame the victim for their behaviors; in such instances, your message should be loud and clear—"hitting does not solve problems, it often destroys families."

Complaints related to illness or stress are more common than complaints related to injuries. Abused women are more likely to present with vague medical complaints, sexual problems, depression, or anxiety.

Presentations common in the ED include:

- Acute pain with no visible injuries, chronic pain, and pain due to diffuse trauma without visible evidence
- History of multiple traumatic and nontraumatic visits to the ED
- A substantial delay between time of injury and presentation for treatment
  - May stem from ambivalence about acknowledging the real cause of the injury
  - May result because victim was unable to leave the house or did not have independent means of transportation
- Noncompliance with treatment regimens, missed appointments, and failure to obtain or take medications
  - May be due to a lack of access to money or telephones, indicating abuser's attempts to exercise control over victim
- Victim and/or partner may deny injury or minimize the incident(s)

Psychiatric Assessment

Patients with psychiatric complaints, especially suicide attempts, ideation, or gestures, always should be questioned about current or past domestic violence.

Partner abuse may be a factor in up to 25% of suicide attempts in women. Of pregnant women who are abused, 20% attempt suicide. When inquiring about the reason for the suicide attempt, it is important to clarify the events that lead to the attempt.

Patients presenting with sleep or eating disturbances should be questioned about current or past abuse and depression.

Symptoms related to stress are common, including anxiety, panic attacks, other anxiety symptoms, and PTSD. Fatigue and chronic headaches also may be noted. There is frequent use of anxiolytic or pain medications.

Abuse of alcohol and other drugs is a correlate of partner abuse. Because substance abuse may develop or worsen as a result of domestic violence, it is appropriate to consider domestic violence when evaluating a patient for alcohol intoxication, drug toxicity, or drug overdose.

A family history of alcohol and drug abuse or similar history in the patient's partner is common.

Screening for Partner Abuse
The Women-Validated Partner Violence Screen (PVS)

The PVS poses the following questions:
1. Have you been hit, kicked, punched, or otherwise hurt by someone in the past year?
2. Do you feel safe in your current relationship?
3. Is there a partner from a previous relationship who is making you feel unsafe now?

A positive screen for intimate partner violence is answering "Yes" to any of these three questions.

The Mnemonic SAFE

The mnemonic **SAFE** directs inquiry into partner abuse.

S = Stress/safety: What stress do you experience in your relationship? Do you feel safe in your relationships (marriage)? Should I be concerned for your safety?

A = Afraid/abused: What happens when you and your partner disagree? Do any situations exist in your relationship in which you have felt afraid? Has your partner ever threatened or abused you or your children? Have you been physically hurt by your partner? Has your partner forced you to have unwanted sexual relations?

F = Friends/family (assessing degree of social support): If you have been hurt, are your friends or family aware of it? Do you think you could tell them if it did happen? Would they be able to give you support?

E = Emergency plan: Do you have a safe place to go and the resources you (and your children) need in an emergency? If you are in danger now, would you like help in locating a shelter? Do you have a plan for escape? Would you like to talk with a social worker, counselor, or physician to develop an emergency plan?

ED Interventions

Facilitating Independence
The ED clinician's role in cases of partner abuse must be that of facilitator rather than rescuer. It is important to assist the victim in regaining a sense of both control and self-direction. Clinicians can be easily frustrated when victims do not take immediate action to remove themselves or their children from a dangerous situation. Dependence on the abuser for shelter, financial support, and other necessities is often a reality for the victim and may take time to overcome.

Formulating an Exit Plan
Once the victim confirms abuse, the ED clinician can suggest resources for obtaining help and encourage formulation of an exit plan. This plan may include packing a suitcase with such necessities as clothing, extra keys, and medicines and leaving it with a neighbor or friend. Financial and identification records, such as checkbook, automobile title, and birth certificates, can be included. This strategy is of particular importance for victims whose abusers have threatened to commit suicide, because suicidal intent of the abusers may unpredictably quickly change to homicidal intent.

Patient Education
Providing basic knowledge about domestic violence may help promote the willingness of the victim to seek help. In addition, the ED clinician may provide education related to these facts:
- Domestic violence occurs often in our society.
  - It continues over time and increases in frequency and severity.
  - It may well have damaging long-term effects on children who are hurt or who witness violence.
- Domestic violence is a crime.
- Resources are available to help.

Counseling and Support Groups
Use of these resources should be encouraged, because they foster a sense of self-esteem and decisiveness to resolve the situation. Contact with spouse abuse centers is strongly recommended,

as is consultation with legal or law enforcement authorities when indicated.

Spouse abuse shelters offer safe accommodations, peer group support, and advice on a range of legal, financial, and personal issues. In overtly dangerous cases, the victim is advised to obtain a court-ordered, emergency "no contact warrant" to prevent further association with the abuser. It may be advisable in these circumstances for the victim to move out of the home, perhaps to live with a friend or relative.

Abuse victims should receive a list of emergency numbers, including the name and telephone number of the local crisis intervention center. General referral cards that have several emergency telephone numbers not limited to agencies dealing with abuse may be kept safely by the patient.

Offer a written list of resources each visit. Post informational brochures, for example, in the women's bathroom, out of sight of an abusive (male) partner. These brochures may provide information about women's shelters and group homes for victims of domestic abuse.

The toll-free number of the National Coalition Against Domestic Violence is 1-800-799-7233. The toll-free number of the National Domestic Violence Hotline is 1-800-799-7233.

Refer victims of cyberstalking to the local police or sheriff's department, the district or state attorney, and/or the FBI. WHOA (Working to Halt Online Abuse) and Cyber Angels also offer help for victims of cyberstalking.

Specific Psychiatric Treatment

Avoid giving sedating medications that impair victims' ability to flee or to defend themselves. Be cautious when prescribing medications for symptomatic relief of anxiety, panic, or chronic pain syndromes because they may be somatic manifestations of abuse.

If suicidal or homicidal ideations or intentions are emerging, psychiatric hospitalization should be considered. Also, consider hospital admission if a safe place has not been found.

Initiate treatment for abuse of alcohol and other drugs, which is often a consequence of being abused.

Follow-up visits and a therapeutic relationship with the ED clinician enhance the likelihood that the abused person will seek greater safety. Consult local laws to determine which circumstances require reporting to adult protective services. If the victim is disabled, the ED clinician must always alert the local adult protective service agency. Many communities offer counseling services to the perpetrators of violence within the legal system or in certain mental health clinics.

Interventions for Rape Victims

Providing medical and psychological care for the rape victim is the first concern. Whenever possible, the victim should be treated in a rape treatment center that is separate from the ED and staffed by trained, concerned support personnel.

Medical Assessment

Because rape is a crime, there are certain requirements for medical evaluation and record keeping, including detailed history and physical examination with the gathering of forensic evidence. The examination report may include a brief account of the attack in the victim's own words and a statement of the physician's clinical determination of injuries and sexual activity. Stating whether rape occurred is not necessary because that is a legal determination, but the diagnosis should be recorded, including all probable or possible physical and psychological complications.

Although most injuries are minor and can be treated conservatively, severe injuries can occur and may require surgical repair. Laceration of the upper vagina may require laparoscopy to determine the depth of the injury, especially in children.

Some rape victims are males. Rape of males is not limited to those in prison. The male victim is more likely than the female to have physical trauma, to have been victimized by several assailants, and to be unwilling to report the crime. A few cases of female rapes of males have also been reported.

Because the risk of becoming infected with a sexually transmitted disease such as gonorrhea, chlamydia, syphilis, human immunodeficiency virus (HIV), and hepatitis is always a concern, preventive measures are required. If the rapist's hepatitis B status is unknown, an initial dose of hepatitis B vaccine should be given, along with instructions for follow-up treatment.

The risk of pregnancy as a result of rape is estimated to range from 2% to 5%; female patients of childbearing age should be offered medications for prophylaxis after current pregnancy status has been determined. Patients should be informed that this treatment is 75% effective and that a repeat pregnancy test should be performed if menstruation does not occur within 21 days.

Prophylactic emergency treatment for HIV should be administered. Because the protocols for such treatments continue to be refined as more is learned about this virus, it is essential that treatment is initiated after consultation with an infectious disease expert.

General medical information, including information about physical illnesses, past or present psychiatric disorders, allergies, current pregnancy status, and date of last menstrual period, if applicable, should be documented. A family history of psychiatric disorders is important, because such a history may be predictive of future mental health complications related to the rape.

Psychiatric Assessment

Once the medical and forensic evaluations are completed, a psychiatric assessment should be made.

Rape presents psychological and social problems for the victims, who must handle their own feelings as well as face the often negative reactions of friends, family, and officials. For both male and female perpetrators, rape is an expression of aggression, anger, or the need for power; it is a violent as much as a sexual act and hence can lead to long-term as well as immediate psychological reactions.

Common immediate reactions include fear and anger; the victim's responses may range from talkativeness, tenseness, crying, and trembling to shock and disbelief, with dispassion and acquiescence. The latter responses rarely indicate lack of concern; rather, they may be avoidance reactions or may reflect physical exhaustion or coping styles that require control of emotion. Usually, patients are severely frightened and embarrassed and feel degraded. The anger felt by many victims may be displaced onto ED staff members, who should be aware of this process and not be troubled by it.

Long-range effects of rape include re-experiencing the assault, aversion to sex, anxiety, phobias, suspiciousness, depression, nightmares and other sleep disorders, somatic symptoms, and social withdrawal. Some women may become promiscuous and act out of character. This may lead to a cycle of further victimization, abuse, and demoralization. Guilt and shame occur when patients feel that somehow they provoked or should have prevented the attack or that the attack was a punishment for some wrongdoing.

Overall, the psychosocial aspects are the most potentially damaging and require sophisticated management. It is important to treat victims with respect, ensure that they are not left alone and assure them that they are safe; demonstrate understanding and empathy by your tone and demeanor and take the time to explain in detail how the evaluation will proceed.

The ED clinician's unhurried, nonjudgmental, willing-to-listen attitude can be therapeutic. Because victims have been traumatized and may be embarrassed by disclosing details, they often omit important data. Therefore, specific details of the assailant's aggression, threats, and violent behavior and of the sex acts committed must be elicited by careful questioning. Empathy can be shown by acknowledging that the questions may be embarrassing or may exacerbate the patient's fears. Properly done, such a potentially distressing interview may begin the therapeutic process.

During the initial interview, explain possible psychological and social consequences of the rape. An appointment with a person trained in rape crisis intervention should be arranged.

Because the full psychological effect of rape cannot be ascertained during an initial interview, follow-up visits must be scheduled. If the patient's acute stress reactions do not subside or if long-range psychological problems seem likely, psychiatric reevaluation may identify the emergence of PTSD (also see Chapter 20).

Family members or friends should be contacted, with the patient's consent, to provide additional support. If consent is obtained, the ED clinician must assess the ability of the family member or friend to intervene and to provide support.

If the patient is unwilling to have family or friends contacted, the ED clinician should explore the reason for this, because the cause may be a sense of shame induced by the rape or the fact that a family member or friend was the perpetrator.

Psychiatric Interventions
Emergency intervention involves restoring the patient to psychological safety, providing information, correcting false attributions, and restoring and supporting effective coping. These psychiatric interventions are summarized in Table 19-1.

Ensuring Social Support
A discussion of the impact of rape on intimacy and the potential for sexual touching to trigger fears and anxiety helps

Table 19–1

Psychiatric Interventions for the Rape Victim

Intervention Goals	Objectives
Restoring psychological safety	Helping patients identify and recognize the safety of the medical environment; if patients are sensitive to power and control issues, a calm, respectful approach will help them to develop a sense of safety.
Providing information	Informing victims about their current medical status; addressing worries about future health problems, including pregnancy, sexually transmitted diseases, and HIV infection; educating victims about the legal system, the role of the police, and the need for evidence collection, in cases when the victim decides to pursue legal charges
Correcting false attributions	Victims of rape commonly and erroneously blame themselves for what happened and often develop fears of a catastrophic nature, such as a belief that being out in the dark or out alone will result in further attacks; helping the victim to define the rape experience more realistically
Restoring and supporting effective coping	Providing psychoeducation about normal responses and common symptoms after rape, such as irritability, sleep problems, intrusive thoughts, nightmares, avoidance, and numbing; helping to restore psychological competence; helping victims to recognize the catastrophic nature of their post-rape beliefs; initiating interventions to decrease anxiety, guilt, and anger; allaying fears on the part of family, friends, and the victims themselves that they are "going crazy" or have "lost control"

Compiled from Osterman JE, Barbiaz J, Johnson P: Emergency psychiatry: Emergency interventions for rape victims. Psychiatr Serv 2001;52:733-740.

patients and their sexual partners understand that these post-rape responses are common and do not reflect on the partner. Such a discussion may prevent the partner from responding negatively to what is perceived as rejection, thus avoiding the development or the escalation of PTSD symptoms. Family and friends must be taught how to listen supportively to the patient; they can do this only if they control their feelings when they are with the patient.

The SANE Program

Many emergency services use the Sexual Assault Nurse Examiner (SANE) program, which involves collaboration with nurses, physicians, hospital administrators, district attorneys, local police, and rape crisis advocates. Although the central focus of the SANE program is on proper evidence collection, its broader goal is to facilitate the return of the victims to their pre-trauma functioning status and to involve the victims in medical decisions. SANE serves as an advocate for the rape victim and provides evidence if the victim wishes to pursue criminal charges. Components of the SANE program are collection of forensic evidence, expert testimony, treatment for sexually transmitted diseases, pregnancy prevention, and psychological counseling. This program encourages rape victims to be active in determining their medical and mental health care.

Medical Treatment

Medication undoubtedly has a place in the aftermath of rape, perhaps more so than in other sexual abuse. In the presence of preexisting psychiatric conditions, medications already prescribed for these conditions may need to be adjusted or modified. In addition adequate follow-up care should be instituted.

Some victims may experience acute anxiety or panic. For these patients, a small amount of a benzodiazepine such as lorazepam (1 mg bid) or diazepam (5 mg bid) may be beneficial in the first few days following the rape incident. However, benzodiazepines should not be prescribed for long-term treatment and are contraindicated in patients with alcohol or substance abuse disorders.

Long-term Care

A support network of health care workers, friends, and family in combination with long-term care is vital. Long-term care may require referral to rape crisis intervention centers. Ongoing community and family support will help to promote recovery. Emergency funds may be needed.

Elder Abuse

Elder abuse is a growing problem that occurs daily in every community. Abuse can involve physical harm, financial exploitation, emotional or verbal abuse, neglect (including self-neglect) or abandonment. All forms of abuse are devastating and often occur in isolation, making it difficult to identify the need for help.

People are living longer because of ongoing medical advances and healthier life styles. As a result, the number of elder abuse cases will increase, and the impact of elder abuse as a public health issue will grow. Aging adults involved in abusive relationships often visit the ED for treatment.

The terminology used to describe elder abuse is not consistent. Terms vary among researchers, and usage is not consistent in the laws of different states. Even the age at which a person is considered elderly, usually 60 or 65 years, is debatable. Seven categories of elder abuse have been described by the National Center on Elder Abuse (NCEA), (formerly the National Aging Resource Center on Elder Abuse). Categories of elder abuse are summarized in Box 19-3.

ED Assessment

Detecting misconduct toward the elderly presents a great challenge. The diagnosis is complicated when the patient is debilitated, has impaired cognitive function, shows self-neglect, or denies abuse because of fear of retribution or of being removed from the home. There is no one simple explanation for elder abuse and neglect. Elder abuse is a complex problem that can emerge from several different causes, and that often has roots in multiple risk factors, including physical and mental impairment, caregiver issues, and cultural issues.

Physical and mental impairment appear to play an indirect role in elder abuse, decreasing seniors' ability to defend themselves or to escape, thus increasing vulnerability.

Caregiver issues include personal problems of the caregiver that can lead to abusing a frail older person, such as stress, mental or emotional illness, dependence on alcohol or other drugs, job loss or other personal crises, and financial dependence on the older person.

Box 19–3. Categories and Characteristics of Elder Abuse

Physical Abuse

Physical abuse includes slapping, hitting, bruising, beating, or any other intentional act that causes someone physical pain, injury or suffering. Physical abuse also includes excessive forms of restraint used to confine someone against their will such as tying, chaining or locking someone in a room, or excessive use of sedating medications.

Psychological/Emotional Abuse

Psychological/emotional abuse includes the infliction of anguish, pain, or distress through verbal and nonverbal acts. Psychological/emotional abuse includes but is not limited to verbal assaults, insults, threats, intimidation, humiliation, and harassment. Some legal definitions require identification of at least 10 episodes of this type of behavior within a single year to constitute psychological/emotional abuse.

Other examples of psychological/emotional abuse are treating elderly persons like infants; isolating them from their family, friends, or regular activities; giving them the "silent treatment"; and subjecting them to enforced social isolation.

Financial Abuse or Exploitation

Financial abuse is the misuse of an elderly person's money or assets for personal gain. Acts such as stealing money, social security checks, and possessions, and coercion such as changing a will or assuming power of attorney all constitute financial abuse.

Neglect

Neglect is the failure of a caregiver to provide an elderly person's basic needs. As in the previous examples of abuse, neglect can be physical, emotional, or financial. Physical neglect is failure to provide eyeglasses or dentures, preventive health care, safety precautions, or basic hygiene. Emotional neglect includes failure to provide social stimulation. Financial neglect involves failure to use the resources available to restore or maintain the elderly person's well-being.

Continued

> ### Box 19–3. Categories and Characteristics of Elder Abuse—cont'd
>
> **Abandonment**
> Abandonment is the desertion of an elderly person by an individual who has assumed responsibility for providing care for that person.
>
> **Sexual Abuse**
> Nonconsensual sexual contact, including sexual contact with any person incapable of giving consent, constitutes sexual abuse. It includes, but is not limited to, unwanted touching and all types of sexual assault or battery, such as rape, sodomy, coerced nudity, and sexually explicit pornography.
>
> **Self-Neglect**
> Self-neglect constitutes behaviors in which persons compromise their own health and safety, as when an aging adult refuses needed help with various daily activities. When persons are deemed competent, many ethical questions arise regarding their right of autonomy and the physician's oath of beneficence.
>
> **Miscellaneous**
> This category includes all other types of abuse, including medical abuse and violation of personal rights by failing to respect the elderly person's dignity and autonomy.

Compiled from Director TD, Linden JA: Domestic violence: An approach to identification and intervention. Emerg Med Clin North Am 2004;22:1117-1132; and Steiner RP, Vansickle K, Lippmann SB: Domestic violence: Do you know when and how to intervene? Postgrad Med 1996;100:103-106, 111-114, 116.

Caregiver stress is a significant risk factor for abuse and neglect. When caregivers are thrust into the demands of daily care for an elder without appropriate training and without information about how to balance the needs of the older person with their own needs, they frequently experience intense frustration and anger that can lead to a range of abusive behaviors.

The risk of elder abuse increases when the caregiver is responsible for an older person who is sick or is physically or mentally impaired. Caregivers in such stressful situations often feel trapped and hopeless and are unaware of available resources and assistance. If they have no skills for managing difficult behaviors, caregivers can find themselves using physical force.

Particularly when there is a lack of resources, neglectful situations can arise.

Sometimes the caregiver's own self-image as a "dutiful child" may compound the problem by considering respite or residential care as a betrayal of the older person's trust.

Dependency is a contributing factor in elder abuse. When the caregiver is dependent financially on an impaired older person, there may be financial exploitation or abuse. When the reverse is true and the impaired older person is completely dependent on the caregiver, the caregiver may experience resentment that leads to abusive behavior.

Family violence is a learned behavior that is passed down from generation to generation. Thus, the child who was once abused by the parent continues the cycle of violence when both are older.

Psychiatric conditions play an important role in elder abuse. If the caregivers have drug or alcohol dependence they are more likely to abuse the elderly; conversely, the caregiver-related stress can lead to alcohol or drug dependence. Caregivers with personality disorders may be unable to control their impulses when feeling angry or resentful of the older person. Mental retardation, dementia, and other conditions in the elderly can increase the likelihood of elder abuse. In fact, family members with such conditions are most likely to be primary caretakers for elderly relatives because they are the individuals typically at home due to lack of employment.

Social isolation can be a strategy for keeping abuse secret, or it can be a result of the stresses of caring for a dependent older family member. Isolation is dangerous because it cuts off family members from the outside help and support they need to cope with the stresses of caregiving. Isolation also makes it harder for outsiders to recognize and intervene in a volatile or abusive situation to protect the older person and to offer help to the abuser.

Societal attitudes make it easier for abuse to continue without detection or intervention. Devaluation and lack of respect for the elderly seen in certain cultures may contribute to violence against older people. When older people are regarded as disposable, society fails to recognize the importance of assuring dignified, supportive, and nonabusive life circumstances for every member of that society.

Cultural norms and belief systems sometimes allow for mistreatment of family members, especially women. Those who participate in these behaviors do not consider them abusive. In some cultures, women's basic rights are not honored, and older women in these cultures may not realize they are being abused. They probably could not call for help outside the family and may not even know that help is available.

The idea that what happens at home is "private" can be a major factor in keeping an older person locked in an abusive situation. Those outside the family who observe or suspect abuse or neglect may fail to intervene because they believe "it's a family problem and none of our business" or because they are afraid of misinterpreting a private quarrel. Shame and embarrassment often make it difficult for older persons to reveal abuse. They don't want others to know that such events occur in their families.

Many factors are involved in the management of older persons who have been abused, including immediate care, long-term assessment and care, education, and prevention. Intervention can be a lengthy process, especially in a busy ED.

Since risk increases with dependency on the caregiver, assessment of the elderly patient's functional ability is important. The patient and the caregiver should be interviewed separately and together. Both should be asked to describe a typical day in order to assess the care burden that each perceives. Open discussion about alternative living arrangements or day-care options may be greeted with relief by family and patient alike. Stress management also needs to be discussed.

The following clinical presentations can help the ED clinician detect the presence of various type of elder abuse.

Signs and symptoms of physical abuse include but are not limited to:

- Bruises, black eyes, welts, lacerations, and rope marks
- Bone fractures, broken bones, and skull fractures
- Open wounds, cuts, punctures, untreated injuries in various stages of healing
- Sprains, dislocations, and internal injuries/bleeding
- Broken eyeglasses/frames, physical signs of being subjected to punishment and being restrained
- Laboratory findings of medication overdose or underutilization of prescribed drugs
- The elder's report of being hit, slapped, kicked, or mistreated
- The elder's sudden change in behavior
- The caregiver's refusal to allow visitors to see the elder alone

Signs and symptoms of emotional/psychological abuse include but are not limited to:

- Emotionally upset or agitated
- Extremely withdrawn and noncommunicative or nonresponsive
- Unusual behavior usually attributed to dementia (e.g., sucking, biting, rocking)
- The elder's report of being verbally or emotionally mistreated

Signs and symptoms of neglect include but are not limited to:

- Dehydration, malnutrition, untreated bed sores, and poor personal hygiene
- Unattended or untreated health problems
- Hazardous or unsafe living conditions/arrangements (e.g., improper wiring, no heat, no running water)
- Unsanitary and unclean living conditions (e.g., dirt, fleas, lice on person, soiled bedding, fecal/urine smell, inadequate clothing)
- The elder's report of being mistreated

Signs and symptoms of abandonment include but are not limited to:

- Desertion of the elder at a hospital, nursing facility, or other similar institution
- Desertion of the elder at a shopping center or other public location
- The elder's report of being abandoned

Signs and symptoms of self-neglect include but are not limited to:

- Dehydration, malnutrition, untreated or improperly attended medical conditions, poor personal hygiene
- Hazardous or unsafe living conditions/arrangements (e.g., improper wiring, no indoor plumbing, no heat, no running water)
- Unsanitary or unclean living quarters (e.g., animal/insect infestation, no functioning toilet, fecal/urine smell)
- Inappropriate and/or inadequate clothing, lack of necessary medical aids (e.g., eyeglasses, hearing aids, dentures)
- Grossly inadequate housing or homelessness

Signs and symptoms of financial or material exploitation include but are not limited to:

- Sudden changes in bank account or banking practices (e.g., unexplained withdrawal of large sums of money by a person accompanying the elder)

- Inclusion of additional names on the elder's bank signature card
- Unauthorized withdrawal of funds using the elder's ATM card
- Abrupt changes in a will or other financial documents
- Unexplained disappearance of funds or valuable possessions
- Substandard care being provided or bills unpaid despite the availability of adequate financial resources
- The elder's signature forged on financial transactions or on titles of his/her possessions
- Sudden appearance of previously uninvolved relatives claiming their rights to the elder's affairs and possessions
- Unexplained sudden transfer of assets to a family member or someone outside the family
- Provision of services that are not necessary
- The elder's report of financial exploitation

Signs and symptoms of sexual abuse include but are not limited to:

- Bruises around the breasts or genital area
- Unexplained venereal disease or genital infections
- Unexplained vaginal or anal bleeding
- Torn, stained, or bloody underclothing
- The elder's report of being sexually assaulted or raped

ED Interventions

Immediate care focuses on treating the physical manifestations of abuse and assuring the safety of the patient. This may include the following:

- Admitting the patient to the hospital
- Obtaining a court protective order
- Placing the patient in a safe home
- Permitting return home if the patient is competent and refuses intervention

The goal of intervention is to enable older people to maintain as much independence as safely as possible. The potential efficacy of continence programs, physical therapy, home health aid, and assisted-living devices such as wheelchairs, hearing aids, and glasses should be evaluated, and assistance should be secured, if feasible. Programs such as respite care, adult day programs, and church activities allow the elderly patient and caregiver to spend time away from each other and should be strongly encouraged.

The ED clinician may need to consult with institutions that have developed multidisciplinary teams of social workers, physicians, nurses, and administrators for these situations. The ultimate goal is to provide the aging adult with a more fulfilling and enjoyable life.

Reporting abuse to authorities depends on local laws and on the clinical status and degree of dependency or dysfunction of the victim. Notifying adult protective service agencies can provide both legal remedies and therapeutic options through community social service networks.

Summary

As previously noted, all states require reporting of suspected child abuse, and nearly all states have mandatory notification laws for suspected elder abuse. Disclosure laws regarding partner abuse differ from state to state. Simply discussing the problem openly and alerting others regarding the abuse may have protective benefits, however. At times, the physician may be justified in calling the police immediately about overtly dangerous situations.

Major authorities vary in their recommendations for detection of domestic violence. Because the accuracy of screening has not been validated, the U.S. Preventive Services Task Force does not advocate universal screening for violence among the asymptomatic population that seeks clinical services. This evidence-based screening guideline is currently under review. In the meantime, investigation of suspected abuse is warranted whenever clinically indicated.

The American Medical Association does recommend screening for domestic violence across all population sectors, and it highlights screening for abuse among women and adolescents seeking medical care. The American Academy of Pediatrics recommends that adolescents and their parents be routinely questioned about violence and methods of dealing with anger.

Despite their pivotal role in breaking the "cycle of abuse," ED clinicians often are reluctant to make the diagnosis of abuse. Perhaps the term "diagnosis" should not be used, because it implies a definitive judgment. Instead, ED clinicians should identify the "possibility" of abuse, keeping in mind that "proof" is not necessary. The reasons for suspecting abuse should be clearly documented in a straightforward manner.

ED clinicians can offer the best treatment options for domestic violence by being familiar with local community resources and by encouraging victims to contact child and adult protective service agencies, shelters, counselors for abuse intervention, or geriatric services. When possible, the perpetrators of abuse should also be assessed for needed intervention and treatment. Whenever ED clinicians identify risks of potential domestic abuse, the implementation of a primary preventive approach may be warranted.

Further Reading

American Medical Association. Diagnostic and treatment guidelines on child physical abuse and neglect. Chicago, American Medical Association, 1992.

American Medical Association. Diagnostic and treatment guidelines on child sexual abuse. Chicago, American Medical Association, 1992.

Beebe DK: Sexual assault: The physician's role in prevention and treatment. J Miss State Med Assoc 1998;39:366-369.

Bostock DJ, Brewster AL: Intimate partner sexual violence. Clinics in Family Practice 2003;5:145.

Bulik CM, Prescott CA, Kendler KS: Features of childhood sexual abuse and the development of psychiatric and substance use disorders. Br J Psychiatry 2001;179:444-449.

Cantu M, Coppola M, Lindner AJ: Evaluation and management of the sexually assaulted woman. Emerg Med Clin North Am 2003;21:737-750.

Cole TB: Is domestic violence screening helpful? JAMA 2000;284:551-553.

Director TD, Linden JA: Domestic violence: An approach to identification and intervention. Emerg Med Clin North Am 2004;22:1117-1132.

Dube SR, Anda RF, Felitti VJ, et al: Childhood abuse, household dysfunction, and the risk of attempted suicide throughout the life span: Findings from the Adverse Childhood Experiences Study. JAMA 2001;286:3089-3096.

Feldhaus KM, Koziol-McLain J, Amsbury HL, et al: Accuracy of 3 brief screening questions for detecting partner violence in the emergency department. JAMA 1997;277:1357-1361.

Gracia E: Unreported cases of domestic violence against women: Towards an epidemiology of social silence, tolerance, and inhibition. J Epidemiol Community Health 2004;58:536-537.

Ledray LE: SANE development and operation guide. J Emerg Nurs 1998;24:197-198.

Logan TK, Walker R: Separation as a risk factor for victims of intimate partner violence: Beyond lethality and injury. A response to Campbell. J Interpers Violence 2004;19:1478-1486.

National Institute of Justice: Legal interventions in family violence: Research findings and policy implications. Washington, DC, US Department of Justice, 1998.

Osterman JE, Barbiaz J, Johnson P: Emergency psychiatry: Emergency interventions for rape victims. Psychiatr Serv 2001;52:733-740.

Richardson J, Coid J, Petruckevitch A, et al: Identifying domestic violence: Cross sectional study in primary care. BMJ 2002;324:274-277.

Ruiz-Pérez I, Plazaola-Castaño J: Intimate partner violence and mental health consequences in women attending family practice in Spain. Psychosom Med 2005;67:791-797.

Smith BH, Hannaford PC, Elliott AM, et al: The "number needed to sample" in primary care research. Comparison of two primary care sampling frames for chronic back pain. Fam Pract 2005;22:205-214.

Steiner RP, Vansickle K, Lippmann SB: Domestic violence: Do you know when and how to intervene? Postgrad Med 1996;100:103-106, 111-114, 116.

U.S. Preventive Services Task Force: Screening for family and intimate partner violence: Recommendation statement. Ann Fam Med 2004;2:156-160.

Ziegler MF, Greenwald MH, DeGuzman MA, Simon HK: Posttraumatic stress responses in children: Awareness and practice among a sample of pediatric emergency care providers. Pediatrics 2005;115:1261-1267.

Other Available Resources

Physical and Sexual Abuse in Children

Henry Kemp National Center for the Prevention and Treatment of Child Abuse and Neglect (Tel: 303-321-3963)

National Committee to Prevent Child Abuse (Tel: 312-663-3520)

National Clearinghouse on Child Abuse and Neglect Information (Tel: 703-385-7565)

Partner Abuse

National Domestic Violence Hotline (Tel: 800-799-SAFE)

American College of Obstetricians and Gynecologists (Tel: 202-863-2518)

Elder Abuse

National Center on Elder Abuse (Tel: 202-682-0100)

National Clearinghouse on Elder Abuse (Tel: 302-831-8712)

POSTSCRIPT

To the sick, while there is life there is hope.
　　　　　　　　　　　　　Marcus Tullius Cicero—106–43 BC

Not by might, not by power, but by my Spirit, saith the Lord of hosts.

—Zechariah 4:6

CHAPTER 20

The Patient with Posttraumatic Stress Disorder

Hani R. Khouzam, MD, MPH, FAPA, Tirath S. Gill, MD, and Doris T. Tan, DO

KEY POINTS

- Posttraumatic stress disorder (PTSD) is a chronic anxiety disorder with a relatively high prevalence in the general population.
- PTSD can go unrecognized by the ED clinician if patients present with other symptoms related to medical, psychiatric, and substance abuse disorders.
- Early intervention, treatment, and referral by the ED clinician for patients with PTSD may limit long-term morbidity and complications.
- The treatment of PTSD requires comprehensive pharmacologic, psychosocial, and, in some instances, spiritual interventions.

Overview

PTSD is a syndrome that could develop as a reaction to violent or traumatic events that involve deliberate and destructive behavior (e.g., murder, rape) and events that are prolonged or physically challenging. The event can also be a natural disaster. Such events include, but are not limited to, experiencing or witnessing sexual assaults, accidents, combat, natural disasters (such as earthquakes), or unexpected deaths of loved ones. PTSD may also occur in people who have serious illness and receive aggressive treatment or who have close family members or friends with such conditions. Figure 20-1 illustrates an acutely traumatized patient.

Survivor of trauma/rape

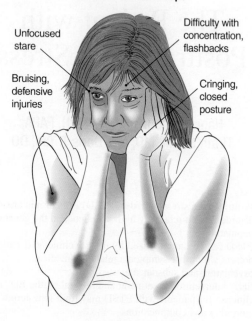

Unfocused stare

Difficulty with concentration, flashbacks

Bruising, defensive injuries

Cringing, closed posture

The Acutely Traumatized Patient

- Anxious, closed posture
- Shell-shocked appearance
- Thousand mile stare
- Emotional numbing
- Bruises, other bodily injuries
- Easy startle response
- Flashbacks
- Cringes on touch

FIGURE 20–1

The acutely traumatized patient.

Witnessing or experiencing such events can lead to the development of abnormal symptoms, including intrusive flashbacks, startle responses, nightmares, and emotional numbing. With immediate intervention, the symptoms can abate and remit in about a month's time. In some cases, however, the symptoms persist beyond this period of time and lead to the development of chronic PTSD. Treatment and clinical intervention are essential in order to limit the suffering of patients with PTSD and to prevent related human costs associated with broken marriages and homes, substance abuse, the development of psychiatric and medical complications, social isolation, and a downward drift to a dysfunctional lifestyle.

Definition

PTSD is a chronic anxiety disorder lasting more than 1 month that may develop in a person who has experienced, witnessed, or learned about a physically or psychologically distressing event. The event may involve death, serious injury, or other threats to a person's physical integrity. The immediate cause of PTSD appears to be the specific stressors associated with the event or events. The severity of the event causes heightened subjective feelings of intense fear, helplessness, and horror. PTSD is considered acute when symptoms last less than 3 months and chronic when symptoms last 3 months or more. Symptoms occurring immediately following the stressors and lasting less than 1 month may be transient and self-limited. Severe symptoms during this time increase the risk of chronic PTSD. When symptoms last 1 to 3 months, active treatment measures may help reduce the otherwise high risk of chronic PTSD, which is associated with comorbid psychiatric disorders.

Epidemiology

A national comorbidity survey found that about 7.8% of American adults suffer from symptoms of PTSD at some time in their lives. The rate is 10.4% in women, more than twice as high as in men, in whom the lifetime prevalence rate is about 5%. Studies estimate a lifetime risk for PTSD in the U.S. population as high as 8%. It is also estimated that 6% to 30% or more of trauma survivors develop PTSD, with children and young people being among those at the high end of the range. The rate is also higher in veterans who have been exposed to combat and have been injured or witnessed injury or death of others. The prevalence rate in Vietnam and other combat veterans is almost three times higher than the general population. The prevalence of PTSD is thought to be in excess of 50% in trauma victims who seek nonpsychiatric medical treatment for the after-effects of the trauma.

Patients with PTSD have high rates of health complaints and medical morbidity and mortality, including diabetes, cardiovascular problems, respiratory difficulties, musculoskeletal problems, and neurologic problems. Patients with chronic PTSD have unusually high rates of associated psychiatric conditions throughout life, including substance abuse and dependence (23%), major depression (20%), alcohol dependence (75%), and personality disorder (20%). Other comorbid psychiatric conditions include panic disorder, agoraphobia, generalized anxiety disorder, social phobia, and bipolar disorder.

Assessment and Diagnosis

When assessing the status of a patient with PTSD, the ED clinician needs to identify the risk factors for this disorder. Although not every person who is exposed to traumatic events will develop PTSD, several risk factors, summarized in Box 20-1, have been identified as predisposing to the development of PTSD.

Certain stressors have been identified that may precipitate the development of PTSD. These include:
• Criminal assault
• Hostage-taking
• Imprisonment
• Military duties
• Natural disaster
• Serious accident
• Sexual or physical abuse
• Torture
• Terrorist attack
• Abortion
• Witnessing or learning about the traumatic events

Factors that are protective against the development of PTSD are outlined in Box 20-2. Complications of untreated PTSD are summarized in Box 20-3. An awareness of these complications may aid in the assessment and diagnosis of the patient with PTSD.

Box 20–1. Risk Factors for Development of Posttraumatic Stress Disorder

- Family history of anxiety
- Childhood history of abuse
- Early separation from parents
- Lack of social support and poverty
- Female gender
- Drug or alcohol abuse
- Preexisting psychiatric disorder, particularly depression, before the traumatic event
- Exposure to prior traumatic events
- Continued likelihood of exposure to the traumatic event
- Sleep disorders such as insomnia and excessive daytime sleepiness as long as a month after the traumatic event
- Sense of helplessness at the time of the traumatic event
- Increased intensity of acute stress reaction
- Traumatic brain injury

Box 20–2. Protective Factors against Development of Posttraumatic Stress Disorder

- Early intervention to provide safe place for person to rest, find a quiet place, sleep
- Early intervention to establish communications with friends and family to provide support
- Helping person make concrete plans to take care of responsibilities for safe care of self and dependents
- Linking with federal and/or local agencies to provide support and sense of empowerment to overcome the situation
- Early medical and psychiatric support and follow-up
- Providing education regarding the normal stress response and offering support and symptomatic treatment for short-term treatment of insomnia to allow sleep and rest
- Reassuring victims of assault that it was not their fault
- Recreational activities and therapy to distract attention from the traumatic event may be helpful in some cases

> **Box 20–3. Complications of Untreated Posttraumatic Stress Disorder**
>
> - Increased divorce rate
> - Increased unemployment
> - Increased likelihood of incarceration
> - Increased likelihood of alcohol and drug dependence
> - Increased incidence of depression
> - Increased incidence of suicide
> - Increased incidence of coronary artery disease
> - Increased incidence of somatic complaints and related disability
> - Emotional numbing, angry outbursts, and social isolation

Clinical Presentation

The patient with PTSD presenting to the ED may exhibit any of the following symptoms:
- Intrusive re-experiencing of the trauma
- Recurrent intrusive thoughts, images, dreams
- Intense distress when remembering the trauma
- Avoidance of reminders of the trauma
- Increased autonomic arousal
- Insomnia
- Irritability or angry outbursts
- Poor concentration
- Hypervigilance
- Exaggerated startle response
- Emotional numbing
- Dissociative symptoms

The mnemonic **TRAUMA** can be used by the ED clinician as a screening tool for identifying PTSD:

T = Traumatic exposure

R = Re-experiencing the event → nightmares, flashbacks, and reminders of the event → emotional effects of distress, fear, and loss of safety

A = Avoidance of reminder places, activities or people, detachment and emotional numbness

U = Unable to function interpersonally, socially, and vocationally

M= Month or longer in duration

A = Autonomic arousal → insomnia, irritability, hypervigilance, exaggerated startle reactions

Interviewing the PTSD Patient

A courteous and attentive approach can help establish trust and rapport during the interview. Avoid any sudden movement or noises during the interview that might evoke a startle response by the patient. Telephones, alarms, and electronic equipment, including computers, should be silenced if possible.

Patients should be allowed to relate their problems at their own pace. The ED clinician may paraphrase and retell a patient's story to facilitate trust and express some understanding of the difficulties that are being experienced. Often, patients may find comfort in knowing that their reactions to extreme trauma are felt by others, and that they are not "going crazy."

The ED clinician should inquire systematically about the constellation of PTSD-associated conditions and comorbidity.

Psychiatric Comorbidity

Persons with chronic PTSD have unusually high rates of associated psychiatric conditions throughout life; usually these conditions were present before the development of PTSD; however, some conditions may have occurred after or coincided with PTSD. Examples of PTSD psychiatric comorbidity include:
- Alcohol and substance abuse and dependence
- Mood disorder, major depression, bipolar disorder
- Personality disorders
- Panic disorder, agoraphobia, generalized anxiety disorder, social phobia

When such conditions are identified and treated, the intensity of PTSD symptoms usually decreases.

Differential Diagnosis

PTSD can be misdiagnosed and inappropriately treated. The ED clinician needs to obtain a detailed history of the onset of symptoms as they relate to traumatic experiences, in order to distinguish PTSD from conditions such as:
- Traumatic head injury and concussion (see Chapter 4)
- Delirium (see Chapters 4, 5, and 17)
- Seizure disorders (see Chapter 16)
- Alcohol and substance abuse with acute intoxication or withdrawal (see Chapters 14 and 15)
- Factitious disorders and malingering (see Chapter 13)

- Personality disorders (see Chapter 12)
- Sleep apnea, which may intensify symptoms of PTSD, including sleeplessness and nightmares
- Acute stress disorder (see Chapter 21)

In some cases, the distinction between comorbid psychiatric conditions and the clinical presentations of PTSD becomes blurred. In these situations consultation with family members and review of other sources of collateral information may be needed in order to differentiate the PTSD symptoms from the symptoms of the comorbid psychiatric conditions.

Treatment

The ED clinician may be the first line of professionals to identify the presence of PTSD in patients presenting with acute symptoms of the illness; in such cases the ED clinician may initiate treatment and plan referral and follow-up care. In other situations, patients with previously diagnosed PTSD may present to the ED because of exacerbation of symptoms. In either case, the treatment of PTSD will include pharmacological and non-pharmacological interventions, with an increased focus on crisis management and problem solving related to any recent stressors.

Pharmacological Treatment

The selection of medication depends on specific symptoms and coexisting psychiatric conditions. Symptoms of PTSD that may respond to pharmacological intervention include anger, hostility, violent impulses, anxiety, poor concentration, sleep disturbances including nightmares, depressed mood, recurrent intrusive recollections (flashbacks), and avoidance behaviors.

Pharmacological therapy for comorbid psychiatric conditions must be carefully selected to complement therapy targeted at PTSD symptoms.

Antidepressants
Selective serotonin reuptake inhibitors (SSRIs), tricyclic antidepressants (TCAs), and other antidepressants can be used for the symptomatic treatment of PTSD (also see Chapter 7).

SSRIs
In general, SSRIs effectively target PTSD symptoms such as intrusive thoughts, flashbacks, hyperarousal, irritability, angry

outbursts, difficulty concentrating, and associated depression and anxiety. SSRIs are also used to treat dissociative symptoms. Their use is encouraged because of their relatively simple dosage regimen (Table 20-1), safety, and favorable outcomes. Sertraline (Zoloft) and paroxetine (Paxil) are approved by the U.S. Food and Drug Administration (FDA) for treatment of PTSD. Another advantage of SSRIs is their effectiveness in treating comorbid depressive and other anxiety disorders. The SSRI fluvoxamine (Luvox) has been used in several countries as an antidepressant but is approved by the FDA only for the treatment of obsessive-compulsive disorder.

The FDA has issued a warning about the risk for suicidal ideation and the occurrence of suicide in children and adolescents maintained on SSRIs. Vigilant monitoring for suicide remains an essential element of treatment of PTSD, especially in patients receiving SSRIs.

Side Effects

The most common side effect of SSRIs is nausea, which is usually mild and occurs in the first weeks of treatment. Dry mouth

Table 20–1

SSRIs for Posttraumatic Stress Disorder

SSRI	Starting Dose (mg/day)	Average Dose (mg/day)	Maximum Dose (mg/day)
Citalopram (Celexa)	20	20-40	60
Escitalopram (Lexapro)	20	10-20	40
Fluoxetine (Prozac, Sarafem)	10-20	20-50	80
Fluvoxamine (Luvox)	50	100-250	300
Paroxetine (Paxil)	10-20	20-50	60
Paroxetine CR (Paxil CR)	25	25-60	62.5
Sertraline (Zoloft)	25-50	50-150	200

SSRIs, selective serotonin reuptake inhibitors.

also may occur. Anxiety is usually transient. Extrapyramidal symptom (EPS) side effects have been reported to cause movement disorders such as tardive dyskinesia, but these side effects are less frequent with SSRIs than with TCAs. Sedation can be a problem; paroxetine appears to be slightly more sedating and to exhibit more anticholinergic side effects among the various SSRIs indicated for depression. Sexual function can be affected by SSRIs; the most common sexual side effects are anorgasmia and delayed orgasm. The sexual side effects may not be volunteered by patients but can contribute to the medication's noncompliance. Abrupt discontinuation or interruption of SSRIs with shorter half-lives such as citalopram, escitalopram, paroxetine, and sertraline can lead to a cluster of withdrawal symptoms known as discontinuation/interruption syndrome that are similar to having a flu infection, with dizziness, fatigue, and nausea.

Potential Drug-Drug Interactions

Individual SSRIs have different effects on the cytochrome P450 (CYP450) system. For example, fluoxetine, sertraline, and paroxetine, but not fluvoxamine, are inhibitors of the 2D6 isoenzyme system, which metabolizes TCAs, type Ic antiarrhythmics, alpha-adrenergic blockers, dextromethorphan, chemotherapeutic agents, and some antipsychotics. Citalopram has minimal inhibitory activity and escitalopram has virtually no inhibitory action on CYP2D6[17].

CYP3A4 metabolizes numerous drugs, including alprazolam, triazolam, carbamazepine, calcium channel blockers, and others. The 3A4 enzymes are inhibited by fluoxetine, sertraline, and fluvoxamine.

CYP1A2 is the liver isoenzyme responsible for dealkylating theophylline, caffeine, and phenacetin. This enzyme system also metabolizes tacrine and clozapine. Of the SSRIs, fluvoxamine is the most potent inhibitor of the 1A2 enzymes, whereas escitalopram is a negligible inhibitor.

CYP2C is a subfamily of isoenzymes that includes 2C9, 2C10, 2C19, and others. This system metabolizes some antidepressants as well as warfarin, phenytoin, and diazepam. Inhibitors of this system include fluvoxamine, fluoxetine, sertraline, and paroxetine.

Concomitant use of serotonin-acting drugs and monoamine oxidase inhibitors (MAOIs) is contraindicated. When used in combination, SSRIs and MAOIs can cause a serotonin syndrome, with potential hyperpyretic crises, seizures, coma, and death. When switching medications, it is important to eliminate any serotonin-acting drug before starting an MAOI.

Tricyclic Antidepressants (TCAs)

TCAs include amitriptyline (daily average dose, 150 mg) nortriptyline (daily average dose, 100 mg), doxepin (daily average dose, 200 mg), and imipramine (daily average dose, 200 mg). These agents have documented some efficacy in the treatment of several PTSD symptoms, including intrusive thoughts, flashbacks, anxiety, panic-related hyperarousal, loss of interest, sleep disturbances, irritability, and depressed mood affecting concentration and contributing to feelings of shame and guilt.

Adverse effects of TCAs include sedation, blurred vision, dry mouth, constipation, urinary retention, postural hypotension, tachycardia, cognitive dysfunction, and weight gain. Interaction with other sedating and anticholinergic medications potentiates their adverse effects. Prior to the development of the newer antidepressants (especially the SSRIs), TCAs were first-line agents for treating PTSD; now they are considered secondary agents because of their potentially life-threatening cardiotoxicity, especially following overdose attempts.

Trazodone

Trazodone is an antidepressant with anxiolytic properties, chemically unrelated to the TCAs. Trazodone can ameliorate chronic insomnia and decrease the intensity of nightmares. It also is effective in the management of aggressive behaviors. Trazodone dosages vary depending on patient's response; the maximum daily dose is 600 mg. Although it possesses minor anticholinergic effects, trazodone is quite sedating, can cause orthostatic hypotension, and in a small percentage of male patients causes priapism requiring surgical intervention. Trazodone is a relatively safe medication in normal, physically healthy individuals and is considered nonlethal unless combined with other sedative or hypnotic medications and alcohol or drugs in intentional and unintentional overdoses.

Atypical Antidepressants

Antidepressants with atypical modes of action can also be considered for the treatment of PTSD in patients unable to tolerate the adverse effects of the other agents discussed here. The role of atypical antidepressants in treating PTSD has not yet been fully studied. These agents include mirtazapine, bupropion, and the serotonin/norepinephrine reuptake inhibitors (SNRIs) venlafaxine and duloxetine.

Mirtazapine

This antidepressant exerts sedating properties that can be beneficial in sleep disturbances and in decreasing hyperarousal in PTSD. Mirtazapine (maximum daily dose, 60 mg) is also an alternative medication for comorbid treatment-resistant depression. Its main side effects are somnolence, dizziness, and increased appetite with weight gain. It can interfere with cognitive and motor performance because of its sedating effects. As with other tetracyclic agents, there is a possible risk of agranulocytosis, so patients should pay particular attention to any flulike or other symptoms suggesting infection.

Bupropion

Bupropion is known to affect the noradrenergic and dopaminergic systems. Its effects on PTSD symptoms are not well understood, but it has shown some beneficial effects in patients with comorbid depression who could not tolerate the adverse effects of other antidepressants. The total daily dose should not exceed 450 mg of the immediate-release formulation or 400 mg of the sustained-release form. The main adverse effects of bupropion include headache, nausea, agitation, and insomnia. Bupropion may be associated with an increased risk of seizures in doses exceeding 300 mg. The single dose of bupropion should also not exceed 150 mg in order to limit the risk of seizures. Bupropion is absolutely contraindicated in patients with seizure disorders and in patients with anorexia and bulimia. Bupropion is marketed under two different trade names: Wellbutrin, indicated for treatment of depression, and Zyban, to be used as an adjunctive pharmacological agent for treatment of smoking cessation.

Venlafaxine

This SNRI antidepressant selectively inhibits serotonin, norepinephrine, and dopamine uptake in order of decreasing potency. It can be used for symptomatic relief of severe depressive symptoms associated with PTSD and for anxiety, phobic reactions, and panic symptoms. The maximum daily dosage of venlafaxine is 225 mg. Side effects include nausea, headache, nervousness, anxiety, anorexia, sweating, and insomnia. At high doses, a small percentage of patients experience increased diastolic blood pressure; a smaller percentage may have increased heart rate and serum cholesterol levels. Venlafaxine, when used as recommended, has no effect on cytochrome P450 isoenzymes.

Duloxetine
This SNRI antidepressant has dual-selective norepinephrine and serotonin effects and, like venlafaxine, can be used for symptomatic relief of severe depressive symptoms and anxiety associated with PTSD. Duloxetine has a daily dose range of 20 to 60 mg. Most patients respond to a 20- to 30-mg dose schedule. One of duloxetine's additional actions is its effect on treating diabetic peripheral neuropathy.

Monoamine Oxidase Inhibitors (MAOIs)
MAOIs are a class of medications that block the degradation of dopamine, norepinephrine, and serotonin (5-hydroxytryptamine, or 5-HT). The MAOI phenelzine has been reported to be effective in decreasing intrusive thoughts and avoidant behaviors and in treatment of atypical depressive symptoms characterized by hypersomnia, hyperphagia, and comorbid symptoms of anxiety. The maximum daily dose is 60 mg, but some patients may tolerate a daily dose of up to 90 mg.

MAOIs are associated with anticholinergic side effects including dry mouth, urinary retention, constipation, and blurred vision. They can also cause orthostatic hypotension and sexual dysfunction. Because of their irreversible inhibitory effects, they can cause a fatal hypertensive crisis if ingested with food containing tyramine. The potential for drug-drug and alcohol interactions with MAOIs precludes their use in PTSD patients with substance abuse comorbidity and in patients using a wide range of other medications including antidepressants and pain medications such as meperidine.

Mood Stabilizers
The mood stabilizers lithium, valproic acid, and lamotrigine have been used successfully in patients with prominent symptoms of hyperarousal, hyperactivity, hostility, irritability, and angry outbursts. These agents can be added in cases with partial response to antidepressants or can be used as first-line treatment for patients having both PTSD and comorbid bipolar disorder.

Lithium
Lithium decreases norepinephrine reuptake and increases serotonin receptor sensitivity. Side effects of lithium include fine

hand tremor, polydipsia, polyuria, nausea, vomiting, drowsiness, muscle weakness, poor coordination, giddiness, ringing or buzzing in the ears, and blurred vision. Because lithium affects the thyroid, monitoring of thyroid function is necessary. Lithium interacts with other medications, including haloperidol, chlorpromazine, TCAs, and calcium channel blockers. Angiotensin-converting enzyme (ACE) inhibitors, nonsteroidal anti-inflammatory drugs (NSAIDs), and diuretics can increase lithium serum levels, resulting in lithium toxicity, manifested by increased tremors, hyperreflexia, alteration in mental state, and delirium. Sodium chloride (NaCl) plays an important role in lithium excretion, so in order to prevent the development of hyponatremia, lithium should not be given with a salt-free diet. Because of the narrow therapeutic/toxic lithium levels, serum lithium levels should be monitored at frequent intervals.

Valproic Acid and Derivatives

This group includes valproic acid, Depakote sprinkles, sodium valproate (the sodium salt), and Divalproex sodium. These anticonvulsants and mood stabilizers increase the levels of gamma-aminobutyric acid (GABA) as well as increasing GABA receptor site sensitivity. The rationale for using them in cases of PTSD is related to limbic kindling. It is hypothesized that increased GABA levels interfere with the kindling process, thus diminishing the clinical symptoms of flashbacks, nightmares, and hyperarousal.

Side effects include gastrointestinal upset and throat or mouth irritation, which occur if the tablets or capsules are chewed. Patients who have difficulty swallowing may benefit from the syrup or the sprinkle forms. Other side effects include indigestion, sedation, sleepiness, weakness, fatigue, skin rash, diarrhea, stomach cramps, and constipation. Valproic acid has been associated with hepatic failure resulting in fatalities, thus monitoring of liver function and liver enzymes is recommended. Problems with muscle coordination, parkinsonian side effects, polycystic ovarian syndrome, hair loss, and weight gain also may occur.

Lamotrigine

This anticonvulsant medication has been approved by the FDA for treatment of bipolar mood disorder type I, especially the depressed phase of this illness; it has shown effectiveness in reducing intrusive thoughts, avoidance, and the numbing symptoms of PTSD.

A frequently reported adverse effect that warranted an FDA warning is lamotrigine's association with the development of potentially life-threatening skin conditions such as toxic epidermal necrolysis and Stevens-Johnson syndrome, reported to occur in 0.1% of adults and 1% to 2% of children.

Carbamazepine

Carbamazepine can be useful in some PTSD patients with sleep disturbances because it decreases sleep latency and is nondisruptive to rapid eye movement (REM) sleep. It is also effective in treating agitation, rage attacks, poor impulse control, and violent behavior including angry outbursts.

Carbamazepine has been reported to modulate the kindling effects that have been documented to occur in PTSD. According to the kindling model, periodic brain stimuli that are initially too low to produce stimulation of the limbic system may progressively induce bioelectrical changes, ultimately leading to abnormal limbic sensitization manifested by periodic mood swings, agitation, and violence.

Side effects of carbamazepine include drowsiness, dizziness, and blurred vision. Carbamazepine is a hepatic enzyme inducer that can initially decrease its own plasma levels and influence the plasma levels of other drugs that are affected by the same hepatic pathways. Severe adverse effects of carbamazepine involve hepatotoxicity and the development of blood dyscrasias, requiring periodic monitoring of liver function and blood counts. It is important to monitor serum carbamazepine levels at intervals of every 3 to 6 months regardless of the patient's stability and absence of adverse effects.

Antianxiety Medications

Antidepressant medications have useful anxiolytic properties, but some PTSD patients may require the adjunctive use of antianxiety agents to treat acute, severe and debilitating symptoms of fear, panic, avoidance, hyperarousal, hypervigilance, startle reactions, and sleep disturbances.

Benzodiazepines

The benzodiazepines are widely used as anxiolytic agents but warrant careful consideration in the treatment of PTSD. In general, the routine use of benzodiazepines to treat PTSD should be avoided because of their potential for inducing physiologic dependence, interdose rebound, and breakthrough anxiety symptoms.

Abuse potential, along with an exacerbation of PTSD symptoms during withdrawal of benzodiazepines, limits their long-term use. When considering benzodiazepines, the clinician should be aware of any comorbid substance abuse disorder and consider the possibility of paradoxical disinhibition, which can precipitate impulsive and hostile behaviors. Depressive symptoms that frequently emerge during PTSD treatment have been associated with benzodiazepines treatment.

Buspirone

Buspirone is a nonbenzodiazepine anxiolytic. It has a high affinity for 5-HT1A receptors. It has no significant affinity for benzodiazepine receptors and does not affect GABA binding. Buspirone has moderate affinity for D2 dopamine receptors and appears to act as a presynaptic dopamine agonist. Because of its efficacy in the management of anxiety disorders, it may play a role in the treatment of hyperarousal and startle responses. Buspirone does not cause sedation or cognitive impairment; however, it can cause dizziness, nausea, headache, fatigue, nervousness, light-headedness, and overexcitement. Patients with PTSD need to be alerted to the possibility of these side effects early in treatment so that they do not interpret these effects as an aggravation of preexisting symptoms. Buspirone has been reported to be effective in the management of the SSRI-induced sexual dysfunction.

Antipsychotic Medications

Traditionally, conventional antipsychotics were generally characterized as being irrelevant in the treatment of PTSD because of their adverse side effects including the potential for inducing tardive dyskinesia. The atypical antipsychotics pose a much lower risk of these side effects, making them useful adjunctive therapeutic agents in the treatment of PTSD, especially in treating comorbid hallucinations and delusions (associated with suspiciousness and paranoia). Irritability, nightmares, and vivid sensory flashbacks with auditory, visual, olfactory, and tactile hallucinations, possibly related to episodes of dissociation and re-experiencing of actual traumatic events, may respond to a short course of treatment with antipsychotics. The association between PTSD and bipolar disorder may indicate the need for adjunctive use of antipsychotics (see Chapter 8).

Adrenergic Medications

These agents primarily act by decreasing autonomic hyperactivity seen in PTSD patients, which manifests as general anxiety, hyperarousal, hypervigilance, and startle reactions. These symptoms may respond to the judicial use of agents such as clonidine, guanfacine, propranolol, and prazosin.

Clonidine and Guanfacine

These alpha 2–adrenergic agonists have been shown to reduce symptoms of hyperarousal and to potentiate the effects of TCAs. The most common side effects are dry mouth, drowsiness, and sedation. Constipation, dizziness, headache, and fatigue are also common but usually diminish within 4 to 6 weeks.

Propranolol

Propranolol is a beta-adrenergic blocker that may have anxiolytic effects in decreasing symptoms of hyperarousal, restlessness, startle reactions, and autonomic hyperactivity. It is usually given in a daily divided dose of 120 to 160 mg and titrated up slowly, starting with 10 mg twice or three times a day, with gradual increase to achieve the desired effects. Other beta-adrenergic blockers such as atenolol and nadolol also have been reported as beneficial. The availability of long-acting propranolol (Inderal LA) in a once-daily dosage formulation offers the advantage of convenient scheduling and better compliance. The main side effects of the beta-adrenergic blockers are tiredness, weakness, bradycardia, dizziness, breathing difficulty, bronchospasm, sleeplessness, and male impotence. Patients maintained on beta-adrenergic blockers require frequent monitoring of blood pressure and pulse rate for early detection of hypotension and bradycardia. A beta-adrenergic blocker given immediately following a traumatic event may be protective against developing PTSD later on.

Prazosin

This alpha 1–adrenergic antagonist has been reported to ameliorate nightmares in combat veterans suffering from PTSD. However, careful monitoring following the first dose is necessary to avoid orthostatic hypotension, dizziness, blacking out, and syncope.

Sedative Hypnotics

The antihistamines and the hypnotic agents zolpidem, zaleplon, and eszopiclone can be used as adjunctive hypnotic agents in the management of chronic sleep disturbances associated with PTSD.

Antihistaminic Agents

Hydroxyzine, diphenhydramine, and cyproheptadine can be used temporarily to induce drowsiness and sleep. Their main side effects include anticholinergic effects such as dry mouth, constipation, urinary retention, and exacerbation of asthma and breathing difficulties. Additive central nervous system (CNS) depressant effects may occur when antihistaminic agents are combined with other sedating pharmacological agents. In some PTSD patients, antihistaminics may cause overstimulation and hyperexcitability.

Hypnotic Agents

Zolpidem

Zolpidem (Ambien) is unrelated to benzodiazepines, barbiturates, and other hypnotic agents but selectively binds to the benzodiazepine type I site. The usual dose is 5 to 10 mg given immediately before bedtime. Downward adjustment of the dose may be necessary when given with other CNS depressants.

Zaleplon

The nonbenzodiazepine hypnotic zaleplon (Sonata) has sedative, anxiolytic, muscle-relaxing, and anticonvulsant properties. The adult dose is 10 mg, and 5 mg for geriatric patients.

Eszopiclone

Eszopiclone (Lunesta) is a newer hypnotic that has shown efficacy in treating insomnia and may subsequently be used in PTSD. In contrast to zolpidem and zaleplon, which are only recommended for short periods of use, eszopiclone can be used for up to 6 months. The average dose is 1 to 3 mg nightly.

Ramelteon

Ramelteon (Rozerem) is a new hypnotic that is a melatonin receptor agonist which contributes to sleep promotion and maintenance of the circadian rhythm underlying the normal sleep-wake cycle. It could be beneficial in PTSD. The adult dose is 4 to 8 mg to be given orally within 30 minutes of bedtime. It should not be administered with or immediately after a high-fat meal.

Nonpharmacological Treatment

The treatment of PTSD requires comprehensive biological, psychological, social, and, in some instances, spiritual interventions. The treatment modalities discussed here can be initiated in the ED with appropriate referral and ongoing follow-up care (also see Chapters 11, 18, and 19).

Cognitive-Behavioral and Supportive Therapy

Cognitive-behavioral and supportive therapy have proved useful for PTSD patients. Eye movement desensitization and reprocessing (EMDR) is a relatively new treatment for traumatic memories that involves elements of exposure therapy and cognitive-behavioral therapy combined with techniques (eye movements, hand taps, sounds) that create an alternation of attention back and forth across the person's midline. While the theory and research are still evolving for this form of treatment, there is some evidence that *alternation*, the therapeutic element unique to EMDR, may facilitate the accessing and processing of traumatic material. Aerobic exercises, dancing, and sports participation have also been reported to be similarly useful.

Group Therapy

Group treatment is often an ideal therapeutic setting because trauma survivors are able to share traumatic material within the safety, cohesion, and empathy provided by other survivors. As group members achieve greater understanding and resolution of their trauma, they often feel more confident and able to trust. As they discuss and share how they cope with trauma-related shame, guilt, rage, fear, doubt, and self-condemnation, they prepare themselves to focus on the present rather than the past. Telling one's story (the "trauma narrative") and directly facing the grief, anxiety, and guilt related to trauma enables many survivors to cope with their symptoms, memories, and other aspects of their lives.

Survival Guilt and Spiritual Intervention

 Survival guilt is one of the associated features of PTSD that may benefit from spiritual and religious intervention in receptive patients. The ED clinician needs to be aware of such individualized treatment options available for patients with PTSD (also see Chapter 24).

Referral for Long-term Treatment

After the initial 3 months of treatment, acute PTSD can be treated with group or individual psychotherapy every 2 to 4 weeks. Patients with chronic PTSD should be followed regularly for at least 6 months with scheduled booster sessions. A small percentage of patients with PTSD, especially those with comorbid psychiatric disorders, remain symptomatic for longer periods of time.

For patients with acute PTSD, medication administration should be continued for 6 to 12 months before considering tapering. Patients with chronic PTSD having a good response, probably should continue treatment for 1 to 2 years, and patients with chronic PTSD with residual symptoms may need to continue treatment for at least 2 years. Some patients will have to be maintained on both pharmacological and nonpharmacological therapy for an extended period beyond 2 years.

Summary

PTSD may cause physical changes in the brain; in some cases the disorder can last a lifetime. Prognosis is usually good when symptoms begin within 6 months of the traumatic event, especially in patients with premorbid psychological stability and with a good social support network. Absence of comorbid medical, psychiatric, or substance-related disorders is also important in predicting the progression of PTSD.

Further Reading

American Psychiatric Association: The Diagnostic and Statistical Manual of Mental Disorders, 4th Ed, Text Revision. Washington, DC, American Psychiatric Association, 2000, pp 429-484.

Chard KM: An evaluation of cognitive processing therapy for the treatment of posttraumatic stress disorder related to childhood sexual abuse. J Consult Clin Psychol 2005;73:965-971.

Fontana A, Rosenheck R: Trauma, change in strength of religious faith, and mental health service use among veterans treated for PTSD. J Nerv Ment Dis 2004;192:579-584.

Friedman MJ: Future pharmacotherapy for post-traumatic stress disorder: Prevention and treatment. Psychiatr Clin North Am 2002;25:427-441.

Grieger TA, Waldrep DA, Lovasz MM, Ursano RJ: Follow-up of Pentagon employees two years after the terrorist attack of September 11, 2001. Psychiatr Serv 2005;56:1374-1378.

Khouzam HR: A simple mnemonic for the diagnostic criteria for post-traumatic stress disorder. West J Med 2001;174:424.

Khouzam HR: Religious meditation and its effects on posttraumatic stress disorder in a Korean war veteran. Clin Gerontologist 2001;22:125-131.

Khouzam HR, Donnelly NJ: Posttraumatic stress disorder. Safe, effective management in the primary care setting. Postgrad Med 2001;110:60-78.

Sawchuk CN, Roy-Byrne P, Goldberg J, et al: The relationship between post-traumatic stress disorder, depression and cardiovascular disease in an American Indian tribe. Psychol Med 2005;35:1785-1794.

Stathis S, Martin G, McKenna JG: A preliminary case series on the use of quetiapine for post-traumatic stress disorder in juveniles within a youth detention center. J Clin Psychopharmacol 2005;25:539-544.

POSTSCRIPT

Worry affects circulation, the heart, and the glands, the whole nervous system, and profoundly affects the heart. I have never known a man who died from overwork, but many who died from doubt.

Charles Horace Mayo—1865-1939

C H A P T E R   2 1

Emergency Psychiatric Care of Survivors of Natural Disasters and Terrorism

Hani R. Khouzam, MD, MPH, FAPA

KEY POINTS

- The reactions of survivors to natural disasters and terrorism may need to be assessed by emergency department (ED) clinicians.
- The scope of emergency psychiatric assessment and treatment will vary depending on the degree, impact, and phase of the survivor's psychological response.
- Normal stress reactions, which may be described as "normal responses to an abnormal situation," are multidimensional and depend on the survivor's developmental level.
- Interventions by ED clinicians following the basics of psychological first aid are needed to dissipate survivors' psychological and physiologic stress reactions.
- ED clinicians need to consider the differential diagnosis of various psychiatric disorders in certain groups of high-risk survivors.
- ED clinicians need to be aware that there is no evidence that psychological debriefing is effective in preventing post-traumatic stress disorder (PTSD) or improving social and occupational functioning; however, debriefing may prevent the development of substance abuse in the survivors.
- Although no medications have been specifically identified that prevent the development of acute stress disorder (ASD) or PTSD in high-risk groups, judicious and appropriate use of medications may provide symptomatic

relief of post-event reactions and help to stabilize pre-existing and post-event–induced psychiatric conditions.
• Natural disasters and terrorist attacks may present a unique opportunity for ED clinicians to teach the goals and objectives of human resilience.

Overview

Natural disasters and terrorism have become all-too-common elements of modern life in the United States and worldwide. Earthquakes, hurricanes, floods, and acts of terrorism are poignant reminders of this fact.

The difference between an act of terrorism and a disaster is one of degree; in a disaster, the social structure and processes are affected sufficiently to threaten the existence and functioning of the community. The resources needed are greater than the resources available. Preparation for a natural disaster is usually the key to survival. However, despite preparation for acts of terrorism, when terrorists strike, panic and anxiety could hamper the prepared plans of action.

Disasters may be categorized as natural (e.g., earthquakes, floods, hurricanes) or man-made (e.g., war, terrorism, industrial accidents). However, this distinction is increasingly difficult to make. The etiology and consequences of natural disasters often are affected by the actions of humans. In some instances the growth of technology has blurred the distinction between natural and man-made disasters. For example, in the earthquakes in Armenia, Iran, India, Pakistan, and Kashmir that claimed so many lives, the majority died because their homes were poorly constructed. Expansion of the world's population and construction in disaster-prone areas are two major factors contributing to the increase in destruction and displacement of huge masses of people, as was demonstrated in the aftermath of the tsunami in Thailand and of the hurricanes Katrina and Rita in the United States. The 9/11 terrorist attack in which the Twin Towers in New York City collapsed and the almost daily suicide bombings in Iraq, Palestine, and Israel are examples of "man-made" disasters.

The prominence accorded to these events on television and in the newspapers does not reflect their complexity and impact on individuals and communities. Nor do the news media typically cover the roles of mental health clinicians in the aftermath of these tragedies.

The effects of chronic stress resulting from exposure to disaster, as seen in toxic accidents such as those at Three Mile Island in Pennsylvania and Chernobyl in the Ukraine have only recently been studied and have been shown to have long-term psychiatric consequences. However, most people exposed to terrorism and other disasters do well over time and do not develop psychiatric complications. The development of these complications depends on the type of disaster, the degree of injuries and death, the duration of community disruption, and the biological, psychological, social, and spiritual vulnerability and resilience of the individuals affected by the event.

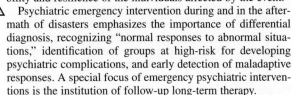

Psychiatric emergency intervention during and in the aftermath of disasters emphasizes the importance of differential diagnosis, recognizing "normal responses to abnormal situations," identification of groups at high-risk for developing psychiatric complications, and early detection of maladaptive responses. A special focus of emergency psychiatric interventions is the institution of follow-up long-term therapy.

Definition

The word "disaster" is derived from the Latin *dis* ("against") and *astrum* ("star"), literally meaning "bad star," and implying that when the stars are in a bad position, a bad event or events will happen. More recently, definitions of disaster have emphasized the social disruption that accompanies the event.

Epidemiology

Today, the world is facing disasters on an unprecedented scale: between 1994 and 2003, an average of more than 255 million people were affected by natural disasters globally each year, with a range of 68 million to 618 million. During the same period, these disasters claimed an average of 58,000 lives annually, with a range of 10,000 to 123,000. In the year 2003, 1 in 25 people worldwide was affected by a natural disaster.

During the last decade, disasters caused damage of an average of $67 billion per year, with a maximum of $230 billion and a minimum of $28 billion. The economic cost associated with natural disasters has increased 14-fold since the 1950s. Scientific evidence indicates that ongoing global climate change will result in an increase in the number of extreme events, creating more frequent and intensified natural hazards such as floods and windstorms.

It is estimated that the lifetime prevalence of exposure to traumatic events in the United States is 39.1%, and that 6% to 7% of the U.S. population is exposed to a disaster or trauma each year, ranging from motor vehicle accidents to hurricanes and tornadoes. It is also predicted that the United States will be subjected to future terrorist attacks. As a result, there is the potential for an increase in the number of people affected by these events and increased need for emergency psychiatric interventions.

Post-Event Psychological and Physiologic Reactions to Natural Disasters and Terrorism

The intensity, timing, and duration of post-event psychological and physiologic responses will vary from person to person. They may be:
- Acute or mild
- Immediate and/or delayed
- Cumulative in intensity

Phases of Post-Event Psychological Reactions

Although individual patterns of survivors' response vary, four phases of psychological response have been identified.

1. The Impact Phase
The first phase, the *impact phase*, occurs immediately following a disaster and has the following qualities:
- Emotions are strong, including feelings of disbelief, numbness, fear, and confusion.
- Panic is usually absent; survivors tend to cooperate, and heroic deeds are witnessed and performed.
- Reactions are best understood as "normal responses to an abnormal event."

2. The Rescue or Crisis Phases
The second phase, the *rescue or crisis phase*, usually lasts from days to several weeks and is characterized by the following:

- Emergency services personnel are available and survivors are willing to take directions from these groups.
- Rescue personnel, family, and neighbors compose the support network most heavily relied on at this time.
- Survivors do what they must to keep themselves and their families safe and alive.
- Survivors increasingly expect rescuers to address their immediate needs and to help them put their lives back together.

3. The Inventory or Resolution Phase

The third phase, the *inventory* or *resolution phase*, lasts from several months up to a year. During this phase:
Survivors assess damage and try to locate other survivors.

- Routine social ties tend to be discarded in favor of more functional social and community relationships.
- Assistance flows in from agencies external to the community, and the cleanup/rebuilding process begins.
- Disappointment and resentment emerge when expectations of aid and restoration are not met during this phase; survivors may believe that rebuilding efforts are not proceeding quickly enough.
- New stressors related to finding temporary living accommodations may cause survivors to pull together against their outside helpers.
- Toward the end of this phase, the strong sense of community may weaken as individuals focus on their personal concerns.

4. The Recovery or Reconstruction Phase

The fourth and final phase, the *recovery* or *reconstruction phase*, may last for years. During this period:

- Survivors gradually rebuild their lives, making homes and finding work.
- Initial psychological and physiologic symptoms are resolved through reappraisal of the event, assignment of meaning, and integration into a new concept of self.
- This phase of adaptation is manifested by denial alternating with intrusive symptoms:
  - Intrusive symptoms generally arise first and consist of unbidden thoughts and feelings, accompanied by autonomic arousal, which could lead later to the development of PTSD.

- Toward the end of the adaptation phase, denial is more prominent.
- An increase in medical visits is common, with complaints of fatigue, dizziness, headaches, and nausea.
- Anger, irritability, apathy, and social withdrawal are often present.

Survivors' reactions may become more intense as the amount of disruption to their lives increases. That is, the more the survivors' lives are disrupted, the greater their psychological and physiologic reactions. Therefore, following the establishment of a recovery environment that provides safety and physiologic recovery, post-event emergency psychiatric interventions should include assessment of normal stress reactions (a normal response to an abnormal situation). These reactions are multidimensional and depend on survivors' developmental level (e.g., whether they are children or adults) and on other factors, such as their occupation (e.g., rescue and relief workers). Possible psychological and physiologic reactions in adult survivors and rescuers are described in Box 21-1. Psychological and physiologic reactions occurring in children and adolescents are summarized in Box 21-2.

Psychological First-Aid Core Interventions

Psychological first-aid core interventions (Table 21-1) constitute the basic objectives of early assistance following terrorist attacks or other disasters. These core interventions should be flexible, using strategies that meet the specific needs of survivors. The amount of time spent on each goal will vary from person to person, according to the circumstances and presenting needs.

Basic Principles of Psychological First Aid for Survivors

- *Time*: Spend as much time as possible with psychologically traumatized individuals.
- *Reassurance*: Reassure safety, including protection from reminders of the traumatic event and ongoing stressors.
- *Assistance*: Offer available assistance even if survivors have not asked for help.
- *Countertransference*: Avoid countertransference by not taking survivors' anger or other feelings personally.

Box 21–1. Psychological and Physiologic Reactions in Adult Disaster Survivors

Emotional Reactions
- Shock, fear, grief, anger, guilt, shame
- Feeling helpless or hopeless, numb, empty
- Diminished ability to feel interest, pleasure, love

Cognitive Reactions
- Confusion, disorientation, indecisiveness, worry
- Shortened attention span, difficulty concentrating, memory loss
- Unwanted memories, self-blame

Physical Reactions
- Tension, fatigue, edginess, insomnia
- Bodily aches or pain
- Startle response, racing heartbeat, nausea
- Change in appetite, change in sex drive

Interpersonal Reactions
- Distrust, conflict, withdrawal
- Work problems, school problems, irritability
- Loss of intimacy, being over-controlling, feeling rejected or abandoned

Adapted from Office of the Surgeon General web site on medical aspects of nuclear, biological, and chemical warfare. http://www.nbc-med.org; and National Center for Post-Traumatic Stress Disorder: Disaster mental health: Dealing with the aftereffects of terrorism. http://www.ncptsd.org/terrorism/index.html

Approaches to Psychological First Aid for Survivors

To assist survivors in dealing with the effects of terrorism or other disaster-related stress, the following approaches may be implemented:

- *Establish rapport*: Listen, talk, and encourage survivors to talk about their feelings as well as their physical needs. Take the time to listen to whatever the survivors are saying.
- *Empathize*: Show through appropriate responses that the survivors' concerns or worries are understood and that such feelings are to be expected.

Box 21–2. Psychological and Physiologic Reactions in Child and Adolescent Disaster Survivors

Young Children (1-6 years)

- Helplessness and passivity; lack of usual responsiveness
- Generalized fear
- Heightened arousal and confusion
- Cognitive confusion
- Difficulty talking about event; lack of verbalization
- Difficulty identifying feelings
- Nightmares and other sleep disturbances
- Separation fears and clinging to caregivers
- Regressive symptoms (e.g., bedwetting, loss of acquired speech and motor skills)
- Inability to understand death as permanent
- Anxieties about death
- Grief related to abandonment by caregiver
- Somatic symptoms (e.g., stomach aches, headaches)
- Startle response to loud or unusual noises
- "Freezing" (sudden immobility of body)
- Fussiness, uncharacteristic crying, and neediness
- Avoidance of or alarm response to specific trauma-related reminders involving sights and physical sensations

School-Aged Children (6-11 years)

- Feelings of responsibility and guilt
- Repetitive traumatic play and retelling
- Feeling disturbed by reminders of the event
- Nightmares and other sleep disturbances
- Concerns about safety and preoccupation with danger
- Aggressive behavior and angry outbursts
- Fear of feelings and trauma reactions
- Concerns about parents' anxieties
- School avoidance
- Worry and concern about others
- Changes in behavior, mood, and personality
- Somatic symptoms (complaints about bodily aches and pains)
- Obvious anxiety and fearfulness
- Social withdrawal
- Specific trauma-related fears; general fearfulness

Continued

Box 21–2. Psychological and Physiologic Reactions in Child and Adolescent Disaster Survivors—cont'd

- Regression (behaving like a younger child)
- Separation anxiety
- Loss of interest in activities
- Confusion and inadequate understanding of the disaster (more evident in play than in discussion)
- Unclear understanding of death and the causes of "bad" events
- Giving magical explanations to fill in gaps in understanding
- Loss of ability to concentrate at school, with lowering of performance
- "Spacey" or distractible behavior

Pre-adolescents and Adolescents (12-18 years)

- Self-consciousness
- Life-threatening reenactment
- Rebellion at home or school
- Abrupt shift in relationships
- Depression and social withdrawal
- Decline in school performance
- Trauma-driven acting out, such as sexual promiscuity and reckless risk-taking
- Efforts to distance oneself from feelings of shame, guilt, and humiliation
- Excessive activity and involvement with others or retreat from others in order to manage inner turmoil
- Accident proneness
- Wish for revenge and action-oriented responses to traumatic event
- Increased self-focusing and withdrawal
- Sleep and eating disturbances, including nightmares

Adapted from the National Center for Post-Traumatic Stress Disorder. Disaster mental health: Dealing with the aftereffects of terrorism; web site:. http://www.ncptsd.org/terrorism/index.html

Table 21–1

Psychological First Aid Core Interventions

Intervention	Goal
Contact and engagement	Respond to contacts initiated by affected persons, or initiate contacts in a nonintrusive, compassionate, and supportive manner
Safety and comfort	Enhance immediate and ongoing safety, and provide physical and emotional comfort
Stabilization	Calm and orient emotionally overwhelmed and distraught survivors
Information gathering	Identify immediate needs and concerns by gathering information, and tailoring it to fit the needs of the individual
Practical assistance	Offer practical help to the survivor in addressing immediate needs and concerns
Connection with social support	Help establish brief or ongoing contacts with primary support persons or other sources of support, including family members, friends, and community helping resources
Information on coping	Provide information about stress reactions and coping to reduce distress and promote adaptive functioning
Linkage with collaborative services	Link survivors with needed services and inform them about available services that may be needed in the future

Adapted from Cloak NL, Edwards P: Psychological first aid: Emergency care for terrorism and disaster survivors. Curr Psychiatry 2004;35:12-23.

- *Provide confidentiality*: Respect the survivors' confidentiality, and do not disclose personal information to others.

By using these approaches you will provide survivors with the initial comfort and support that are needed in taking a first step toward recovery.

Psychological First Aid for Rescuers

To assist rescue workers in dealing with the effects of terrorism or other disaster-related stress, the following approaches should be considered:

- *Briefing*: Explain to rescue personnel before the rescue operation begins what they can expect to see and what they can expect in terms of psychological reactions in themselves and others.
- *Emphasize teamwork*: Sharing the workload and emotional load with team members can help to defuse pent-up emotions. Team members are also encouraged to share their experiences with other rescue workers.
- *Rotate*: Encourage rescuers to rest and regroup to avoid fatigue and exhaustion.
- *Encourage breaks*: Encourage rescuers to take breaks away from affected areas.
- *Provide adequate and proper nutrition*: Ensure that rescuers have adequate food and water; avoid caffeine or high carbohydrate–containing beverages.
- *Gradually phase out rescue personnel*: Abrupt removal of rescuers from their duties could precipitate additional stress. They should be allowed to gradually stand down from the incident by easing from high- to medium- to low-stress situations.

Psychiatric ED interventions other than psychological first aid are not usually needed unless individuals:

- Are a danger to themselves or others
- Exhibit psychotic symptoms
- Lack social support networks
- Are unable to perform activities of daily living that are necessary for self-care
- Have lost the ability to begin the recovery process

Psychiatric Emergency Assessment

Psychiatric emergency providers, including ED clinicians, need to assess the adaptive, psychological, and physiologic responses of survivors so as to intervene appropriately.

Psychiatric Disorders Associated with Disasters

A myriad of psychiatric disorders are associated with disasters. The less severe the disaster or traumatic event, the more important the role of preexisting psychiatric disorders in predicting the outcome; the more severe the stressor, the less important the role of preexisting psychiatric disorders.

Mass Panic

Mass panic is characterized by intense contagious fear whereby individuals behave with reference only to self. There may be flight in a desire to escape, or alternatively, people may become behaviorally "frozen" or paralyzed. Mass panic leads to a loss of social organization and social roles as well as substantial community chaos.

One might anticipate that mass panic would be a common problem after a devastating attack; however, it did not occur after the Sarin gas attack in Tokyo, the Israeli SCUD missile attacks, the Oklahoma City bombing, or following the 9/11 attack on the Twin Towers in New York City. It is not yet clear if a mass panic did occur during the aftermath of hurricane Katrina in New Orleans. Although mass panic does occur, it is actually rare after disasters. Instead, social, adaptive, and helpful behavior is the norm.

Risk factors for mass panic include:
- Belief that there is a minimal chance of escaping
- Perceived high risk
- Unavailability or limited availability of treatment resources
- Perception of ineffective treatment response
- Loss of credibility of authorities

The risk of mass panic is reduced by providing accurate knowledge even if the information is disturbing, and providing advanced training of rescue personnel, with disaster simulation. Mass media communication can be either a vector for propagating distress and misperceptions or an effective tool for educating the public and promoting responsible behaviors. When interviewed by reporters, front-line experts, including medical personnel, may either fuel panic or calm and reassure the public.

Major Depression

Depression is associated with prolonged grief reactions and strongly related to the accumulation of post-event problems. Depressive symptoms include persistent depressed or irritable mood, loss of appetite, sleep disturbances such as early morning awakening, greatly diminished interest or pleasure in life activities, fatigue or loss of energy, feelings of worthlessness or guilt, feelings of hopelessness, and thoughts about suicide.

Demoralization is a common response to unfulfilled expectations about improvement in recovery efforts.

Dissociative Symptoms

Dissociative symptoms such as depersonalization, derealization, fugue, and amnesia may develop. These symptoms need to be differentiated from psychotic symptoms.

Generalized Anxiety Disorder (GAD)

Symptoms of preexisting GAD may be seen; however, post-event new-onset GAD often occurs.

Adjustment Disorders

Adjustment disorders may occur, with symptoms such as anxious and depressed mood or mixed emotions manifested by rage, extreme irritability, intense agitation, extreme numbness, inability to control emotions, persistent problems in work or school, and significant problems in self-care. Adjustment disorders are relatively common during the 6 to 12 months after a disaster and may reflect survivors' reactions to acquired physical injuries.

Phobias

Various phobic symptoms, such as fear of confined places after being trapped in a mining accident or refusal to go indoors following an earthquake, may arise after a disaster. These symptoms require evaluation and intervention to treat the specific phobia and to limit transference to other areas of life.

Traumatic Grief

Traumatic grief is an example of a complicated grief reaction that occurs following the traumatic death of someone close. In traumatic bereavement, the individual is preoccupied with images of the traumatic event, rather than of the person who is deceased, as in normal bereavement. Moreover, the mourning process lasts longer than expected, hindering recovery to normal life functioning.

Somatization

Somatization, a process in which psychological needs are expressed as physical symptoms, is a frequent presentation of anxiety and depression in patients seeking medical care; its recognition can help in the appropriate diagnosis and treatment of these psychiatric disorders, thereby avoiding inappropriate medical treatment.

Psychological Factors Affecting Physical Conditions

Concomitant psychological symptoms are frequently seen in injured victims who may be dealing with the stress of their injury, the loss of family members, and an absence of resources and social support networks with which to plan recovery. The symptoms of fear, demoralization, anxiety, and depression may be exacerbated by continued apprehension about possible risk and may exacerbate the physical condition of the injured.

Acute Stress Disorder (ASD) and Posttraumatic Stress Disorder (PTSD)

These two conditions can occur at higher than average rates. In ASD, symptoms begin within 4 weeks of a traumatic event and last from 2 days to 4 weeks. The symptoms are not due to the direct effects of a substance, a general medical condition, or an exacerbation of a preexisting disorder. The development of ASD may predict an adverse outcome and may be associated with increased rates of somatic complaints. Acute symptoms of intrusion, avoidance, and dissociation, which are part of the symptom complex of ASD, may predict the development of later psychiatric disorders, particularly PTSD. PTSD has been widely studied following both natural and man-made disasters. Table 21-2 compares ASD and PTSD (also see Chapter 20).

Toxic Exposure

Toxic exposure to the various chemical and biological agents described here can have serious psychological effects.

Chemical Agents

- *Organophosphate compounds such as Sarin, Soman VX, and Tabun*: Impaired cognition, depression, anxiety, sleep disturbances, delirium

Table 21–2

Comparison of ASD and PTSD

Clinical Presentation	PTSD	ASD
Nature of Trauma/Reaction to Trauma		
Individual experienced, witnessed, or was confronted with event that involved actual or threatened death or serious injury or a threat to the physical integrity of self or others	Present	Present
Individual's response involved intense feelings of fear, horror, or helplessness	Present	Present
Symptom Criteria		
Persistent re-experiencing of trauma	Present	Present
Avoidance of reminders of trauma	Present	Present
Physical symptoms of hyperarousal	Present	Present
Symptoms of dissociation during or immediately after trauma	Absent	Present
Clinically significant distress or impairment	Present	Present
Time Requirements		
Duration of symptom constellation	>1 month	2 days to 4 weeks
Onset of symptoms in relation to trauma	Any time following trauma	Within 4 weeks of trauma

ASD, acute stress disorder; PTSD, post-traumatic stress disorder.
Adapted from Ursano RJ, Fullerton CS, Norwood AE: Psychiatric dimensions of disaster: Patient care, community consultation, and preventive medicine. Harv Rev Psychiatry 1995;3:196-209.

- *Atropine*: Blurred vision, tachycardia, impaired cognition, psychosis, delirium
- *Cyanide*: Anxiety, confusion, giddiness, hyperventilation
- *Blistering agents such as mustard gas and phosgene*: Psychological distress due to disfigurement such as blindness and burns

Biological Agents
All biological agents can cause delirium, which should be differentiated from dissociative phenomena.
- *Anthrax*: Meningitis

- *Brucella canis* (Brucellosis): Depression, irritability, headache
- *Coxiella burnetii* (Q fever): Malaise, fatigue, hallucinations
- Botulinum toxin: Depression due to the long recovery time
- *Viruses causing encephalitis*: Impaired cognition and depression.

Reactions to Attacks Using Chemical and Biological Agents

Several unique features of chemical and biological agents make them especially terrifying. Like radiation, they are frequently invisible and odorless. Individuals exposed to or infected with certain agents may initially develop symptoms of common illnesses and therefore escape early detection. Many of these agents may be unfamiliar to American physicians and treatment may not be readily available. Some agents cause gross deformities such as the lesions of smallpox and the severe blisters of mustard gas.

The unseen and mysterious nature of these agents may lead to mass panic, such as the so-called gas hysteria seen during World War I. During that time, there were twice as many cases of gas hysteria as there were actual cases of gas exposure. Similar syndromes include conversion reactions with respiratory features and gas mask phobia, which was a significant problem during the Persian Gulf War. The protective gear worn during chemical and biological attacks increases one's sense of isolation, decreases intragroup communication, and may increase the incidence of psychiatric casualties.

The behavioral response to biological agents differs from that to chemical agents. There is usually a time delay between initial exposure to a biological agent and the development of symptoms. The first responders to a biological attack will include ED personnel and public health officials; firemen and emergency medical technicians (EMTs) usually are the first responders to a chemical attack.

If the attack is covert, it may initially appear to be a natural outbreak. On the other hand, terrorists may claim responsibility for a natural outbreak to further their agenda.

People may have unfounded fears about the contagious spread of disease across a region or nation, especially when there is uncertainty about the attack or questions about the effectiveness of treatment. Attempted quarantine, infection control, vaccination, and treatment programs may be accompanied by negative rumors, which can do real harm by creating a public opinion backlash against government and public health officials.

Other Causes of Psychiatric Disorders Associated with Disasters

⚠ Medically induced mental disorders often are overlooked after a terrorist attack or other disaster. Any physical injury can increase the risk of psychiatric disorders. These include central nervous system (CNS) disorders attributable to head trauma and metabolic disturbances following crush injuries and burns.

Responses to medications used for resuscitation or pain control, such as atropine, epinephrine, lidocaine, and morphine, can lead to alterations in mental status.

Infections due to lack of appropriate sanitation and destruction of sewage systems can cause rapidly progressing meningitis, with psychiatric symptoms such as lethargy, confusion, coma, and seizures.

When resources are limited and employment and financial resources are scarce in the community, as is frequently the case following a natural or man-made disaster, family violence (including spouse, child, and elder abuse) increases, with high morbidity and significant mortality. Hostility, with its accompanying social disruption, feelings of frustration, and perception of chaos, is common. Overt and ongoing hostility in patients presenting to the ED should remind the ED clinician to assess for the risk of family violence and substance abuse.

Factors That Affect the Development of Psychiatric Disorders in Survivors

Factors that influence the development of psychiatric disorders in disaster survivors include:
- Previous experience with a similar event
- Intensity of the disruption
- Length of time that has elapsed between the event occurrence and the present circumstances
- Feeling that there is no escape, setting the stage for the development of ASD and/or PTSD
- Pre-event psychological and social functioning

High-Risk Groups
The following groups have been identified as being at greater risk for traumatic stress-related reactions.

Rescue Workers

Disaster and rescue workers often develop PTSD and other stress-related disorders. They are repeatedly exposed to mutilated bodies, mass destruction, and life-threatening situations while performing physically demanding work that in itself entails fatigue, sleep loss, and dangerous risks. Despite their training and experience, rescuers may be overwhelmed by the scale of destruction and the technical difficulties that complicate rescue procedures. Under such circumstances, they may experience persistent feelings of guilt, helplessness, and incompetence.

"Hidden" Workers

Hidden workers, such as those who handle telephone hot lines, are also at risk for stress-related disorders, despite their relative distance from the events.

Injured Survivors

Survivors who have been injured and those who have the perception of being at high risk for death or injury are at high risk for adverse psychological responses.

Heroes

Heroes are part of every disaster. Empirical observations suggest that they are often overlooked as a highly stressed group. Heroes are isolated by the burden of idealization placed on them by the community. They are often expected to travel and give talks, to be upbeat and inspiring, and always to be good. Seldom are they encouraged to express their own feelings of despair, worry, and fear, nor are they afforded the privacy and time to recall these feelings, which they ignored while performing their heroic acts.

Medical Personnel

In addition to performing medical interventions, medical personnel handle the personal effects of the injured and dead, such as wallets, photographs, and jewelry. This is particularly stressful, because they are reminders of the lives of deceased victims.

Leaders

Leaders experience great stress because often they must make rapid decisions with little or no information and must instill hope in others despite their own fears.

Individuals Deemed Responsible for a Disaster

Individuals considered responsible for a disaster are vulnerable to feelings of guilt, anger, and resentment toward self. They may be at risk of social withdrawal and isolation. Intense self-blame and self-criticism as well as criticism by the community may predispose these individuals to suicidal ideation and acts.

The Elderly

Preexisting problems in the elderly such as chronic illness and medication use, memory disorders, and limited mobility may be exacerbated in the aftermath of a disaster or may be secondary to injury occurring during evacuation.

Children

Children may manifest a wide array of post-event symptoms, including depression, sleep disturbances, anxiety, trauma-specific fears, behavioral problems, and somatic disorders. The level of distress in children tends to increase with the age of the child and with preexisting health problems of the parents or child. The child's exposure to a disaster as well as the parents' reactions are prominent predictors of morbidity.

Interventions with parents and families are directed at (1) assisting children to regain a sense of safety; (2) validating children's emotional reactions rather than discouraging or minimizing them; (3) anticipating and providing additional support during times of heightened distress, such as anniversaries of the event; and (4) minimizing secondary stresses.

Single Parents

Single parents often have fewer resources than couples, and they may have lost some of the social support network that could have helped with recovery plans.

Ethnic Groups

Certain ethnic groups are particularly susceptible to the stress of disasters. These include immigrants and refugees, many of whom had left their country of origin because of natural disasters or man-made atrocities. PTSD caused by pre-migration trauma may become exacerbated by the recent disaster experience. Older immigrants, who had difficulty with acculturation and language acquisition, are particularly susceptible to stress.

Overall, groups in lower socioeconomic levels and at-risk populations such as refugees will experience a greater level of psychological and physiologic distress from disasters. Under-standing the culture of a community is necessary in order to intervene effectively in that community.

Bereaved Individuals

Individuals who have lost a loved one such as a family mem-ber, friend, or pet are at high risk for adverse psychological reactions. Actually witnessing the loss increases the risk.

Media Representatives

Media representatives are under constant pressure to report the latest developments following a disaster, thereby com-pounding the stress inherent in the disaster itself.

Predisposing Conditions for Developing Psychiatric Complications

These may include the following:

- *Threat*: The higher the perception of threat of death or injury, the more likely that an adverse psychiatric response will develop.
- *Physical harm or injury*: Crush injuries, burns, and later illnesses resulting from the breakdown of sanitation systems lead to an increase in destructive impact.
- *Exposure to traumatic scenes*: Viewing dead or mutilated victims of a disaster increases the risk of psychiatric illness, especially in emergency personnel, rescue workers, firemen and police officers.
- *Sudden, violent loss of a loved one*: The unexpected, violent death of a family member or friend is especially difficult and gives rise to bereavement issues. The bereaved survivor may experience intrusive images surrounding the circumstances of the death.
- *Witnessing or learning of violence to a loved one*: This can lead to the development of intrusive thoughts related to the violent event.
- *Learning of exposure to a noxious agent*: Exposure to toxins and/or radiation often goes undetected, sometimes for decades. Revelation of the exposure, and the threat of illness, injury, or death, can create severe stress.
- *Causing death or severe harm to another*: Technological disasters such as plane crashes, which are often caused by human error, can precipitate psychiatric distress in the people who committed the error. The stress and distress is

compounded by the belief that the disaster could have been prevented.

- *Intentional injury/harm*: Perpetrating deliberate injury and massive death, as in the Oklahoma City bombing and the 9/11 terrorist attack, can provoke strong emotions, thoughts, and behaviors in survivors and eye-witnesses.

ED Psychiatric Intervention

ED psychiatric intervention includes psychiatric therapy, psychological debriefing, psychoeducation and support, and pharmacological treatment. See earlier section on Psychological First-Aid Core Interventions for initial treatment strategies.

Psychiatric Therapy

Initiation or referral for treatment of psychiatric disorders, especially in high-risk groups, is advisable. Appropriate treatment for these disorders includes psychosocial support and interventions to deal with post-event stressors.

Psychological Debriefing

Psychological debriefing provides education about trauma experiences, It is an early intervention originally developed for rescue workers that has been widely applied in the aftermath of potentially traumatic events.

Critical Incident Stress Debriefing (CISD)

CISD is a structured, one-session group intervention in which survivors' experiences and emotional reactions are discussed and education and follow-up recommendations are provided. The usual practice is for the debriefer to provide educational information about stress management and the normal psychological/physiologic response to acutely stressful situations. Although it is common for group participants to express profound feelings about an incident they have witnessed or experienced, CISD is not a group psychotherapy session. Feelings expressed are acknowledged but not probed by the group leader.

When properly structured and facilitated, these sessions result in participants feeling that they are experiencing normal reactions to an abnormal event and have the tools needed to manage their stress. In some cases CISD affords the debriefer the opportunity to identify individuals who need follow-up assistance such as referral for psychotherapy.

The formal CISD process consists of seven standard phases:

1. *Introductory phase*: In this phase of debriefing, the team leader introduces the CISD process and approach, encourages participation by the group, and sets the ground rules by which the process will operate.
2. *Fact phase*: During this phase, group members are asked to describe briefly their job or role during the incident and, from their own perspective, some facts regarding what happened.
3. *Thought phase*: In this phase, the CISD leader asks the group members to discuss their first thoughts during the critical incident.
4. *Feeling or reaction phase*: This phase is designed to move the group participants from the predominantly cognitive level of intellectual processing to the emotional level of processing. Group participants discuss their feelings about the incident. Listening to the others talk about their feelings during this phase of the debriefing is beneficial in and of itself. Many participants will discover that the reactions they had or are currently experiencing are similar to the feelings and reactions of other group members.
5. *Symptom phase*: This phase begins the movement back from the predominantly emotional processing level toward the cognitive processing level. Participants are asked to describe the physical, cognitive, emotional, and behavioral signs and symptoms of distress that they experienced (1) at the scene, (2) within 24 hours of the incident, and (3) a few days after the incident, and (4) that they are still experiencing at the time of the debriefing.
6. *Teaching phase*: Information is exchanged about the nature of the stress response and the expected psychological and physiologic reactions to critical incidents. The process of critical-incident stress, stress reactions, and techniques to decrease stress are explored. This serves to normalize the stress and coping response, and provides a basis for questions and answers.
7. *Re-entry phase*: This is a wrap-up in which any additional questions or statements are addressed, referrals for

individual follow-ups are made, and general group solidarity and bonding are reinforced.

ED clinicians need to be aware that there is no evidence that psychological debriefing is effective in preventing PTSD or improving social and occupational functioning. In some instances, debriefing may increase symptoms, especially when used with groups of unknown individuals with widely varying trauma exposures or when administered early after trauma exposure before safety and decreased arousal are established. Psychological debriefing, however, may be beneficial in decreasing or preventing the development of substance abuse in survivors.

Psychoeducation and Support

Early interventions with psychoeducation and support appear to be helpful in reducing the psychological complications of exposure to mass violence or disaster.

When access to expert care is limited by environmental conditions or reduced availability of medical resources, rapid dissemination of educational materials may help many survivors to deal effectively with subsyndromal manifestations of traumatic exposure.

Early supportive interventions, psychoeducation, and case management appear to be helpful in acutely traumatized individuals because they promote engagement in ongoing care and may facilitate entry into evidence-based psychotherapeutic and psychopharmacological treatments.

Encouraging acutely traumatized persons to rely on their inherent strengths, their existing support networks, and their own judgment may reduce the need for further intervention.

Pharmacological Treatment

General Guidelines

Although no medications have been specifically developed to prevent ASD or PTSD in high-risk groups, use of certain medications may stabilize symptoms within the first 48 hours of the event.

Sedating medications may affect neurologic assessment of the injured, thus hindering ongoing monitoring and follow-up plans. Medications should be used judiciously; if indicated, anxiolytics, antidepressants, and sleep medications can be effective. When patients are acutely psychotic or agitated or if their behavior endangers themselves or others, medication may be necessary.

Medications for Agitation and Psychosis

Medications for agitation and psychosis include fast-acting benzodiazepines and antipsychotic agents. The ED clinician should always provide structure and supervision for medicated patients.

Option 1

The amount needed to calm a patient is roughly the same amount needed for the next 24 hours.

- Haloperidol, 5 mg intramuscularly (IM), orally (PO), or as a concentrate every 30 min until patient is calm
- Lorazepam 1 to 2 mg IM or PO every 4 hours as needed for anxiety
- Benztropine,1 mg PO or IM, or diphenhydramine, 50 mg PO or IM, can be given along with any haloperidol dose that exceeds 10 mg to prevent the possible emergence of dystonic reactions

Option 2

Option 2 is a combination antipsychotic and benzodiazepine. For fewer side effects, use less of each type of medication.

- Haloperidol, 5 mg IM, PO, or as a concentrate every 30 minutes until patient is calm
- Alternate with lorazepam, 2 mg IM, PO, or concentrate every 30 minutes prn until patient is calm

Option 3

- Chlorpromazine, 25 mg IM; never give more than a total of 50 mg IM because of the risk of severe hypotension; avoid use in the elderly and debilitated

Adjunctive antipsychotic medications are summarized in Table 21-3.

Medications for Sleep Disturbances

Patients with persistent sleep disturbances not responding to relaxation therapy, implementation of sleep hygiene techniques, or reconditioning may benefit from temporary use of hypnotic medications such as benzodiazepines until a normal sleep rhythm is established. Commonly prescribed benzodiazepines for sleep disturbances are flurazepam (Dalmane), estazolam

Table 21–3

Adjunctive Antipsychotic Treatments

Medication	Type of Medication	Daily Dose Range	Comments
Haloperidol	High-potency conventional antipsychotic	10-20 mg	Available as tablet, liquid concentrate, and short- and long-acting injectable formulations
Perphenazine	Medium-potency conventional antipsychotic	4-60 mg	Available as oral and injectable short-acting formulations
Chlorpromazine	Low-potency conventional antipsychotic	300-1000 mg	Available as tablets or oral concentration; may cause hypotension and sedation
Risperidone	Atypical antipsychotic	1-8 mg	Available as oral formulation, liquid concentrate, disintegrating tablet, and injectable long-acting formulations
Olanzapine	Atypical antipsychotic	5-10 mg	Available as disintegrating tablet and oral and injectable short-acting formulations
Ziprasidone	Atypical antipsychotic	20-80 mg	Available as oral and injectable short-acting formulations

(ProSom), temazepam (Restoril), and triazolam (Halcion). This group of drugs can be effective in inducing and maintaining sleep, relieving both nighttime and daytime symptoms. The most common side effects of these drugs are residual daytime drowsiness and withdrawal symptoms, including rebound insomnia if these agents are abruptly discontinued. The development of tolerance and dependence limits the use of benzodiazepines as long-term treatment for sleep disturbances. Another group of hypnotics, including zolpidem (Ambien) and zaleplon (Sonata), can be used for short-term treatment. Eszopiclone (Lunesta) can be used for a long-term period of up to 6 months.

Antidepressants, especially sedating antidepressants such as trazodone, can also be used in small doses for temporary relief of sleep disturbances. Although not generally characterized as hypnotics, the sedative effects of antihistamines such as diphenhydramine products can be used if no other agents are available for inducing drowsiness and sleep. Patients should be strongly advised against the use of alcohol and other sedative/hypnotic medications when taking medications for sleep. Table 21-4 summarizes some of the medications used for treatment of sleep disturbances.

Medications for Anxiety Disorders, ASD, PTSD, and Depression

Table 21-5 lists various pharmacological interventions that may be used for the treatment of anxiety disorders, depression, ASD, and PTSD.

Although no medications are available that will prevent the development of ASD or PTSD, certain medications can stabilize various anxiety disorders and provide symptomatic relief of ASD and PTSD.

Selective serotonin reuptake inhibitors (SSRIs), antidepressants, buspirone, and benzodiazepines offer effective treatment interventions for anxiety disorders. SSRIs and other antidepressants represent reasonable clinical interventions for ASD. SSRIs are recommended as first-line treatment for PTSD because they have relatively few side effects and they ameliorate the three PTSD symptom clusters—re-experiencing, avoidance/numbing, and hyperarousal. Also, SSRI therapy may reduce clinical symptoms of suicidality, impulsivity, and aggressive behaviors that often complicate management of PTSD (also see Chapter 20).

Text continues on page 509.

Table 21-4

Medications for Sleep Disturbances

Medication	Class	Properties	Daily Dose Range	Comments
Triazolam	Benzodiazepine	Short-acting	0.124-0.25 mg	Anterograde amnesia and rebound insomnia may occur with high doses; this medication has been banned in some countries
Estazolam	Benzodiazepine	Intermediate-acting	1-2 mg	Withdrawal symptoms may occur after discontinuation of long-term use
Lorazepam	Benzodiazepine	Intermediate-acting	1-4 mg	Withdrawal symptoms may occur after discontinuation of long-term use
Temazepam	Benzodiazepine	Intermediate-acting	15-30 mg	Because of slow absorption, sleep-onset insomnia may not respond
Clonazepam	Benzodiazepine	Long-acting	0.5-2.0 mg	Beneficial effects on restless legs syndrome
Flurazepam	Benzodiazepine	Long-acting	15-30 mg	Active metabolites lead to morning residual effects
Quazepam	Benzodiazepine	Long-acting	7.5-15 mg	Accumulation of side effects could occur with chronic dosing

Medication	Class	Properties	Daily Dose Range	Comments
Zolpidem	Hypnotic	Short-acting	5-10 mg	Minimal next-day residual effects; daytime drowsiness occasionally occurs; withdrawal symptoms, such as nausea, may occur if abruptly discontinued; long-term use may lead to loss of hypnotic effects
Zaleplon	Hypnotic	Short-acting	5-10 mg	Minimal next-day residual effects such as daytime drowsiness occasionally occur; withdrawal symptoms, such as nausea, may occur if abruptly discontinued; long-term use may lead to loss of hypnotic effects
Eszopiclone	Hypnotic	Short-acting	1-3 mg	Hypnotic effects may last for 6 months
Trazodone	Antidepressant	Short- and long-acting	50-150 mg	Induces sleep through sedation; daytime drowsiness, hypotension, and priapism are rare complications
Diphenhydramine, hydroxyzine, and others	Antihistamines	Vary	Varies	Because of sedative effect, may be prescribed for sleep disturbances; side effects include daytime sleepiness, cognitive impairment, dry mouth, and elevated blood pressure; long-term use is not recommended
Ramelteon	Hypnotic	Short-acting	4-8 mg	Effective for chronic and transient insomnia characterized by difficulty with sleep onset; decreases mean latency to persistent sleep; it is a non-controlled substance; can cause drowsiness, dizziness, headache

Table 21–5

Pharmacological Interventions for Depression, Anxiety, ASD, and PTSD

Agent (Oral Dose Range)	Absolute and Relative Contraindications	Adverse Events	Remarks
Selective Serotonin Reuptake Inhibitors (SSRIs)			
Fluoxetine (20–60 mg/d) Paroxetine (20–60 mg/d) Sertraline (50–200 mg/d) Fluvoxamine (50–150 mg bid) Citalopram (20–60 mg/d) Escitalopram (10–40 mg/d)	MAOI use within past 14 days; hypersensitivity	Nausea, headache, sexual dysfunction, hyponatremia, SIADH	Avoid abrupt discontinuation of all agents except fluoxetine; citalopram and sertraline are less likely to be involved in hepatic enzyme drug interactions; fluoxetine and fluvoxamine are generically available
Tricyclic Antidepressants			
Imipramine (150–300 mg/d) Amitriptyline (150–300 mg/d) Desipramine (100–300 mg/d) Nortriptyline (50–150 mg/d) Protriptyline (30–60 mg/d) Clomipramine (150–250 mg/d)	MAOI use within past 14 days; acute myocardial infarction within past 3 months; coronary artery disease; prostatic enlargement; clomipramine contraindicated for patients with history of seizure disorders	Anticholinergic effects; orthostatic hypotension; tachycardia; increased heart rate; ventricular arrhythmias	Desipramine and nortriptyline have lower rate of anticholinergic and hypotensive effects; nortriptyline has a therapeutic blood level

Table 21-5

Pharmacological Interventions for Depression, Anxiety, ASD, and PTSD—cont'd

Agent (Oral Dose Range)	Absolute and Relative Contraindications	Adverse Events	Remarks
MAOIs			
Phenelzine (target, 1 mg/kg/d) Tranylcypromine (target, 0.7 mg/kg/d)	All antidepressants within past 7 days of start of MAOI, except fluoxetine (within past 5 weeks); CNS stimulants and decongestants	Hypertensive crisis with drug/tyramine interactions; bradycardia; orthostatic hypotension; insomnia	Patient must maintain tyramine-free diet; doses should be taken in the morning to reduce insomnia
Antihypertensive Agents			
Beta-adrenergic blocking agents: Propranolol (10-120 mg/d)	Propranolol: sinus bradycardia, congestive heart failure	Propranolol: hypotension, bronchospasm, bradycardia	Propranolol has only been used in a single dose for prevention of PTSD
Alpha-adrenergic agonists: Clonidine (0.5 mg PO qd; increase by 0.5 mg q3-4d until dose reaches 0.1-0.3 mg/d PO divided tid) Guanfacine (0.5 mg PO qd; increase by 0.5 mg q3d until desired effect is reached)	Clonidine and guanfacine: documented hypersensitivity; cardiovascular disease; depressive symptoms		

Continued

Table 21–5

Pharmacological Interventions for Depression, Anxiety, ASD, and PTSD—cont'd

Agent (Oral Dose Range)	Absolute and Relative Contraindications	Adverse Events	Remarks
Alpha-adrenergic blockers:			
Prazosin (target, 6–10 mg/d; start with 1 mg at bedtime and increase as blood pressure allows)		Prazosin: first-dose syncope/sudden loss of consciousness (in 1% of patients given 2 mg or greater)	Prazosin is primarily used for management of recurrent distressing dreams
Novel Antidepressants			
Mirtazapine (15–60 mg/d)	MAOI use within past 14 days	Mirtazapine: sedation, increased appetite, weight gain, agranulocytosis (rare)	Give bupropion in regular-release single doses >150 mg/d and total daily dose >450 mg/d; reduce dose in low-weight patients
Bupropion (150–450 mg/d)	Bupropion contraindicated for patients with seizure disorders, anorexia/bulimia		
Nefazodone (300–600 mg/d)		Trazodone and nefazodone: sedation, priapism (rare)	Taper down venlafaxine to prevent rebound signs/symptoms; obtain baseline and periodic LFTs when treating with nefazodone; nefazodone not recommended as initial
Trazodone (300–600 mg/d)			
SNRIs:			
Venlafaxine (150–375 mg/d)	Duloxetine has not been used yet for treatment of PTSD	Venlafaxine: hypertension in patients with and without preexisting hypertension	
Duloxetine (20–60 mg/d)			

Agent (Oral Dose Range)	Absolute and Relative Contraindications	Adverse Events	Remarks
			treatment but can be given for patients already maintained on it who have not developed hepatotoxicity; duloxetine also indicated for treatment of diabetic peripheral neuropathy; this group has a lower rate of sexual dysfunction compared with SSRIs
		Nefazodone: hepatotoxicity (not recommended as initial treatment. Can be given for patients already maintained on it who have not developed hepatotoxicity	
Anticonvulsants/Mood Stabilizers			
Carbamazepine (target, 400-1600 mg/d)	Bone marrow suppression, particularly leukopenia	Leukopenia, SIADH, drowsiness, ataxia	Therapeutic blood levels not established but blood level monitoring may be useful in cases of suspected toxicity with carbamazepine; if given with valproate, max dose of lamotrigine is 200 mg
Gabapentin (target, 300-3600 mg/d)	Renal impairment	Sedation, ataxia	
Lamotrigine (target, 25-500 mg/d; start at 25 mg qod for 2 weeks, then	Increased rash when administered with valproate or other anticonvulsants	Stevens-Johnson syndrome, fatigue	

Continued

Table 21-5

Pharmacological Interventions for Depression, Anxiety, ASD, and PTSD—cont'd

Agent (Oral Dose Range)	Absolute and Relative Contraindications	Adverse Events	Remarks
25 mg qd for 2 weeks, then 25-50 mg qd for 1-2 weeks, up to 400 mg/d or as tolerated)			
Topiramate (target, 200-400 mg/d)	Hepatic impairment	Angle closure glaucoma, sedation, dizziness, ataxia, kidney stones	
Valproate (target, 10-15 mg/kg/d)	Impaired liver function, thrombocytopenia	Nausea/vomiting, sedation, ataxia, thrombocytopenia, weight gain, hepatotoxicity	
Benzodiazepines Clonazepam (0.25 mg bid; increase 0.25 mg q1-2d divided bid) Lorazepam (1-10 mg/d divided bid/tid) Alprazolam (1.5-6 mg/d) Diazepam (10-40 mg/d)	Use with caution in elderly patients and patients with impaired liver function; risk of abuse in patients with history of substance abuse	Sedation, memory impairment, ataxia, dependence	Tolerance, withdrawal; lethal if overdosed with alcohol or other CNS depressants

Agent (Oral Dose Range)	Absolute and Relative Contraindications	Adverse Events	Remarks
Typical Antipsychotics (Neuroleptics, Conventional Antipsychotics, Major Tranquilizers)			
Chlorpromazine (100–800 mg/d)	Parkinson's disease QTc prolongation	Sedation, orthostatic hypotension with chlorpromazine and thioridazine; akathisia, dystonia, drug-induced parkinsonism; tardive dyskinesia may occur with all antipsychotics with long-term use; NMS and also QTc changes could occur	Therapeutic doses not established; use should be well justified because of the risk of tardive dyskinesia, retinitis pigmentosa, and NMS; thioridazine is rarely used as a first-line treatment but can be given for patients already maintained on it
Haloperidol (2–20 mg/d)			
Thioridazine (100–800 mg/d)			
Atypical Antipsychotics			
Olanzapine (5–20 mg/d)	Parkinson's disease	Sedation, weight gain, NMS; higher doses may cause akathisia, drug-induced parkinsonism, especially with risperidone doses >6 mg/d	Therapeutic doses not established; weight gain occurs with all agents; however, olanzapine produces significantly greater gain; relative risk of tardive dyskinesia compared with
Quetiapine (300–800 mg/d)			
Risperidone (1–6 mg/d)			

Continued

Table 21-5

Pharmacological Interventions for Depression, Anxiety, ASD, and PTSD—cont'd

Agent (Oral Dose Range)	Absolute and Relative Contraindications	Adverse Events	Remarks
			typical antipsychotics has not been established; monitor for development of diabetes and hyperglycemia
Non-benzodiazepines			
Hypnotics: Zaleplon (5-10 mg/d) Zolpidem (5-10 mg/d)	Use with caution in patients with alcohol/drug abuse history, in elderly patients, and in patients with liver dysfunction	Sedation, ataxia; rebound insomnia may occur	Abuse can occur, resulting in withdrawal reactions
Anti-anxiety agents: Buspirone (20-60 mg/d)	MAOI use within past 14 days	Nausea, headache	

ASD, acute stress disorder; CNS, central nervous system; LFTs, liver function tests; MAOIs, monoamine oxidase inhibitors; NMS, neuroleptic malignant syndrome; PTSD, posttraumatic stress disorder; SIADH, syndrome of inappropriate antidiuretic hormone; SNRIs, serotonin/norepinephrine reuptake inhibitors.

Adapted from Khouzam HR, Donnelly NJ: Posttraumatic stress disorder. Safe, effective management in the primary care setting. Postgrad Med 2001;110:60-78.

SSRIs are effective treatments for psychiatric disorders that are frequently comorbid with PTSD, including depression, panic disorder, social phobia, and obsessive-compulsive disorder.

Tricyclic antidepressants (TCAs) and monoamine oxidase inhibitors (MAOIs) may also be beneficial. Minimal evidence is available to recommend the use of other antidepressants such as venlafaxine, mirtazapine, bupropion, trazodone, and nefazodone. Trazodone may be beneficial for sleep difficulties.

Benzodiazepines may be useful in reducing anxiety and improving sleep. Their efficacy in preventing PTSD or treating the core symptoms of PTSD has not been established or adequately evaluated. Concerns about addictive potential in individuals with comorbid substance use disorders warrants caution regarding the use of benzodiazepines. Worsening of symptoms with benzodiazepine discontinuation has been reported.

Anticonvulsant/mood stabilizers such as carbamazepine, valproate, topiramate, and lamotrigine may be beneficial in treating symptoms related to re-experiencing of trauma.

Second-generation atypical antipsychotic medications such as olanzapine, quetiapine, and risperidone may be helpful in patients with comorbid psychotic disorders or when first-line approaches have been ineffective in controlling symptoms.

Alpha-adrenergic agents and beta-adrenergic blockers may be helpful in treating specific symptom clusters in individual patients.

SSRIs, TCAs, MAOIs, selective serotonin/norepinephrine reuptake inhibitors (SNRIs), and other antidepressants may be useful in treating depression.

Legal and Ethical Considerations

Post-disaster and terrorist attack scenes are chaotic and stress-provoking. ED clinicians may be called upon to provide general support and information rather than specific clinical interventions. These encounters require flexibility and decisiveness in regard to the nature of the clinician-patient (survivor) relationship.

The ED clinician-patient relationship is established whenever diagnosis or treatment is discussed. Once that happens, documentation, even if it is brief, should include
- Signs and symptoms
- Working diagnosis
- Suicide or homicide potential

- Emergency psychiatric treatment
- Follow-up plans

Although preserving confidentiality may be difficult, permission before sharing information is required unless the survivor's situation is a dire emergency.

Long-Term Treatment and Interventions

Long-term interventions include continued outreach and education and needed follow-up services. Existing structures may provide effective follow-up, but additional resources are often needed.

Federal Programs

Following a presidential declared disaster, the Federal Emergency Management Agency (FEMA) provides funding for crisis counseling. Programs are typically funded for 9 to 15 months and administered through the emergency services and disaster relief branch of the Substance Abuse and Mental Health Services Administration (SAMHSA) and community mental health organizations.

Psychotherapy

For survivors with acute stress disorder, various psychotherapies, especially cognitive-behavioral therapy (CBT), provided by trained therapists may prevent PTSD and other traumatic complications such as depression, generalized anxiety disorder, and substance abuse. CBT interventions may begin as early as 2 weeks after trauma and focus sequentially on anxiety management, cognitive restructuring, exposure therapy, and relapse prevention.

Teaching relaxation techniques and encouraging acquisition of new responses to trauma reminders may be helpful components of behavioral psychotherapies for PTSD. Exposure therapy and stress inoculation training are two specific types of cognitive-behavioral therapies with demonstrated efficacy in treating PTSD.

Eye movement desensitization reprocessing (EMDR) has not shown consistent benefit in studies. Studies have suggested that effective behavioral exposure therapies should control the duration of emotional exposure and avoid unstructured processing of painful emotions, which may be harmful to trauma victims.

Individuals and families affected by traumatic stress may have mistaken beliefs about "those responsible" for the disaster; the ramifications of these beliefs may include self-blame, the shattering of previous assumptions about human nature, and rage. Survivors may feel angry, guilty, or anxious and may experience reduced awareness, numbness, helplessness, hopelessness, or a sense of not being part of the world.

Psychotherapy may be initiated to assist survivors in modifying distorted and unrealistic expectations of how they might have acted to prevent or mitigate the traumatic event. Some of these events will be more likely to shatter the belief in a just and safe world than others and therefore may require more challenging interventions. Various psychotherapeutic techniques may initiate relaxation intervention for managing symptoms of hyperarousal. Similarly, supportive psychotherapy may facilitate the mourning process to deal with issues of death and dying.

Therapeutic Aspects of the Human and Pet Bond
The intricate relationship between humans and their pets needs to be considered as an important component in healing the trauma associated with natural disasters and terrorism. The reestablishment of the human-animal bond is a critical element in promoting resilience of individuals and communities. The survivors may forego rescue efforts in order to find and save their pets. On the other hand, search and rescue teams with canine units confront physical and emotional demands that affect both handler and animal. A familiarity with these issues is important for psychiatrists and other mental health professionals who are providing relief in disaster situations.

Assessing and Teaching Resilience
Each disaster and terrorist attack may present unique challenges to providers of mental health services. Approaches that are flexible, imaginative, proactive, and assertive minimize the negative impact of disasters on the rescuers and the survivors. Long-term intervention can include the teaching of resilience; and coping skills. The objectives and goals of resilience are summarized in Table 21-6.

Planning Ahead
Because some cases of PTSD and other emotional complications of trauma may be long-term, clinicians involved in mental health administration after a disaster should identify potential

Table 21-6

Objectives and Goals of Resilience

Objective	Goals
Maintaining interpersonal and spiritual connections	1. Keeping in touch with family, friends, and others 2. Connecting with people who provide social support and who strengthen resilience 3. Connecting with a higher power, whether through religious or spiritual beliefs or privately
Helping others	1. Performing volunteer work at a community organization 2. Helping families of the police, rescuers, active reservists, or military personnel involved in the recovery efforts can be empowering for the helpers
Maintaining a daily routine	1. Keeping daily routine of work, errands, household chores, and hobbies to provide a feeling of stability in the face of chaos 2. Daily routine can be comforting for children as well
Self-care	1. Appropriating time to eat, exercise, and rest 2. Scheduling time for social activities and hobbies 3. Making time for relaxing activities to maintain balance and to improve coping with stressful environment

Objective	Goals
Time out from "the news"	1. Controlling the amount of time spent watching TV news reports (e.g., a limit of 1 hour a day) 2. Considering a limit on reading newspaper reports 3. Avoiding watching TV news reports right before bedtime
Planning	1. Devising an emergency plan to gain control and to prepare for the unexpected 2. Spelling out the details of facing a crisis in the plan, including a list of items needed for an emergency 3. Establishing a calling list to clarify the chain of calling family, agencies, and emergency personnel 4. Making a plan for the pets' disposition
Preparing a security kit	1. Including in an emergency kit those things that give a sense of comfort and security, such as a favorite book, a journal, pictures of loved ones 2. Recording a list of loved ones' phone numbers in order to reestablish connections as soon as possible
Improving self-image	1. Recalling past experiences with successful coping with hardships 2. Utilizing coping skills to meet current challenges 3. Regaining trust in problem-solving and in making appropriate decisions

Continued

Table 21-6

Objectives and Goals of Resilience—cont'd

Objective	Goals
Maintaining long-term perspective	1. Remembering that dire situations will change and circumstances can ultimately improve
	2. Being inspired by examples of others who have faced similar events and turned them into opportunities to prosper and flourish
Maintaining hope	1. Focusing on personal strengths and qualities rather then weakness and deficiencies
	2. Appreciating the steps of nurturing and maintaining hope

Adapted from the Office of the Surgeon General web site on medical aspects of nuclear, biological, and chemical warfare. http://www.nbc-med.org; and National Center for Post-Traumatic Stress Disorder: Disaster mental health: Dealing with the aftereffects of terrorism. http://www.ncptsd.org/terrorism/index.html

sources of funding for long-term treatment of disasters and terrorism. Identifying federally funded grants and funding through professional or charitable organizations is an important aspect of planning for mental health treatment needs in the wake of natural disasters and terrorist attacks.

A lack of social preparedness makes community chaos and behavioral problems more likely, as was evident in the aftermath of hurricane Katrina. Hospitals and communities should develop emergency and disaster plans and repeatedly practice them. These plans should be adequately funded and should include realistic scenario simulation and robust and redundant communication systems. Such efforts will reduce a community's sense of helplessness before and after the occurrence of a terrorist attack or natural disaster. If leaders, first responders, and other members of the community are prepared for their roles before these events, then available resources can be directed at providing social support for victims and survivors rather than being hampered by bureaucratic procedures for deciding and sorting out roles and responsibilities during the post-event stages of confusion.

Outreach

Outreach in the form of additional community and regional resources will be required. These resources include the Red Cross, community mental health centers, social services, and hospice care providers. Schools, churches, synagogues, and mosques may serve as locations for psychosocial treatment. Incorporation of these resources into the response plan strengthens the community's social organization, enlists a larger portion of the community in social behavioral responses, and decreases the burden on primary care facilities.

In addition, by including these agencies in the post-event planning process, the confusion that arises when well-intentioned but poorly trained volunteers arrive on the scene is minimized. Such offers of help can unintentionally create more confusion and make an already difficult situation worse. In addition to personal liaison with various agencies, several Internet sites provide useful information.

Prevention of Psychiatric Complications in Caregivers and ED Staff

Caregivers and ED staff, including clinicians, are considered survivors. The following principles of coping are particularly relevant to them during and following natural disasters and terrorist attacks.

- Maintain interpersonal ties and connection with family and friends.
- Get adequate rest, food, exercise, and relaxation.
- Encourage talking about events and feelings only if this feels comfortable and helpful; staff should be allowed to defuse their feelings following troubling incidents and following each shift.
- Implement psychoeducational sessions related to understanding common cognitive distortions, such as survivor guilt and fears that the world is totally unsafe.
- Intervene when chaos and confusion result in conflicts between the various professional disciplines and groups that are participating in emergency care.
- Develop a system of support and encouragement among coworkers.
- Return to normal routine as much as possible.
- Avoiding exposure to trauma cues, including TV images.
- Workers assigned in transporting the dead may lessen the effects of such a traumatizing experience by avoiding a direct examination of the faces of the deceased.
- Reach out to others who need assistance.
- Promote faith, spirituality, and religious practices in those who rely on these beliefs in their normal healing processes.

The following warning signs should alert caregivers and ED staff about the need to seek psychiatric interventions:

- Development of abnormal reactions such as psychotic episodes, suicidality, risky behaviors including substance abuse, and symptoms suggesting ASD or PTSD
- Persistence of normal stress reactions such as insomnia, anxiety, and mild dissociation for longer than 2 months
- Exacerbation of preexisting conditions in those at high risk for persistent reactions such as bereavement, injury, prior trauma or psychiatric disorder, and lack of a social support network

Summary

Psychiatrists and other mental health professionals can assist survivors and communities to recover from natural disasters and acts of terrorism. The majority of individuals who are exposed to these traumatic events eventually recover without the development of psychiatric illness. Disaster survivors may experience normal reactions to such events, and these reactions may need to be assessed by the ED clinicians. Treatment of disaster survivors may vary according to their developmental level.

The provision of psychological first aid is a necessary and crucial intervention for coping with various stress reactions. The development of psychiatric problems depends on pre-existing psychiatric conditions, the degree of physical injury, the actual and the perceived threat to life, and the duration of community disruption.

Emergency psychiatric intervention is based on the identification of high-risk groups, assistance in community recovery, and minimization of social disruption. Critical incident debriefing, psychotherapy, and psychopharmacological interventions may also be beneficial in the treatment of ASD, PTSD, depression, and anxiety disorders. The ED clinician may also initiate long-term treatment plans toward assessing and teaching the principles of human resilience.

Further Reading

American Academy of Child and Adolescent Psychiatry: Talking to children about terrorism and war (2003). http://www.aacap.org/publications/factsFam/87.htm

American Psychiatric Association: Diagnostic and statistical manual of mental disorders. 4th ed, Text Revision. Washington, DC, American Psychiatric Association, 2000, pp 181-190, 429-481.

Amir M, Weil G, Kaplan Z, et al: Debriefing with brief group psychotherapy in a homogeneous group of non-injured victims of a terrorist attack: A prospective study. Acta Psychiatr Scand 1998;98:237-242.

Armstrong K, O'Callahan W, Marmar CR: Debriefing Red Cross disaster personnel: The multiple stressor debriefing model. J Trauma Stress 1991;4:581-593.

Barker SB, Barker RT: The human-canine bond: Closer than family ties? J Ment Health Couns 1988;10:46-56.

Barker M: Calming the aftershocks. Occup Health Saf 2001;70:28-33.

Bisson JI: Single-session early psychological interventions following traumatic events. Clin Psychol Rev 2003;23:481-499.

Brady K, Pearlstein T, Asnis GM, et al: Efficacy and safety of sertraline treatment of posttraumatic stress disorder: A randomized controlled trial. JAMA 2000;283:1837-1844.

Braun P, Greenberg D, Dasberg H, Lerer B: Core symptoms of posttraumatic stress disorder unimproved by alprazolam treatment. J Clin Psychiatry 1990;51:236-238.

Brumback R: Post-traumatic stress disorder in law enforcement (2000). http://acs.eku.edu/~stubrumb/

Bryant RA, Harvey AG, Dang ST, et al: Treatment of acute stress disorder: A comparison of cognitive-behavioral therapy and supportive counseling. J Consult Clin Psychol 1998;66:862-866.

Centers for Disease Control and Prevention. http://www.cdc.gov/

Cloak NL, Edwards P: Psychological first aid: Emergency care for terrorism and disaster survivors. Curr Psychiatry 2004;3:12-23.

Critical Incident Stress Emergency (2000). http://www.geocities.com/CapitolHill/Lobby/3082

Davidson JR: Pharmacotherapy of posttraumatic stress disorder: Treatment options, long-term follow-up, and predictors of outcome. J Clin Psychiatry 2000;61(Suppl 5):52-56.

DiGiovanni C Jr: Domestic terrorism with chemical or biological agents: Psychiatric aspects. Am J Psychiatry 1999;156:1500-1505.

Dishion T, McCord J, Poulin F: When interventions harm. Am Psychol 1999;54:755-764.

Engel CC Jr: Outbreaks of medically unexplained physical symptoms after military action, terrorist threat, or technological disaster. Mil Med 2001;166(Supp 12):47-48.

Fullerton CS, Ursano RJ: Health care delivery in the high-stress environment of chemical and biological warfare. Mil Med 1994;159:524-528.

Glass TA, Schoch-Spana M: Bioterrorism and the people: How to vaccinate a city against panic. Clin Infect Dis 2002;34:217-223.

Greenough PG, Kirsch TD: Hurricane Katrina public health response—assessing needs. N Engl J Med 2005;353:1544-1546.

Hall MJ, Ng A, Ursano RJ, et al: Psychological impact of the animal-human bond in disaster preparedness and response. J Psychiatr Pract 2004;10:368-374.

Holloway HC, Norwood AE, Fullerton CS, et al: The threat of biological weapons: Prophylaxis and mitigation of psychological and social consequences. JAMA 1997;278:425-427.

International Critical Incident Stress Foundation, Inc. CISM information pamphlet. Ellicott City, MD, Chevron Publishing, 2000.

Jones FD: Neuropsychiatric casualties of nuclear, biological, and chemical warfare. In Zajtchuk R, Bellamy RF (eds): Textbook of Military Medicine: Part I. War Psychiatry. Washington, DC, Office of the Surgeon General, U.S. Department of the Army, TMM Publications, 1995, pp 85-111.

Khouzam HR: A simple mnemonic for the diagnostic criteria for post-traumatic stress disorder. West J Med 2001;174:424.

Khouzam HR, Donnelly NJ: Posttraumatic stress disorder. Safe, effective management in the primary care setting. Postgrad Med 2001;110:60-78.

Lacy TJ, Benedek DM: Terrorism and weapons of mass destruction: Managing the behavioral reaction in primary care. South Med J 2003;96:394-399.

Mayou RA, Ehlers A, Hobbs M: Psychological debriefing for road traffic accident victims. Three year follow-up of a randomised controlled trial. Br J Psychiatry 2000;176:589-593.

Mitchell JT: Crisis intervention and CISM: A research summary (2003). www.icisf.org/articles/cism_research_summary.pdf

National Center for Post-Traumatic Stress Disorder. Disaster mental health: Dealing with the aftereffects of terrorism (2003). http://www.ncptsd.org/terrorism/index.html

NIMH: Mental Health and Mass Violence: Evidence-Based Early Psychological Intervention for Victims/Survivors of Mass Violence: A Workshop to Reach Consensus on Best Practices. Warrenton, VA, Oct 29-Nov 1, 2001.

Pynoos RS: Grief and trauma in children and adolescents. Bereave Care 1992;11:2-10.

Raphael B: Conclusion: Debriefing—science, belief and wisdom. In Raphael B, Wilson JP (eds): Psychological Debriefing: Theory, Practice and Evidence. New York, Cambridge University Press, 2001, pp 351-359.

Red Cross. http://www.redcross.org/

Ritchie EC: Psychological problems associated with mission-oriented protective gear. Mil Med 2001;166(Suppl 2):83-84.

Shalev AY: Acute to chronic: Etiology and pathophysiology of PTSD—a biopsychosocial approach. In Fullerton CS, Ursano RJ (eds): Posttraumatic Stress Disorder. Washington, DC, American Psychiatric Press, 1997, pp 209-240.

Ursano RJ, Fullerton CS, Norwood AE: Psychiatric dimensions of disaster: Patient care, community consultation, and preventive medicine. Harv Rev Psychiatry 1995;3:196-209.

Ursano RJ, McCaughey BG, Fullerton CS: The structure of human chaos. In: Ursano RJ, McCaughey BG, Fullerton CS (eds): Individual and Community Responses to Trauma and Disaster: The Structure of Human Chaos. London, Cambridge University Press, 1994, pp 3-27.

Young BH, Ford JD, Ruzek JI, et al: Disaster mental health: A guidebook for clinicians and administrators. Washington, DC, National Center for Post-Traumatic Stress Disorder (1998). http://ncptsd.org/publications/disaster/index.html

POSTSCRIPT

You are my hiding place from every storm of life; you preserve me from trouble; you surround me with songs of deliverance . . .

Psalm 32:7

CHAPTER 22

Emergency Psychiatry and Medications

Tirath S. Gill, MD

KEY POINTS

- Psychiatric medications are prescribed by many different specialties to treat anxiety, mood disorders, and other psychiatric symptoms.
- Drug interactions can occur due to displacement of the free drug or to inhibition or induction of metabolic enzymes.
- Enzymatic inhibitors are more likely to precipitate acute emergencies.
- Additive effects of different medications can precipitate toxic syndromes.

Overview

Psychiatric and other medications are being prescribed more frequently than in the past, and many patients are taking 10 or more different medications. The increased number of medications increases the risk for adverse reactions, interactions, and other side effects. This chapter attempts to summarize the possible interactions associated with psychiatric medications that may be a cause for an emergency department (ED) presentation.

The chapter is divided into two sections. The first section discusses some common complications of psychiatric medication treatment; the second lists currently used psychiatric medications, listed alphabetically by their generic names, with a concise description of each drug.

Complications of Psychiatric Medication Treatment

Akathisia

This is a distressing side effect of antipsychotic medications that block dopamine receptors. It is frequently noted with conventional antipsychotics such as haloperidol, fluphenazine, trifluoperazine, and the more potent atypical antipsychotics such as risperidone.

Clinical Presentation

The patient is often noted to be pacing or walking in place. The patient may appear agitated and report a subjective sense of restlessness. Untreated akathisia can result in violence toward self and others. It is associated with high rates of noncompliance and consequent exacerbation of the primary underlying illness.

Management

Akathisia can be treated with diphenhydramine, 50 mg by the intramuscular (IM) route or by mouth (PO). Alternatively, give lorazepam, 1 to 2 mg PO, or propranolol, 10 mg two to three times a day or benztropine, 1 to 2 mg PO or IM, can be used. If propranolol is used, symptoms of dizziness related to decreased blood pressure may occur and vitals may need to be monitored.

Psychosis and/or Hallucinations Induced by Antiparkinsonian Medications

Antiparkinsonian medications such as bromocriptine, amantadine, and levodopa may induce hallucinations, delusions, and agitation and precipitate a manic episode. Treatment consists of reducing the dose of the dopamine agonists and adding an antipsychotic such as quetiapine, which has low extrapyramidal syndrome (EPS) side effects. The addition of clozapine or olanzapine are other options for patients who require dopaminergic medications and control of iatrogenic psychosis. If the symptoms suggest a more manic presentation, it may be helpful to add mood stabilizers such as divalproic acid or carbamazepine. Anticholinergics such as benztropine and trihexiphenidyl used to treat parkinsonism may also lead to a toxic confusional state as well.

Amoxapine-Induced Disorders

Amoxapine is a unique antidepressant that also has antipsychotic properties. It was used in the 1980s, but appears to have fallen out of favor due to a high incidence of abnormal involuntary movement and Parkinsonian side effects. If a patient is prescribed amoxapine and develops tardive dyskinesia (TD) or Parkinsonian side effects, the medication should be tapered and eventually discontinued, and a suitable antidepressant and atypical antipsychotic substituted. If this is done early in the course of the emergence of these side effects, the tardive dyskinesia symptoms may gradually disappear. The patient and family should be informed about the high risk for tardive dyskinesia and other effects, and informed consent should be obtained for use of this and all other psychiatric medications.

Complications of Treatment with Amphetamine and Other Sympathomimetic Drugs

Amphetamines may be prescribed for the treatment of attention deficit hyperactivity disorder (ADHD), narcolepsy, anergia, and depression in the elderly. However, they may induce delirium and delusional states, including hallucinations, in susceptible individuals. If such symptoms occur, the amphetamine or sympathomimetic should be withdrawn, and a low dose of an atypical antipsychotic such as quetiapine, 12.5 to 25 mg twice a day, or risperidone, 0.5 to 1 mg twice a day, may be used for 7 to 10 days until the condition is resolved.

Analgesic Abuse

This is often a hidden problem that goes unsuspected and unrecognized. The use of aspirin, acetaminophen, and other non-steroidal anti-inflammatory drugs (NSAIDs) can have serious consequences over the long term. Analgesic abuse is five to six times more common in women than in men and often is associated with symptoms of fatigue and bodily aches that may have a psychosomatic origin. These patients are at higher risk for emergence of overt illnesses such as depression, hypochondriasis, personality disorders, and paranoia. If the liver enzymes are elevated or the patient presents with atypical symptoms and recurrent headaches, referral should be made for psychiatric assessment. Treatment of the psychiatric disorder may prevent the abuse and toxicity related to analgesic abuse.

Anticholinergic Toxicity

A large number of medications have anticholinergic side effects. These medications may be added inadvertently to a patient's drug regimen without recognizing the additive effect with other agents that also have anticholinergic side effects. Some common medications that may cause toxicity are benztropine (Cogentin), tricyclic antidepressants, phenothiazines, clozapine, olanzapine, and other low-potency first-generation antipsychotics. Some cough mixtures may contain anticholinergic medications such as scopolamine. Antispasmodic medications such as dicyclomine, eye drop preparations, and nonprescription asthma remedies may also contain anticholinergic agents. The list of anticholinergic medications includes newer agents used for urinary frequency such as oxybutynin and tolterodine and other agents including propantheline, diphenoxylate, cyclobenzaprine, promethazine, ipratropium, trihexyphenidyl, amantadine, chlorpheniramine, diphenhydramine, hydroxyzine,

---

Box 22–1. Common Agents That Inhibit Metabolism of Other Drugs, Leading to Toxicity

Amantadine
Amiodarone
Amphotericin
Antifungals such as fluconazole and itraconazole
Antimalarials
Calcium channel blockers
Disulfiram
Grapefruit juice
Isoniazid
Macrolide antibiotics such as erythromycin and azithromycin
Nefazodone
Phenothiazine
SSRIs
Valproic acid
Protease inhibitors such as ritonavir, saquinavir, and indinavir

SSRIs, selective serotonin reuptake inhibitors.

cyproheptadine, loratadine, fexofenadine, cetirizine, carbamazepine, procainamide, and quinidine. Some uncommon sources
include disopyramide, antiemetics prochlorperazine, and meclizine. Digoxin is also reported to have some anticholinergic properties and may add to the anticholinergic load of the patient.

Clinical Presentation

The patient presents with dilated pupils, dry and hot skin, a
flushed face and exhibits signs of agitated delirium. Other
symptoms may include tachycardia due to vagal blockade, dry
mouth, and urinary retention. The classic presentation of
anticholinergic toxicity can be remembered as "hot as a hare,
blind as a bat, red as a beet, dry as a bone, and mad as a hatter."
If the patient has been receiving multiple anticholinergic
medications and presents with delirium, the transit time in the
gastrointestinal tract is often prolonged, and ammonia levels
may also be elevated.

Treatment

Physostigmine, 0.5 mg to 2 mg, given by the IM or intravenous
(IV) route, can reverse the anticholinergic syndrome. IV physostigmine should be given slowly at a rate of no more than
1 mg per minute. Repeated doses in 30 minutes to an hour may
be required in view of the drug's short half-life. Cholinergic
toxicity may occur, marked by diarrhea, abdominal pain, and
excessive salivation. Because of the risk of arrhythmia, vital
signs should be carefully monitored.

The patient who is delirious should be protected from accidental injury such as falls and dislodgment of IV lines. If the
patient has cardiac conduction problems, supportive measures
while awaiting the gradual clearance of anticholinergic medications may be necessary. Anxiolytics and antipsychotics such
as haloperidol or fluphenazine may help to calm the patient.

Anticonvulsant Toxicity

Anticonvulsant toxicity may occur due to drug interactions with
phenytoin, primidone, carbamazepine, clonazepam, and valproic
acid and various enzyme inhibitors. The usual physical signs
of toxicity such as lethargy, dysarthria, nystagmus, and ataxia
are not always present. Lamotrigine levels may be elevated in
the presence of valproic acid, and dose reduction during initial

titration is recommended to decrease the risk associated with initial high doses, such as skin rashes and Stevens-Johnson syndrome.

Although phenytoin and carbamazepine generally tend to induce metabolic enzymes and lower the level of other anticonvulsants, valproic acid may raise the levels of other agents. Phenytoin has a relatively narrow therapeutic window and levels may become toxic when enzyme inhibitors such as the antifungal agents ketoconazole, itraconazole, and fluconazole are added. Macrolide antibiotics such as azithromycin and erythromycin may also result in phenytoin toxicity. Carbamazepine and oxcarbazepine have been associated with the syndrome of inappropriate diuretic hormone (SIADH), and the development of hyponatremia may result in an altered mental status. Valproic acid and topiramate use has been associated with cases of hyperammonemia, and this should be looked for in patients with altered mental status.

Lithium Toxicity

Lithium has a narrow therapeutic index, and levels may become toxic in the presence of medications such as NSAIDs, angiotensin-converting enzyme (ACE) inhibitors, diuretics used for hypertension, and tetracycline. Lithium used over the long term may impair kidney function and cause a rise in its own levels due to decreased excretion. A low-sodium diet, if a patient is taking lithium, can precipitate lithium toxicity, as can fluid loss due to excessive sweating, diarrhea, or vomiting. In the United States, 4000 to 5000 poisonings related to lithium occur every year. Lithium toxicity may occur after an acute overdose or build up gradually due to the factors mentioned previously. A serum lithium concentration greater than 1.5 mEq/L may be associated with toxicity.

Symptoms of lithium toxicity include nausea, tremor, drowsiness, thirst, behavioral changes, and muscle irritability. More severe poisoning produces coarse tremor, dysarthria, muscle fasciculations, twitching, rigidity, hyporeflexia, seizures, hyperpyrexia, decreased alertness, seizures, and coma.

While treating the patient for lithium toxicity, cardiac monitoring is warranted to assess for bradycardia, conduction blocks, and arrhythmias. The sodium and water balance should be restored using gentle rehydration with normal saline. If the lithium level is greater than 4 mEq/L, hemodialysis is indicated.

Neurologic consequences may resolve slowly after the lithium levels have returned to normal range.

Opioid Overdose

Opioid overdose can produce sedation, cyanosis, pinpoint pupils, and shallow respiration or respiratory arrest. The use of opioid antagonist naloxone may reverse the respiratory suppression and other symptoms. If naloxone is not immediately available, assisted respiration may be needed.

Benzodiazepine Toxicity

Benzodiazepines are used widely and often are taken in overdose; about 50,000 overdoses are reported yearly. Benzodiazepines are rarely fatal if taken alone but may be lethal if they are taken with other sedative/hypnotics. Flumazenil can be used to treat toxicity if the patient is not benzodiazepine-dependent. However, there is a risk for seizures, increased anxiety and agitation, and dysrhythmias in some patients.

Barbiturate Toxicity

Barbiturates are rarely prescribed now, but when taken in overdose, can cause a serious poisoning risk requiring artificial respiratory support. If the agent is phenobarbital, urinary alkalinization is necessary to enhance secretion. Multiple-dose activated charcoal therapy may be considered.

Acetaminophen Toxicity

Acetaminophen overdose is responsible for more deaths than any other chemical substance. After ingestion, the patient may exhibit symptoms for the first 24 hours that seem benign, such as mild gastrointestinal distress. After 24 to 48 hours, however, the patient begins to suffer from hepatic damage, and subsequent renal failure may occur within 96 hours. Because patients are not actively symptomatic during the first few hours, it is important to monitor acetaminophen levels to ascertain the risk of liver toxicity.

N-acetylcysteine (Mucomyst) is an antidote to acetaminophen-induced toxicity. The recommended regimen is 140 mg/kg as a loading dose, followed by 70 mg/kg every 4 hours for 17 additional doses. It should be started as soon as possible after acetaminophen ingestion, although even if given later, it may have a protective effect upon the liver.

Aspirin Poisoning

Salicylate poisoning is common; about 25,000 overdoses are reported every year. Symptoms may include increased respiratory rate, agitation, ringing in the ears, fever, and seizures. Other findings may include pulmonary edema, renal failure, nausea and vomiting, acid-base disturbances, and cardiac arrhythmias. Treatment involves cardiac monitoring and use of activated charcoal. Alkalinization of the urine should be initiated with IV sodium bicarbonate, 1 to 2 mEq/kg, followed by IV infusion of 100 to 150 mEq of sodium bicarbonate per liter of D5W 1.5 times the maintenance fluid rate to target a urine pH of 7.5. Potassium supplementation is generally required with urinary alkalization to prevent arrhythmias. Hemodialysis may be necessary in some patients to prevent renal failure and death.

Drug-Associated Impaired Pain Control

Paroxetine and fluoxetine may inhibit the conversion of codeine to its active metabolite and impair the control of pain by some medications containing codeine. Codeine is broken down to its active metabolite, morphine. Due to inhibition of the metabolic pathway, the active metabolite levels may fall, resulting in loss of pain control.

Serotonin Syndrome

If a patient taking a selective serotonin reuptake inhibitor (SSRI) or a serotonin/norepinephrine reuptake inhibitor (SNRI) develops confusion, diarrhea, fever, and brisk reflexes and is also taking another serotonergic agent or a monoamine oxidase inhibitor (MAOI), this can indicate the development of serotonin syndrome, which has a high risk of lethality. MAOIs may interact with meperidine to produce a syndrome akin to serotonin syndrome. Tramadol, which also has serotonergic properties, should also be avoided, although it has rarely caused problems. MAOIs should never be used with other MAOIs, SSRIs, or atypical antidepressants such as nefazodone or mirtazapine. The use of L-tryptophan, dextromethorphan, sumatriptan,

Table 22–1

The Relative Enzyme Inhibition of Some SSRIs

SSRI	Enzyme			
	3A	2C	2D6	1A2
Fluoxetine	2 to 3+	2+	4+	
Sertraline	2	1	1	
Paroxetine			4	
Fluvoxamine	3	2		4
Citalopram			1	
Effexor			1	
Duloxetine			3	

SSRIs, selective serotonin reuptake inhibitors.

Box 22–2. Agents That Can Induce the CYP450 System

Barbiturates
Carbamazepine
Chronic alcoholism
Cigarette smoke
Phenytoin
Rifampin
Some antiretrovirals such as efavirenz and abacavir
St. John's wort

CYP450, cytochrome P450.

sibutramine, buspirone hydrochloride, carbamazepine, lithium, dihydroergotamine, and St. John's wort should be avoided because these drugs are also considered serotonergic agents.

Serotonin syndrome is often precipitated by an increase in the dose of serotonergic agent or by the addition of another agent. Three of the following symptoms usually are sufficient to confirm the diagnosis of serotonin syndrome: mental status changes, diaphoresis, agitation, diarrhea, myoclonus, incoordination, tremor, fever, shivering, and hyperreflexia. Treatment includes the serotonin antagonist cyproheptadine, supportive care, and withdrawal of the offending agent(s). If needed, activated charcoal may be useful.

A waiting period of suitable duration should elapse after the use of an SSRI before an MAOI is introduced. In the case of fluoxetine, this may be up to 5 weeks or more. The duration may be shorter when using an SSRI with a shorter half-life. At least five half-lives should be allowed to expire before an MAOI is started. One must also be careful when using selegiline, which is an MAOI, in doses greater than 10 mg/day.

Fluvoxamine and other 3A4 enzyme inhibitors such as the azole antifungal agents and human immunodeficiency virus (HIV) protease inhibitors (ritonavir, indinavir, and saquinavir) may raise the level of other agents that are metabolized by this enzyme system; such as clozapine, pimozide, theophylline, ranitidine, and prednisone. Medications that affect the levels of clozapine, theophylline and lithium, which have a narrow therapeutic window, must be monitored carefully when other medications are added that may affect their metabolic pathway or excretion (see Box 22-1).

Manic Switch

Antidepressant medications may induce a manic episode in a patient who has not manifested a manic episode in the past and who is not known to be bipolar. If this should occur, the antidepressant should be withdrawn and antimanic agents should be added. Agents with a high to low risk, respectively, for inducing manic episodes are MAOIs, tricyclic antidepressants, SSRIs, and bupropion.

Carbamazepine-Associated Problems

Carbamazepine may cause hyponatremia, cardiac conduction delay, aplastic anemia, and fatal hepatotoxicity. It also may interact with other medications and reduce their levels by induction of the CYP-450 enzyme system. Monitoring of patients taking carbamazepine should include electrolytes, a complete blood count (CBC), liver function tests (LFTs), and electrocardiography (ECG).

Neuroleptic Malignant Syndrome

This infrequent syndrome can develop in patients taking antipsychotic medications. As the name implies, it is a malignant and serious condition that can progress to muscle breakdown, renal shutdown, disseminated intravascular coagulation, cardiac arrhythmias, and death. The patient usually is a young male in a relative state of dehydration. Sometimes the condition is associated with iron deficiency. The reaction appears to be idiosyncratic in nature, and once it develops, the patient should not be rechallenged with the same medication. Treatment may require an ICU admission and consists of the muscle relaxant dantrolene, the D_2 agonist bromocriptine, and anticholinergic medications. Maintain normal body temperature by cooling, and monitor vital signs. Transfer to an intensive care unit is warranted in many cases.

Adverse Reactions to Medications in the Elderly (see also Chapter 17)

It is better to start with low doses when prescribing medications for the elderly, because liver and kidney function are decreased and other physiologic changes may alter the pharmacokinetics of medications. The half-lives of medications are generally prolonged in the elderly, and too brisk a titration in dosage may result in increased plasma levels and toxicity. Older patients are especially sensitive to side effects such as sedation, urinary retention, orthostasis, and delirium. Sedation, dizziness, or altered mental status can result in falls and hip fractures. Such an outcome carries a grave prognosis in the elderly due to further complications related to their bedridden status, such as osteoporosis and decubitus ulcers.

Drug-Induced Leukopenia and Agranulocytosis

Psychotropic agents such as clozapine, carbamazepine, valproic acid, mirtazapine, and the first-generation antipsychotics have the potential for causing bone marrow toxicity. Transient leukopenia may be noted with initiation of carbamazepine therapy. A more severe bone marrow reaction that results in agranulocytosis appears to be an idiosyncratic reaction that cannot be predicted by monitoring of white blood cell (WBC) and platelet counts. Clozapine may cause a dose-related toxic reaction in the bone marrow; regular WBC monitoring can help to prevent more severe bone marrow suppression by cutting back or withholding the dose if the WBC count decreases to less than 3000 or the absolute neutrophil count falls below 1500. The risk of agranulocytosis tends to be higher in Jewish women and tends to occur less frequently after the first six months on the medication. Clozapine may cause elevation of liver enzymes and cardiomyopathy; patients should be monitored for any symptoms related to weakness, shortness of breath, congestive heart failure, or arrhythmias. Seizures are also a risk with higher doses of clozapine.

Hypertensive Crisis

There is a high risk of hypertensive crisis when MAOIs are used with tyramine-containing foods or sympathomimetics. Treatment includes alpha blockers such as phentolamine and monitoring in the ICU to prevent complications such as hypertensive bleeding or stroke. Clonidine, 0.2 mg, may be provided to a patient prescribed MAOIs. It can be given as an initial one-time dose to begin the blood pressure stabilization of a patient in a hypertensive crisis, while they are being brought to the ED. Repeat doses and more vigorous measures using phentolamine can be initiated by the emergency room physician to control this dangerous adverse reaction. Patients should be informed about side effects related to sedation and should be cautioned not to drive if sedated with clonidine.

Cardiac Arrhythmias

Some psychotropic medications affect cardiac conduction and may exacerbate any underlying cardiac conduction problems. With QT_C prolongation greater than 480 msec, the risk of arrhythmias begins to increase. There is a high risk with QT_C prolongation for a particularly lethal ventricular arrhythmia called torsades de pointes. Medications that prolong cardiac conduction include tricyclic antidepressants, lithium, pimozide, and high doses at risperidone, ziprasidone, and haloperidol. The risk of arrhythmia may be further increased if the patient is taking an adrenergic agent such as a bronchodilator in the context of severe chronic obstructive pulmonary disease (COPD), asthma, or other conditions that result in a state of relative hypoxemia.

Disorders Associated with Atypical Antipsychotics

A growing body of literature has expressed concerns about adverse metabolic effects associated with the use of atypical antipsychotics. One serious effect is metabolic syndrome, characterized by unintended weight gain, elevated blood pressure, abnormal triglyceride and fasting blood glucose (sugar) levels, and abnormal high-density lipoprotein (HDL) levels. The presence of any three of these abnormalities in a person confirms the diagnosis of metabolic syndrome, a cluster of symptoms that increases the risk for developing heart disease, diabetes, and stroke.

Monitoring of weight and waistline is advisable for patients at risk for metabolic syndrome. A baseline glucose level and lipid profile should be repeated at 3 months and on a yearly basis. If there is significant weight gain, a glucose level less than 60 or greater than 300, or a fasting glucose greater than 120 mg/dL, a review of the medication regimen is indicated in order to select an alternative antipsychotic.

Medications frequently associated with weight gain and the metabolic syndrome are clozapine and olanzapine. Other atypical agents have been implicated, but to a lesser degree.

Risperidone appears to be effective in treating the more florid symptoms of psychotic illness but has a tendency to cause a marked increase in prolactin levels. Quetiapine tends to cause some orthostatic symptoms, and doses of 600 mg or more are required for efficacy, which may not be comparable to other agents.

Some Common Psychiatric Medications

The past two decades have seen the introduction of many new pharmaceutical agents. Many are commonly in use. They are listed alphabetically here by their generic names. Information about each drug includes indications for use; cautionary statements about side effects, drug interactions, and other restrictions; available forms (tabs = tablets; caps = capsules; conc = concentrate; DR = delayed-release; inj = injectable form; sol = solution; supp = suppository; susp = suspension; syr = syrup; XR = extended-release); usual dosage; and Federal Drug Administration (FDA) pregnancy category (Table 22-2), if available.

The following points should be kept in mind when administering these agents:
- Use adequate doses for adequate duration for the right diagnosis for optimum results.
- It is acceptable to titrate the dosage upward slowly to avoid side effects and consequent noncompliance.

- Informed consent is mandatory for all prescribed medications.
- Prescribing medications involves a working knowledge of many aspects of human physiology and pathology. It is a mistake to seek advice about psychotropic medications from therapists and other clinicians who are not trained in the field of medicine and psychiatry.
- It is important to rule out pregnancy in women of child-bearing age. Risks to the fetus and the mother should be

Table 22–2

FDA Pregnancy Categories and Their Interpretation

Category	Interpretation
A	Adequate, well-controlled studies in pregnant women have not shown an increased risk of fetal abnormalities to the fetus in any trimester of pregnancy.
B	Animal studies have revealed no evidence of harm to the fetus; however, there are no adequate and well-controlled studies in pregnant women. OR Animal studies have shown an adverse effect, but adequate and well-controlled studies in pregnant women have failed to demonstrate a risk to the fetus in any trimester.
C	Animal studies have shown an adverse effect, and there are no adequate and well-controlled studies in pregnant women. OR No animal studies have been conducted and there are no adequate and well-controlled studies in pregnant women.
D	Adequate well-controlled or observational studies in pregnant women have demonstrated a risk to the fetus. However, the benefits of therapy may outweigh the potential risk. For example, the drug may be acceptable if needed in a life-threatening situation or serious disease for which safer drugs cannot be used or are ineffective.
X	Adequate well-controlled or observational studies in animals or pregnant women have demonstrated positive evidence of fetal abnormalities or risks. The use of the product is contraindicated in women who are or may become pregnant.

FDA, Federal Drug Administration.

discussed should the woman become pregnant while receiving treatment.
- If pregnancy is planned, a low-risk agent or a drug holiday should be considered for the first three months of the pregnancy.

Alprazolam (Xanax)

Indications: Generalized anxiety disorder; panic disorder with or without agoraphobia.

Caution: May be addictive in the abuse-prone individual; sudden cessation may cause withdrawal seizures and rebound anxiety; can impair motor performance by sedation. Ketoconazole, itraconazole, fluvoxamine, and other cytochrome P450-3A4 inhibitors may significantly raise levels of alprazolam.

Available Forms: Tabs 0.25, 0.5, 1, and 2 mg; also available in Xanax-XR form.

Usual Dosage: Dose for anxiety tends to be lower—0.25-0.5 mg PO bid to tid; dose for panic disorder tends to be higher—2-6 mg/d divided doses. Titration is required on the way up and on the way down to avoid side effects and complications such as intoxication, delirium, and withdrawal seizures.

Amantadine (Symmetrel)

Indications: Extrapyramidal reactions when anticholinergic side effects are undesirable; parkinsonism; antiviral.

Caution: May exacerbate manic, psychotic symptoms in some individuals; dose may need reduction in patients with compromised renal function.

Available Forms: Caps 100 mg; syr 50 mg (5 mL).

Usual Dosage: 100 mg PO once or twice/d; elderly patients may do better with syrup, 50 mg (5 mL) bid.

FDA Pregnancy Category: C.

Amitriptyline (Elavil, Endep, Enovil, Levate)

Indications: Depression; sometimes used for neuralgic pain in low doses.

Available Forms: Tabs 10, 25, 50, 75, 100, 150 mg; IM inj 10 mg/mL.

Caution: Strong anticholinergic, antihistaminic, and peripheral alpha blockade; may predispose to delirium because of side effects. Quinidine-like effects may be additive with other agents that cause prolongation of cardiac conduction times.

Usual Dosage: Starting dose, 25 mg in adult; 10 mg in patients with kidney dysfunction; not recommended for use in elderly patients; lower doses, 10-50 mg at bedtime. are usually sufficient for neuropathic pain. Maximum adult dosage is 150-300 mg/d. Metabolism can vary widely and is affected by enzyme inhibitors and inducers and individual genetics.

FDA Pregnancy Category: C.

Aripiprazole (Abilify)

Indications: Schizophrenia, bipolar disorder.

Available Form: Tabs 2, 5, 10, 20, 30 mg.

Caution: Some reports indicate exacerbation of psychosis at higher doses; is sedating, has long half-life, and may be more useful for borderline personality and other neurotic disorders rather than for major psychotic illness.

Usual Dosage: Starting dose 5-10 mg/d; maximum dose varies, 10-40 g/d. There is limited real world experience with this medication, which seems like the perfect antipsychotic in theory, but this has not been translated into success in patient outcomes.

FDA Pregnancy Category: C.

Atomoxetine (Strattera)

Indication: ADHD.

Available Form: Tabs 10, 18, 25, 40, 60 mg.

Caution: Significant gastrointestinal side effects; some cases of hepatotoxicity reported. Has received a black box warning because of hepatic failure in some cases.

Usual Dosage: Start with 10 mg bid and gradually increase dose to 60-120 mg.

FDA Pregnancy Category: C.

Benztropine (Cogentin)

Indications: Parkinsonism; EPS side effects.

Caution: May lead to anticholinergic toxicity or related side effects if combined with other agents with anticholinergic effects.

Available Forms: Tabs 0.5, 1, 2 mg; IM inj 1 mg/mL.

Usual Dosage: 1 mg bid or tid; dosage range is 1-6 mg/d.
FDA Pregnancy Category: C.

Buprenorphine (Buprenex, Subutex, Suboxone)

Indications: Opioid detoxification; long-term maintenance for opioid dependence and detoxification in outpatient office setting.

Available Form: Sublingual tabs 2, 8 mg; inj 0.3 mg/mL.

Caution: Some risk of abuse; outpatient form is combined with naloxone to prevent overdose by parenteral use (Subutex).

Usual Dosage: Adult maintenance dose, 4-24 mg/d; for detoxification give 2 mg q8h for 2 days and then decrease to 1 mg q8h for 2 days; give additional dose of 2 mg q4-6h for breakthrough symptoms for the first 72 hours. In patients using 1 gram or less of heroin, this will usually suffice and provide a safe and comfortable detoxification.

FDA Pregnancy Category: C.

Buspirone (BuSpar)

Indications: Generalized anxiety disorder; sometimes used to augment antidepressant response.

Available Form: Tabs 5, 10, 15 mg (may be bisected or trisected).

Usual Dosage: 10 mg PO bid; increase after 2-3 days to 15 mg PO bid. Allow 2 weeks for therapeutic response; if none is seen, increase dosage by 15 mg every 2 weeks up to 60 mg to obtain a response. Patience is required by the patient and the physician. In the meantime, a benzodiazepine, which can be tapered later, may be used for the short term.

FDA Pregnancy Category: B.

Carbamazepine (Tegretol, Carbatrol)

Indications: Tonic-clonic, psychomotor, and mixed seizures; trigeminal neuralgia; bipolar disorder and schizoaffective disorder.

Caution: Induces CYP450 enzyme system and may induce its own metabolism and that of other medications such as oral contraceptives, thus lowering their efficacy; risk (rare) of causing aplastic anemia; associated with transient suppression of WBC count initially; hepatitis is a risk with long-term use. May initially cause sedation and dizziness. Implicated in causing hyponatremia by SIADH effect in geriatric population.

Available Forms: Chewable tabs 100 mg; tabs 200 mg; XR tabs 100, 200, 400 mg; susp 100 mg/5 mL.

Usual Dosage: Start slowly on 100 mg once or twice a day and gradually increase dose q3-4d by 100 mg to achieve initial stabilization dose of 400-600 mg/d. Tends to induce its own metabolism, so dose may have to be increased to maintain the same plasma levels.

FDA Pregnancy Category: D.

Chlordiazepoxide
(Librium, Libritabs, Mitran)

Indications: Alcohol withdrawal; short-term treatment of anxiety.

Caution: Additive effect with other sedating agents; long half-life and possible cumulative risk of increasing sedation. Not recommended for elderly patients because of long half-life, active metabolites, and cumulative toxicity.

Available Forms: Caps 5, 10, 25 mg; tabs 5, 10, 25 mg; powder for IM inj 100 mg ampule.

Usual Dosage: 10-25 mg once or twice a day to treat mild anxiety symptoms; dose may be titrated up to control symptoms; to stabilize alcohol withdrawal symptoms, give 75-200 mg/d initially, then taper by 20-25% to detoxify.

FDA Pregnancy Category: D.

Chlorpromazine (Thorazine, Largactil)

Indications: Psychotic disorders, mania; intractable hiccups, nausea and vomiting; possible role in low doses for parkinsonism patient who is also psychotic. Frequency of EPS side effects such as rigidity and tremor is low.

Caution: Many side effects including anticholinergic, orthostatic hypotension, and sedation; dose must be titrated up slowly. Not recommended for elderly patients because of orthostatic and anticholinergic side effects.

Available Forms: Tabs 10, 25, 50, 100, 200 mg; XR caps 30, 75, 150 mg; syr 10 mg/5mL; conc 30, 100 mg/mL; supp 25, 100 mg; IM/IV inj 25 mg/mL.

Usual Dosage: Small dosages (25-150 mg) recommended for neurotic conditions such as borderline and schizotypal personality disorders; larger doses recommended for control of major psychotic disorders, 600-800 mg titrated up 100-200 mg every day or every other day. Not recommended for elderly patients because of risk of falls due to blood pressure drop with change of body position and anticholinergic side effects that confound cognitive problems.

FDA Pregnancy Category: D.

Citalopram (Celexa)

Indications: Depressive disorders, anxiety disorders; PTSD.

Caution: Should not be used with an MAOI because of risk of cumulative serotonin toxicity; some evidence that SSRIs such as citalopram may induce or worsen suicidal ideations in some patients; close monitoring is indicated.

Available Form: Tabs 20, 40 mg.

FDA Pregnancy Category: Not available; appears safe, but clinical experience lacking.

Clomipramine (Anafranil)

Indication: Obsessive-compulsive disorder.

Caution: Should not be used with an MAOI; avoid use in early recovery from myocardial infarction. Do not use in children less than 10 years of age.

Available Form: Tabs 25, 50, 75 mg.

FDA Pregnancy Category: C.

Clonazepam (Klonopin)

Indications: Lennox-Gastaut syndrome; absence (petit mal), akinetic, and myoclonic seizures; restless legs syndrome; bipolar disorder, generalized anxiety disorder, and panic disorder.

Caution: Do not use with valproic acid for absence seizures; Additive sedative effect with other agents; not recommended for elderly patients because of long half-life. May increase carbamazepine levels.

Available Form: Tabs 0.5, 1, and 2 mg.

FDA Pregnancy Category: D.

Clozapine (Clozaril)

Indications: Refractory schizophrenia; schizoaffective disorder.

Caution: May cause bone marrow suppression in 1/100 persons; monitor WBC count weekly for first 6 months and then every 2 weeks. May cause seizures at higher doses. Because of risk for myocarditis, monitor creatine kinase levels and obtain ECG if patient complains of malaise and tiredness or shortness of breath. IM lorazepam has been associated with respiratory arrest when used with clozapine.

Available Form: Tabs 25, 100 mg.

FDA Pregnancy Category: B.

Desipramine (Norpramin, Pertofrane)

Indication: Depressive disorders.

Caution: Tricyclic with minimal anticholinergic, orthostatic side effects. Has quinidine-like effects like other tricyclics.

Available Form: Tabs 10, 25, 50, 75, 100, 150 mg.

FDA Pregnancy Category: C.

Diazepam (Valium, Vivol, Diastat)

(Controlled Substance Schedule IV)

Indications: Generalized anxiety disorder; acute alcohol withdrawal; status epilepticus.

Caution: Addictive liability in abuse-prone patients. Not recommended for elderly patients because of long half-life.

Available Forms: Tabs 2, 5, 10 mg; XR caps 15 mg; IM/IV inj 5 mg/mL; oral sol 5 mg/5mL; rectal pediatric gel 2.5, 5, 10 mg; adult supp 10, 15, 20 mg.

FDA Pregnancy Category: D.

Diphenhydramine (Benadryl, Siladryl)

Indications: Parkinsonism; EPS side effects, akathisia, motion sickness; allergic reactions.

Caution: Not recommended for elderly patients because of antihistaminic, anticholinergic side effects.

Available Forms: Caps 25, 50 mg; soft-gel caps 25 mg; tabs 25, 50 mg; chewable tabs 12.5 mg; elixir 12.5 mg/5 mL; syr 12.5 mg/mL; IM/IV inj 10, 50 mg/mL; liquid 6.25, 12.5 mg/mL; sol 12.5 mg/5 mL.

FDA Pregnancy Category: C.

Disulfiram (Antabuse)

Indication: Chronic alcoholism; used in concert with psychosocial program. Decreased cocaine use has been reported.

Caution: Ingestion of alcohol may lead to a severe disulfiram reaction; may interact with metronidazole and isoniazid, causing psychosis and optic neuritis. May worsen hepatitis; monitoring of liver function is recommended. Do not administer to an individual who has imbibed alcohol in the last 12 hours. May exacerbate psychosis in patients with preexisting psychotic illness.

Available Form: Tabs 250, 500 mg.

FDA Pregnancy Category: X.

Donepezil (Aricept)

Indication: Mild to moderate dementia of Alzheimer's type.

Caution: May exacerbate peptic ulcer disease, asthma, and COPD; may cause aggression, dizziness, insomnia, psychosis in some individuals; may exacerbate effects of succinylcholine. Ketoconazole may increase levels and side effects of donepezil; NSAIDs may exacerbate gastrointestinal side effects.

Available Form: Tabs 5, 10 mg.

FDA Pregnancy Category: C.

Doxepin (Sinequan)

Indications: Depressive disorders; sometimes used for pruritus; H_2 blockade may be beneficial in treatment of dyspepsia and peptic ulcer disease.

Caution: Strong anticholinergic; antihistaminic at H_1 and H_2 receptors; orthostatic side effects. Not recommended for elderly patients due to orthostatic and anticholinergic side effects.

Available Forms: Caps 10, 25, 50, 75, 100, 150 mg; oral conc 10 mg/mL.

FDA Pregnancy Category: C.

Duloxetine (Cymbalta)

Indications: Depressive disorders; peripheral neuropathic pain.

Caution: Some reports of hepatotoxicity; risk of toxicity to immature fetal liver. Limited clinical experience at this time.

Available Form: DR caps 20, 30, 60 mg.

FDA Pregnancy Category: C.

Estazolam (Prosom)

(Controlled Substance Schedule IV)

Indication: Insomnia.

Available Form: Tabs 1, 2 mg.

FDA Pregnancy Category: X.

Escitalopram (Lexapro)

This is an isomer of citalopram and essentially has the same profile.

Available Forms: Tabs 5, 10 mg; oral conc 5 mg/5 mL.

Flumazenil (Romazicon, Anexate)

Indication: Benzodiazepine overdose.

Caution: May precipitate seizures if the patient is dependent on benzodiazepines. Keep IV diazepam or lorazepam available in case a withdrawal seizure occurs.

Available Forms: IM inj 0.1 mg/mL in 5- and 10-mL vials.

Fluoxetine (Prozac)

Indications: Depressive disorders; obsessive compulsive disorder; bulimia nervosa, anorexia nervosa; premenstrual disorders

Caution: As with all SSRIs, should not be used within 14 days of last use of an MAOI. MAOIs should not be used for 5 weeks after last dose of fluoxetine due to the long half-life of active metabolites.

Available Forms: Tabs 10 mg; DR once-weekly caps 90 mg; pulvules 10, 20, 40 mg; liquid 20 mg/5 mL.

Fluvoxamine (Luvox)

Indication: Obsessive-compulsive disorder.

Caution: Inhibits several CYP 450 isoenzymes and can significantly raise levels of Haldol, terfenadine, astemizole, theophylline, alprazolam, warfarin, TCAs, beta blockers, diltiazem, leading to possible toxic effects of these agents.

Available Form: Tabs 25, 50, and 100 mg.

FDA Pregnancy Category: C.

Gabapentin (Neurontin)

Indications: Adjunctive therapy for partial seizures; no proof of efficacy for bipolar disorder but may be useful for anxiety states; some efficacy with peripheral neuropathy reported.

Caution: Do not use in children less than 12 years of age. Avoid sudden cessation to prevent withdrawal seizures.

Available Forms: Caps 100, 300, 400 mg; tabs 600, 800 mg; oral sol 250 mg/5 mL.

Galantamine (Reminyl)

Indication: Mild to moderate dementia of Alzheimer's type.

Caution: Use with caution in individuals with heart block or peptic ulcer disease. May cause gastrointestinal side effects, agitation, and worsening of depression.

Available Forms: Tabs 4, 8, 12 mg; oral sol 4 mg/mL.

Haloperidol, Haloperidol Decanoate (Haldol, Haldol Decanoate)

Indications: Schizophrenia and other psychotic disorders; Tourette's syndrome.

Caution: May cause parkinsonian side effects, dystonia, and akathisia in doses greater than 5 mg if given to young individuals without an anticholinergic agent. People of Asian descent may be more susceptible to EPS side effects. May exacerbate parkinsonian features in the elderly, increasing risk for falls. High doses may be associated with prolonged QTc interval and resultant arrhythmias.

Available Forms: Tabs 0.5, 1, 2, 5, 10 and 20 mg; conc 2 mg/mL; IM inj 5 mg/mL; decanoate 50, 100mg/mL.

Hydroxyzine (Vistaril, Atarax)

Indications: Anxiety; nausea; some antihistaminic, anticholinergic effects.

Caution: May have additive sedative effect with other sedating agents.

Available Forms: Tabs 10, 25, 50, 100 mg; caps 25, 50, 100 mg; syr 10 mg/5 mL; oral susp 25 mg/5 mL; IM inj 25, 50 mg/mL.

FDA Pregnancy Category: C.

Imipramine (Tofranil)

Indications: Depressive disorders; enuresis in children; panic disorder.

Caution: Anticholinergic side effects may be troublesome, especially in older individuals; constipation and urinary retention possible.

Available Forms: Caps 75, 100, 125, 150 mg; tabs 10, 25, 50 mg; IM inj 12.5 mg/mL; pamoate salt (XR caps) 75, 100, 125, 150 mg.

FDA Pregnancy Category: C.

Lamotrigine (Lamictal)

Indications: Bipolar disorder; adjunctive treatment for partial seizures.

Caution: Do not use during lactation; do not use in patients with impaired hepatic, renal, or cardiac function. Risk for serious skin rash and Stevens-Johnson syndrome. Titration up should be done slowly. It may be less likely to cause birth defects compared with other anticonvulsants.

Available Form: Tabs 25, 100, 150, and 200 mg.

FDA Pregnancy Category: C.

Lithium Carbonate (Eskalith, Eskalith CR)

Indications: Bipolar disorder, intermittent explosive disorder, schizoaffective disorder; augmenting agent for refractory depressive state.

Caution: Narrow therapeutic index; levels may be raised by diuretics, low-sodium diet, tetracycline, NSAIDs, and ACE inhibitors; may prolong conduction delay and decrease thyroid function. Because of risk of renal complications with long-term use, monitor ECG, CBC, basic metabolic panel along with thyroid profile at baseline and periodically. Educate patient about signs of lithium toxicity.

Available Forms: Caps 150, 300, 600 mg; tabs 300 mg; DR tabs 300 mg; syr 300 mg/5 mL (as citrate).

FDA Pregnancy Category: D.

Lorazepam (Ativan)

Indications: Anxiety; status epilepticus.

Caution: Use with caution in elderly or debilitated patients to avoid risk of sedation and falls. Do not give by IM route if patient is taking clozapine.

Available Forms: Tabs 0.5, 1, 2 mg; IM/IV inj 2, 4 mg/mL; oral sol 2 mg/mL.

FDA Pregnancy Category: D.

Memantine (Namenda)

Indications: Alzheimer's disease; used off-label to treat spasticity, parkinsonism, neuropathic pain.

Caution: *N*-methyl-D-aspartate (NMDA) receptor blocker with a long half-life; titration is required. May have additive effect with dextromethorphan, amantadine, and ketamine; can cause hallucinations in some patients.

Available Form: Tabs 5, 10 mg.

Methadone (Dolophine)

(Controlled Substance Category II)

Indications: Pain; methadone maintenance; opioid detoxification in certified programs.

Caution: Methadone doses should be confirmed by the prescribing agency because overdose can lead to respiratory arrest. This can be reversed by naloxone but repeated doses will be needed due to the short half-life of naloxone.

Available Forms: Tabs 5, 10 mg; oral sol 5, 10 mg/5 mL, 10 mg/10 mL; dispersible tabs 40 mg; oral conc 10 mg/mL; subcutaneous IM inj 10 mg/mL.
FDA Pregnancy Category: C.

Methohexital (Brevital)

Indication: General anesthesia for electroconvulsive therapy (ECT).

Caution: Ultra short-acting barbiturate, highly lipophilic; onset in 10-15 sec and duration of 5-7 min. Succinylcholine is then administered and artificial respiration is provided prior to ECT. Rare cases of bronchospasm, laryngospasm reported.

Available Forms: Powder for IV inj: ampules 2.5, 5 gm; vials 500 mg/50 mL, 2.5 g/250 mL, 5 g/500 mL.

Methylphenidate (Ritalin, Concerta, Ritalin LA, Metadate ER, Metadate CD, Methylin, Methylin ER)

(Controlled Substance Schedule II)

Indications: ADHD; narcolepsy; anergic depression of the elderly.

Caution: May exacerbate tics, lower seizure threshold, and exacerbate psychosis. Do not give within 14 days of use of an MAOI.

Available Forms: Tabs 5, 10, 20 mg; Ritalin LA, caps 20, 30, 40 mg; Concerta, tabs 18, 27, 36, 54 mg; Methylin, tabs 5, 10, 20 mg; Methylin ER and Metadate ER, tabs 10, 20 mg; Metadate CD, caps 20 mg.

FDA Pregnancy Category: C.

Mirtazapine (Remeron)

Indications: Depression; especially useful for patients with insomnia and decreased appetite. Sometimes used for SSRI-induced sexual dysfunction.

Caution: May cause weight gain by increasing appetite. Monitor for increase in suicidal ideation, especially early in recovery or with change of dosage.

Available Form: Tabs 15, 30, 45 mg; orally disintegrating tabs 15, 30, 45 mg.

FDA Pregnancy Category: C.

Modafinil (Provigil)

Indications: Narcolepsy; used off-label for ADHD.

Caution: May cause headache, nausea, and anxiety; may increase levels of phenytoin, diazepam, and propranolol; risk of psychological dependence. Real world experience is limited.

Available Form: Caps 100, 200 mg.

FDA Pregnancy Category: C.

Molindone (Moban)

Indication: Psychotic disorders.

Caution: May cause EPS side effects. Risk for tardive dyskinesia with long-term use, as with all typical dopamine-blocking antipsychotics, but less likely to cause weight gain.

Available Forms: Tabs 5, 10, 25, 50, 100 mg; oral conc 20 mg/mL.

FDA Pregnancy Category: C.

Naloxone (Narcan)

Indication: Narcotic-induced respiratory depression.

Caution: Short half-life; requires repeated doses to prevent relapse into respiratory arrest. May induce acute opioid withdrawal in opiate-dependent individual.

Available Forms: IM/IV inj, subcutaneous 0.02, 0.04, 1 mg/mL.

Naltrexone (Revia, Trexan)

Indications: Treatment of alcohol dependence during maintenance phase; narcotic addiction.

Caution: May have to be initiated at a low dose because of significant gastrointestinal side effects. Monitor liver function if initially elevated. Injectable naltrexone has become available. It is given in the dose of 380 mg IM per month.

Available Form: Tabs 50 mg; injectable suspension (Vivitrol) 380 mg/vial.

FDA Pregnancy Category: C.

Nortriptyline (Pamelor)

Indications: Depression, anxiety disorders; tinnitus; peripheral neuropathy.

Caution: May cause cardiac conduction delay like other tricyclics; anticholinergic side effects and risk of orthostasis in elderly patients.

Available Forms: Caps 10, 25, 50, 75 mg; sol 10 mg/5 mL.

FDA Pregnancy Category: C.

Olanzapine (Zyprexa, Zydis)

Indications: Schizophrenia; schizoaffective disorder; bipolar disorder.

Caution: May cause weight gain; insulin resistance is significant. May have additive sedative effect with other sedating agents.

Available Forms: Tabs 2.5, 5, 7.5, 10, 15, 20 mg; orally disintegrating tabs 5, 10, 15, 20 mg.

FDA Pregnancy Category: C.

Oxazepam (Serax)

Indications: Anxiety states; alcohol withdrawal.

Caution: May have additive sedative effect with other agents. Not recommended for elderly patients because of risk of falls due to sedation.

Available Forms: Caps 10, 15, 30 mg; tabs 15 mg.

FDA Pregnancy Category: D.

Paroxetine (Paxil)

Indications: Depression; panic disorder, social anxiety disorder, obsessive-compulsive disorder.

Caution: Contraindicated with MAOIs; be cautious of additive effects with other serotonergic agents. May cause disturbance of orgasmic response and diminished libido.

Available Forms: Tabs 10, 20, 30, 40 mg; susp 10 mg/5 mL.

FDA Pregnancy Category: D.

Perphenazine (Trilafon)

Indication: Psychotic disorders.

Caution: As with other typical dopamine-blocking agents, may produce EPS side effects and tardive dyskinesia with long-term use.

Available Forms: Tabs 2, 4, 8, 16 mg; conc 16 mg/5 mL; IM inj 5 mg/mL.

FDA Pregnancy Category: C.

Phenelzine (Nardil)

Indication: Atypical depression.

Caution: Do not give with meperidine, SSRIs, or adrenergic agents; risk for hypertensive response and serotonin syndrome.

Available Form: Tabs 15 mg.

FDA Pregnancy Category: C.

Pimozide (Orap)

Indication: Tourette's syndrome, delusional disorders, somatoferm disorder.

Caution: Risk for EPS symptoms, conduction delay.

Available Form: Tabs 2 mg.

FDA Pregnancy Category: C.

Propranolol (Inderal)

Indications: Akathisia; stage fright; organic impulsivity.

Caution: May induce hypotension, bradycardia, and worsening of asthma; do not use concurrently with vasodilating agents; contraindicated for patients who are dehydrated, hypotensive, or with obstructive airway disease such as asthma. In higher doses it may induce depressive symptoms.

Available Forms: XR caps 60, 80, 120, 160 mg; tabs 10, 20, 40, 60, 80, 90 mg; IM inj 1 mg/mL; oral sol 4, 8 mL; conc oral sol 80 mg/mL.

FDA Pregnancy Category: C.

Protriptyline (Vivactil)

Indications: Depression; tends to have an activating effect; sometimes used to suppress REM sleep and associated nightmares or sleep apnea–related problems.
Available Form: Tabs 5, 10 mg.
FDA Pregnancy Category: C.

Quetiapine (Seroquel)

Indications: Schizophrenia; psychosis; bipolar disorder. Some efficacy reported in treating insomnia and nightmares associated with PTSD.
Caution: Gradually titrated higher dose required for schizophrenia and bipolar disorder.
Available Form: Tabs 25, 100, 200, 300 mg.
FDA Pregnancy Category: C.

Risperidone (Risperdal, Risperdal Consta)

Indications: Psychosis; Tourette's syndrome and other tic disorders; bipolar disorder; aggressive behaviors in developmentally disabled patients. It is an effective antipsychotic and may have greater efficacy for positive symptoms of schizophrenia.
Caution: Can delay cardiac conduction, especially at higher doses. If titration is rapid, patient may experience dizziness due to low blood pressure with change of body position. Associated with elevated prolactin levels which may disrupt the menstrual cycle and cause galactorrhea.
Available Forms: Tabs 0.25, 0.5, 1, 2, 3, 4 mg; oral sol 1 mg/mL; rapid dissolving tabs 0.5, 1, 2 mg; long-acting inj 25, 37.5, 50 mg/vial given every 2 weeks. Oral Risperdal should be continued for 3 weeks after giving first injection of Risperdal Consta. At that time, significant blood levels of risperidone from the injection become available, and oral tablets can be discontinued.
FDA Pregnancy Category: C.

Rivastigmine (Exelon)

Indication: Alzheimer's disease.
Caution: Agitation, as with other ACH inhibitors.

Available Forms: Caps 1.5, 3, 4.5, 6 mg; oral sol 2 mg/mL.
FDA Pregnancy Category: B.

Sertraline (Zoloft)

Indications: PTSD; depression; panic disorder, obsessive-compulsive disorder, premenstrual dysphoric disorder; premature ejaculation.

Caution: Titrate dose up slowly; may cause significant gastrointestinal side effects, including nausea, anorexia, asthenia, and diarrhea. SSRIs such as sertraline are strictly contraindicated with the concurrent use of MAOIs.

Available Forms: Tabs 50, 100 mg; oral conc 20 mg/mL.
FDA Pregnancy Category: B.

Thiothixene (Navane)

Indication: Psychotic disorders.

Caution: Side effects as with other conventional antipsychotic agents.

Available Forms: Caps 1, 2, 5, 10, 20 mg; oral conc 5 mg/mL; IM inj 2 mg/mL.

FDA Pregnancy Category: C.

Topiramate (Topamax)

Indications: Reports of some success promoting alcohol abstinence along with psychosocial interventions; used in obese patients with bipolar disorder as an adjunctive agent.

Caution: This mild carbonic anhydrase inhibitor may cause electrolyte imbalance and paresthesias; other side effects include elevated ammonia levels and hyponatremia, kidney stones, and cognitive dulling.

Available Forms: Caps 25, 100, 200 mg; sprinkle caps 15, 25 mg.

FDA Pregnancy Category: C.

Tranylcypromine Sulfate (Parnate)

Indication: Atypical depression.
Caution: May precipitate onset of mania.
Available Form: Tabs 10 mg.
FDA Pregnancy Category: C.

Trazodone (Desyrel)

Indications: Depression; insomnia.

Caution: May cause hypotension, cardiac arrhythmia (rare), priapism (risk about 1/8000; risk increased if used with other vasodilating agents).

Available Form: Tabs 50, 100, 150, 300 mg.

FDA Pregnancy Category: C.

Trifluoperazine (Stelazine)

Indication: Psychosis.

Caution: May cause acute dystonic reactions in young patients and patients of Oriental descent. Strong D_2 blockade; other side effects include EPS and akathisia. Risk of tardive dyskinesia with long-term use.

Available Forms: Tabs 1, 2, 5, 10 mg; oral conc 10 mg/mL; IM inj 2 mg/mL.

FDA Pregnancy Category: C.

Trihexyphenidyl (Artane)

Indications: Parkinsonism; EPS side effects associated with the use of antipsychotic agents.

Caution: Risk for addiction; has some mood-elevating effects. May increase digoxin levels.

Available Forms: Tabs 2, 5 mg; slow-release caps 5 mg; elixir 2 mg/5 mL.

FDA Pregnancy Category: C.

Valproic Acid (Depakote, Depakote ER, Depakene)

Indications: Bipolar disorder, intermittent explosive disorder, and other impulse control disorders; generalized and partial seizures. The once-a-day ER formulation is convenient. The dose may have to be raised by 10 to 20% to achieve equivalent levels to twice-a-day formulations.

Caution: If liver function tests indicate active hepatitis, use alternative agent or use with caution; hyperammonemia, hepatotoxicity, and acute pancreatitis have been reported. Associated with polycystic ovary syndrome and obesity. Valproic acid tends to cause more gastrointestinal side effects compared with the delayed-release formulations.

Available Forms: Caps 250 mg; syrup 250 mg/mL; sprinkle caps 125 mg; delayed-release tabs (Depakote) 125, 250, 500 mg; extended-release tabs (ER) 500 mg for once daily dosing; inj 100 mg/mL.

FDA Pregnancy Category: D.

Venlafaxine (Effexor, Effexor XR)

Indications: Depression; generalized anxiety disorder, social anxiety disorder, and panic disorder.

Caution: May cause hypertension; monitor blood pressure at each visit. Use is strictly contraindicated with MAOIs. Side effects include initial nausea and gastrointestinal distress; Using the XR form, tapering the dose up slowly, and giving with meals may limit these symptoms. May be associated with abnormal ejaculation, anorgasmia, and decrease in sexual drive.

Available Forms: Tabs 25, 37.5, 50, 75, 100 mg; XR caps 37.5, 75, 150 mg.

FDA Pregnancy Category: C.

Zaleplon (Sonata)

Indication: Insomnia.

Caution: Risk of additive sedation and associated falls. Underlying causes of insomnia should be investigated, including faulty sleep hygiene.

Available Form: Caps 5, 10 mg.

FDA Pregnancy Category: C.

Ziprasidone (Geodon)

Indication: Psychosis; schizophrenia; acute agitation (IM form).

Caution: The efficacy of oral ziprasidone for schizophrenia is contested by some clinicians.

Available Forms: Caps 20, 40, 60, 80 mg; MI inj 20 mg.

Zolpidem (Ambien)

Indication: Insomnia.
Caution: Should be taken immediately before going to bed.
May induce psychological dependence. Sedative effect may
be additive with other sedating agents.
Available Form: Tabs 5, 10 mg.
FDA Pregnancy Category: B.

Caution about New Medications

 The ED clinician should exercise due diligence and caution
regarding new drugs. They are advertised and promoted vigor-
ously by the pharmaceutical industry, and the clinician should
never rely on the drug representative when making decisions
about choice of drugs. The pharmaceutical industry is immensely
powerful in its influence over the FDA, the medical publishing industry, and individual physicians. Although there are
scrupulous bureaucrats, researchers, and editors of reputable
journals out there, one cannot ignore the recent revelations
regarding the withholding or falsification of critical data about
Vioxx and Celebrex. The astute ED clinician must be patient
and allow enough real world experience to accumulate before
trying out newly touted panaceas on their patients.

Further Reading

2005 PDR Physician's Desk Reference. Montvale, NJ,
    Thomson Healthcare, 2005.
Nestler EJ, Hyman SE, Malenka RC: Molecular Basis of
    Neuropharmacology: A Foundation for Clinical
    Neuroscience. New York, McGraw-Hill, 2001.
Schatzberg AF, Cole JO, DeBattista C: Manual of Clinical
    Psychopharmacology. Washington, DC, American
    Psychiatric Press, 2003.
Spratto GR, Woods AL: PDR Nurse's Drug Handbook. New
    York, Delmar, 2005.
Stahl SM, Grady MM: Essential Psychopharmacology: The
    Prescriber's Guide (Essential Psychopharmacology Series).
    New York, Cambridge University Press, 2006.

C H A P T E R   2 3

Medical and Legal Aspects of Emergency Psychiatry

Hani R. Khouzam, MD, MPH, FAPA

Key Points

- Emergency department (ED) clinicians need to be keenly aware of the criteria for legal commitment and involuntary hospitalization.
- ED clinicians should protect patients' confidentiality and be aware of the grounds for confidentiality exceptions.
- Each emergency intervention, after careful assessment of its benefits and risks, should be implemented without committing acts of negligence.
- Informed consent, assessing competence, initiating restraints, and instituting appropriate disposition are some of the challenges facing ED clinicians.
- Ethical standards are essential when making emergency interventions.

Overview

ED clinicians are often confronted with medical and legal challenges during emergency assessment due to the following factors:

- Unavailable medical/psychiatric history and inability of patient to provide accurate and urgently needed information.
- Absence of previously established professional relationship between patients receiving emergency treatment and providers of such treatment.
- Despite the presenting emergency, refusal by patients to comply with ED treatment recommendations.

An understanding of the basic medical and legal principles of ED treatment allows clinicians to intervene effectively even when on-site immediate legal consultations are not available.

In general, the focus should be on the urgency of the clinical presentation and prompt intervention based on what is judged to be the patient's best interests.

Basic Medical and Legal Principles of ED Treatment

The Duty to Warn in High-Risk Emergency Situations

In most states, when a patient expresses the intention to harm a particular person, the evaluating clinician is required to warn the intended victim and notify a specified law enforcement agency. Specific requirements vary by state. Typically, state regulations also require reporting of suspected abuse of children, the elderly, and spouses.

Involuntary Hospitalization

Criteria and procedures for involuntary hospitalization vary by jurisdiction. Usually, certification for commitment must state that the patient is a danger to self or others and refuses treatment. The criteria for commitment usually include:

- *Harm to self*: Substantial risk of serious harm indicated by threats (written or verbal) or attempts to commit suicide or inflict other physical harm to self.
- *Harm to others*: Behavior that has caused harm to others or places others in reasonable fear of sustaining harm. The behavior may be written, verbalized, or expressed as an actual act of assault.
- *Property damage*: Behavior that has caused substantial loss or damage to the property of others.
- *Gravely disabled*: Behavior that may cause serious physical harm resulting from neglect of basic health and safety needs; or deterioration in routine functioning evidenced by repeated and escalating loss of control over actions, with subsequent neglect of basic health and safety needs.

Confidentiality

Confidentiality is the ethical principle or legal right that a physician or other health professional will hold secret all information relating to a patient, unless the patient gives consent permitting disclosure. As such, it follows that breaching confidentiality can result in "harm" to the relationship between the receiver and the provider of emergency care.

The first federal privacy standards to protect patients' medical records and other health information provided to health plan staff, doctors, hospitals, and other health care providers took effect on April 14, 2003. Developed by the Department of Health and Human Services (DHHS), these new standards give patients access to their medical records and more control over how their personal health information is used and disclosed. The standards represent a uniform, federal floor of privacy protection for consumers across the country. Patients' privacy protections are part of the Health Insurance Portability and Accountability Act (HIPAA) of 1996. The HIPAA act includes provisions designed to encourage electronic transactions and also requires new safeguards to protect the security and confidentiality of health information. ED clinicians need to be familiar with all the HIPAA regulations related to confidentiality when intervening during an emergency.

Confidentiality Exceptions

Because confidentiality is such a critical issue, exceptions to confidentiality must also be considered during an emergency. Some examples of confidentiality exceptions are given here.

When Disclosure Is Required to Prevent Clear and Imminent Danger to Patients

The complexities surrounding confidentiality are brought to the forefront when dealing with a suicidal or potentially suicidal patient. Any decision to breach confidentiality should be made with careful consideration. The difficulty in making a decision, even in cases of suicide risk, lies in assessing "clear and imminent danger." Determining that a patient is at risk of committing suicide leads to actions that can be exceptionally disruptive to the patient's life. Just as clinicians can be accused of malpractice for neglecting to take action to prevent harm when a patient is determined to be suicidal, they also can be accused of wrong-doing if they overreact and precipitously take actions that violate a patient's privacy or freedom when there is no basis for doing so.

When Suicidal Patients Are Transferred from the ED Setting to Another Facility

Confidentiality exceptions allow the transferring ED clinician to forward pertinent information that is crucial to initiate treatment in the receiving facility.

To Prevent Possible Harm to a Potential Victim

Breaching of confidentiality is allowed to fulfill the responsibility of warning an intended victim of possible harm.

Negligence

Negligence in the ED may result from a wrongful intervention subsequently leading to an "injury" to the patient receiving the intervention. As a general legal principle, in order to accuse an ED clinician with negligence, a court of law must find evidence of the following infractions:

1. A duty was owed by the ED clinician to the patient.
2. The duty owed was breached.
3. There is sufficient legal causal connection between the breach of duty and the patient's injury.
4. Injury or damages were suffered by the patient.

The following questions are related to negligence in assessing the benefits and risks of the emergency intervention:

1. Was the ED clinician aware or should the clinician have been aware of the risk?
2. Was the ED clinician thorough in assessment of the patient's suicide risk and the urgency of the intervention?
3. Did the ED clinician make "reasonable and prudent efforts" to collect sufficient and necessary data to assess risk?
4. Were the assessment data misused, thus leading to a misdiagnosis where the same data would have resulted in appropriate diagnosis by another ED clinician?
5. Did the ED clinician mismanage the case, being "unavailable or unresponsive to the patient's emergency situation"?
6. Was the ED clinician negligent in ways in which the intervention was carried out after assessing risk?

7. Did the ED clinician make adequate attempts to keep the patient safe (e.g., set up a plan of contingencies with appropriate resources, phone numbers)?
8. Did the ED clinician remove the means to be used by the patient in the suicide attempt?
9. In cases involving minors, were parents or caregivers informed of the minor's potential risk?

Informed Consent

Patients requiring emergency treatment must be given sufficient and accurate information to make an informed decision about the treatment. Treating without consent or exceeding the limitations of the consent may make the ED clinician liable for lack of informed consent. Although obtaining a written consent is wise, this is not legally necessary.

When obtaining informed consent, it is important to give the patient the opportunity to ask questions about significant risks, benefits, and alternatives. Documentation is crucial, because patients may not remember the informed consent if adverse events occur.

Relatively few malpractice verdicts are based solely on lack of informed consent. The issue becomes more of a factor when patients experience an unexpected complication. ED clinicians should not be concerned about frightening patients if they discuss all possible risks associated with an emergency intervention. It is better to give full information about possible risks than face future negligence claims.

Competence to Consent to Treatment

Under certain circumstances, there are exceptions to the informed consent rule. The most common exceptions are:

- An emergency in which medical care is needed immediately to prevent serious or irreversible harm
- Incompetence—that is, someone is unable to give permission (or to refuse permission) for testing or treatment.

The Right to Refuse Treatment

Except for involuntary treatment, patients who are declared legally competent to make medical decisions and who are judged by the ED clinician to have decision-making capacity have the legal right to refuse any or all treatment, even though their decisions may result in serious disability or even death.

Refusing a test, procedure, or recommended treatment does not necessarily mean that patients are refusing all care. An alternative treatment should always be offered to anyone who refuses the initially recommended treatment.

Signing Out Against Medical Advice

Signing out against medical advice (AMA) is often an indication of lack of communication between the receiver and provider of emergency care. There may be several reasons for AMA, including fear, anger, and psychosis.

Patients who leave AMA often return for needed emergency treatment, unless the ED has explicitly denied them further care. Patients who are considered competent have the right to sign out against medical advice, and they are not required to sign an AMA form before leaving the ED. If they refuse to sign the form, their refusal is documented in their medical records. If they leave without signing the form, although they did not actually refuse to do so, this also needs to be documented.

Assessment of Competence

Whether a patient is competent to accept or refuse emergency treatment depends on the following factors:
1. The capacity to understand and make decisions about the provided information
2. Recognition of the presence of a condition requiring emergency treatment
3. Understanding the risks and benefits of the treatment, alternatives to the treatment, and refusing the treatment
4. Making the decision voluntarily and without coercion

Incompetence

Patients who are considered incompetent to make informed decisions in regard to treatment may require surrogate decision-makers. State laws differ on the necessity for this requirement. In some states the patient's family may be allowed to fulfill this role; in others further legal procedures may be needed; for example, a guardian may be appointed by the court to make decisions. In the case of minors, parents or legal guardian may assume this role.

Methods for Controlling Potential or Actual Violence

Many EDs have implemented security protocols to prevent violence that jeopardizes the safety of patients and staffs. In most states, ED clinicians can restrain patients for the purpose of assessment and examination pending commitment and involuntary hospitalization. However, before recommending restraint or seclusion, ED clinicians need to be knowledgeable about the various local and state involuntary commitment laws.

Methods for controlling potential and actual violence include physical restraints, chemical (pharmacological) restraints, and verbal management techniques.

Physical Restraints

ED clinicians are legally and ethically required to clearly state the reason for restraint, even if the patient is unable to hear or to understand the explanation. Physical restraints are not applied unless they are determined to be absolutely necessary in order to prevent the patient from causing serious injury to self or others or if they are necessary to attend to the patient's medical treatment. After 24 hours, the ED clinician involved in the care and treatment of a restrained patient must make a new determination before the restraint can be continued.

Use of a restraint and the reasons for it are noted in the patient's clinical records. A copy of each entry or a summary of such entries is forwarded to the chief medical officer for review. A patient placed in physical restraint is checked at least every 30 minutes by staff trained in the use of restraints, and a written record of such checks is documented.

When the application of a restraint is necessary in emergency situations to protect the patient from immediate injury to self or to others, restraints may be authorized by attending staff, who must immediately report the action taken to the ED clinician involved in the care and treatment of that patient. The ED must have written policies and procedures that govern the use of restraints and that clearly delineate, in descending order, the personnel who can authorize the use of restraints in emergency situations.

All orders for physical restraints must be in writing and state the time and the reasons restraints were applied. Criteria for removal of restraints need to be established before the written order expires; these criteria must be based on the staff's clinical evaluation that restraints are no longer necessary.

Once restraints are applied, any injury or harm to the patient is de facto evidence of negligence.

If physical restraints are instituted but commitment or involuntary treatment is not accomplished, clinicians are not considered liable, provided that good faith and reasonable causes justified the application of restraints.

Chemical (Pharmacological) Restraints

Chemical restraints are considered by many to be more humane than physical restraints.

Since 1991, the laws governing the use of chemical restraints have been modified several times, and they vary among the different states. In general, amendments to the law make it possible for a hospital to medicate patients committed involuntarily with short-term (up to 30 days) pharmacological therapy if a second, concurring medical opinion has approved use of the medication. For treatment extending beyond 30 days, a special court hearing is required to determine if there is legal justification for continuing administration of the medications. The advantages and disadvantages of chemical restraints are summarized in Table 23-1.

Medications may be given orally, intramuscularly, or intravenously, alone or in combination, and adjusted as needed. No single medication is appropriate for every situation. Details of the pharmacological management of violent agitated patients are discussed in several chapters throughout this book.

Verbal Management

In many cases, verbal management of violent patients may be as effective as physical or chemical restraints. Some examples of verbal management are shown in Box 23-1.

Verbal management is not effective in patients with florid psychosis, delirium, severe intoxication, or agitation secondary to manic episodes. Such patients may be asked if they wish to be restrained; sometimes they agree because they feel that they are a part of the decision process, which gives them a sense of control.

Limitations in the ED Setting

It is important to recognize and understand the limitations in emergency care. ED clinicians should never be afraid to admit that they do not have all the answers, nor should they be

---

Table 23–1

Advantages and Disadvantages of Chemical Restraints

Advantages	Disadvantages
Control violent behavior and patient agitation without physical force	May result in complications, such as respiratory depression
May reduce need for physical restraints	Paradoxical reactions may occasionally occur, resulting in increased agitation
Facilitate medical examination procedures, such as radiographic imaging	Limit mental status assessment and neurologic examination during episodes of sedation

---

Box 23–1. Examples of Verbal Management of Violent Patients

- Minimize hostility by avoiding direct confrontation.
- Empathize with patients' concerns.
- Involve other ED staff members if necessary.
- Encourage cooperation by offering food and liquids.
- Clarify limits and outline the consequences of violent behavior.

reluctant to request consultation when it may benefit patients. Patients respect this candor and usually will follow recommendations if they are informed that it is in their best interests to seek consultation.

Use of Consultants

All ED clinicians should know to profit from access to consultants and should always inform patients of the intent to obtain input from other caregivers. Explain in lay terms the reasons for the decision to seek consultation and give patients the opportunity to request a specific physician if they so desire. If the consultation concerns an invasive or an extensive procedure, this should be discussed with the patient. When calling a consultant, the specific reason for the call must be clearly stated and documented.

Standard of Care

 The concept *standard of care* is defined as the care a patient can reasonably expect to receive from a provider with comparable experience and training in the same geographic location as the ED. For example, clinicians in a geographic location without access to specialists caring for a patient with an acute episode of agitation will be held to a different standard than clinicians in a location where such specialists are readily available.

It is important for clinicians to know the standard of care for the ED within their specialty and geographical area. For example, if the standard of care in a community includes ED clinicians qualified to perform and interpret neuropsychological tests, performance of these tests by an untrained staff member would be below the standard of care.

End-of-Life Care

 The issues surrounding end-of-life care are difficult ones for most clinicians. It is essential that patients and their families know that ED clinicians are there for them during this time. When the primary care physician may not be intimately involved in a patient's terminal care, the patient and family may seek the clinician's guidance and support.

ED clinicians should never abandon their patients, either physically or emotionally. They should provide the opportunity for the patient and family to ask questions. By establishing a close rapport with patients, clinicians will know when the time is appropriate to recommend ending aggressive measures and providing palliative care.

Basic Standards in Emergency Psychiatry Interventions

 Emergency psychiatry interventions need to be conducted in an appropriate private area of the ED, where patients and family members can be interviewed without distractions. The area should be equipped with communication equipment such as phones, computers, and emergency buttons.

Emergency psychiatric interventions require adequate time to provide a comprehensive assessment and treatment recommendations. Access to laboratory test facilities and medical specialties for consultation should be available to rule out medical conditions, as well as medication to treat those conditions.

Patients requiring emergency psychiatry interventions should be afforded the same standards of treatment as other patients presenting to the ED.

Documentation and Disposition

 ED clinicians should exercise care when documenting data supporting emergency treatment and involuntary commitment. It is especially important to record the reasons for releasing a patient. If a bad outcome occurs, such as suicide, homicide, or assault, a poorly documented note, even if the decision was appropriate, will be judged retrospectively as grounds for negligence.

Further Reading

Beachamp TL, Childress JF: Principles of Biomedical Ethics, 4th ed. New York: Oxford University Press; 1994, pp 132-141, 164-170.

Brennan TA, Sox CM, Burstin HR: Relation between negligent adverse events and the outcomes of medical-malpractice litigation. N Engl J Med 1996;335:1963-1967.

Checkland D: On risk and decisional capacity. J Med Philos 2001;26:35-39.

Citrome L: New treatments for agitation. Psychiatr Q 2004;75:197-213.

COBRA: The Consolidated Omnibus Budget Reconciliation Act. 1987.

Culver C, Gert B: The inadequacy of incompetence. Milbank Q 1990;68:619-643.

Haffey WJ: The assessment of clinical competency to consent to medical rehabilitative interventions. J Head Trauma Rehabil 1989;4:43-56.

Joint Commission on Accreditation of Healthcare Organizations: Comprehensive Accreditation Manual for Hospitals: The Official Handbook (CAMH). Oak Brook Terrace, Ill, 2005-2006.

Jonsen A, Siegler M, Winslade W: Clinical Ethics, 3rd ed. New York, McGraw-Hill, 1992, pp 41-55.

Khouzam HR: Customer service vs patient care. Conn Med 2002;66:161-162.

Khouzam HR: Personal accounts: A touch of dynamic psychiatry. Psychiatr Serv 2000;51:437-438.

Knowles FE 3rd, Liberto J, Baker FM, et al: Competency evaluations in a VA hospital. A 10-year perspective. Gen Hosp Psychiatry 1994;16:119-124.

Levinson W: Physician-patient communication: A key to malpractice prevention [editorial]. JAMA 1994;272:1619-1620.

Mebane A, Rauch H: When do physicians request competency evaluations? Psychosomatics 1990;31:40-46.

Morris CD, Niederbuhl JM, Mahr JM: Determining the capability of individuals with mental retardation to give informed consent. Am J Ment Retard 1993;98:263-272.

Moskop JC, Marco CA, Larkin GL, et al: From Hippocrates to HIPAA: Privacy and confidentiality in emergency medicine—Part I: Conceptual, moral, and legal foundations. Ann Emerg Med 2005;45:53-59.

Moskop JC, Marco CA, Larkin GL, et al: From Hippocrates to HIPAA: Privacy and confidentiality in emergency medicine—Part II: Challenges in the emergency department. Ann Emerg Med 2005;45:60-67.

Puryear DA: Proposed standards in emergency psychiatry. Hosp Community Psychiatry 1992;43:14-15.

Roth LH, Meisel A, Lidz C: Tests of competency to consent to treatment. Am J Psychiatry 1977;134:279-284.

Slusarenko PK: Epidural anaesthesia: Concerns regarding informed consent. Can Anaesth Soc J 1985;32:681-682.

Urofsky R, Sowa C: Ethics education in CACREP-accredited counselor education programs. Counsel Values 2004;49:37-47.

Postscript

The search for truth is more precious than its possession.

John Dryden—1631-1700

C H A P T E R 2 4

Religious and Spiritual Dimensions of Psychiatric Emergencies

Hani R. Khouzam, MD, MPH, FAPA

KEY POINTS

- Religious and spiritual beliefs are an important component in the lives of many people.
- Religious and spiritual problems may be misunderstood and misdiagnosed by both emergency department (ED) clinicians and religious professionals.
- Taking a religious and spiritual history should be an integral component of the emergency psychiatric assessment of patients presenting with religious or spiritual problems.
- The accurate evaluation and assessment of powerful religious and spiritual emergencies can significantly influence the eventual outcome and lead to appropriate disposition.
- Patients' religious and spiritual beliefs are important tools that can be utilized for enhancing coping and problem solving.
- Intervening in religious and spiritual emergencies may be an opportunity for ED clinicians to reflect on and test their own religious and spiritual beliefs.

Overview

Spiritual and religious experiences unfortunately may be misunderstood by ED clinicians and religious professionals, resulting in misdiagnosis. Individuals undergoing powerful religious or spiritual experiences are sometimes at risk for being treated as mentally ill or psychiatrically unstable. An appropriate response on the part of the ED clinician to a person's religious and spiritual problems can determine whether the experience is integrated and used as a stimulus for personal growth or whether it is repressed as a bizarre event that may be a sign of mental instability. Similarly, negative reactions by religious professionals to a religious emergency can intensify the individual's sense of isolation and block his or her efforts to seek assistance in understanding and assimilating the experience.

This chapter addresses the evaluation, assessment, and disposition of psychiatric emergencies related to religious and spiritual problems. Methods for utilizing a patient's personal spiritual and religious beliefs as a coping tool in time of emergencies are summarized and emphasized.

Definition

Religious or spiritual emergencies are crises during which the process of growth and change may become chaotic and overwhelming. In such episodes, individuals often suddenly and dramatically enter into new realms of mystical and spiritual experience. However, they may also become fearful and confused and have difficulty coping with their daily lives, jobs, and relationships. In the fourth edition of the *Diagnostic and Statistical Manual of Mental Disorders*, *Text Revision* (DSM-IV-TR), religious or spiritual problems are defined as distressing experiences that involve a person's relationship with a transcendent being or force but are not necessarily related to an organized church or religious institution.

Religion. Religion is generally regarded as any system of belief regarding humankind's relation to the divine, which includes practices of worship, sacred texts, and, usually, administrative and physical structures to promote the ongoing practice of the religion and member cohesion.

Spirituality. Spirituality can be defined as a belief system focusing on intangible elements that impart vitality and meaning to life events. Spirituality represents the belief that an individual can be affected directly by a transcendent, divine spirit, and that this experience can be facilitated by focused contemplation, meditation, prayer, or other rituals. Often spirituality is expressed through formalized religions.

The distinction between "being spiritual" and "being religious" appears, moreover, to be gaining in prevalence. Although religious and spiritual concepts often now overlap, the meanings of these words continue to evolve, with concepts of religion tending to become narrower over time, whereas those of spirituality tend to broaden.

The interplay of spirituality, religion, and health care has been documented in many research studies; this factor has an impact on the incidences, experiences, and outcomes of several common medical and psychiatric conditions.

Epidemiology

Several epidemiologic studies have shown that 96% of Americans believe in a God or a Universal Spirit, 75% pray regularly, 42% attend religious worship services somewhat regularly, 67% are members of some local religious body, and 67% feel that religion is "very important in their lives." Furthermore, 79% believe spiritual faith can help people with disease and 63% believe that physicians should talk with patients about their spiritual faith.

Approximately 80% of the general U.S. population perceived some overlap between the terms *religion* and *spirituality*. However, the respondents considered spirituality broader and more indicative of a personal connection to a higher power, as opposed to religion, which was linked to more institutional beliefs and practices.

Studies show that people are living longer, often with major chronic diseases, and in their later years are becoming more concerned about spiritual and religious issues.

Studies also report that people born after 1950 are less likely to have had moral, emotional, religious, or spiritual preparation to cope with life in today's technologically fast-paced information culture. A "spiritual hunger" or search for the sacred is often cited to explain why books on spiritual topics become bestsellers.

In today's modern society, in which individualism and personal autonomy are promoted and idealized, people may feel more socially disconnected and more fragmented in their personal lives, with little sense of connectedness or community. Religious and spiritual affiliation offer alternative options to belong and to connect with others.

Assessment of Religious and Spiritual Aspects of Psychiatric Emergencies

The initial clinical assessment of powerful spiritual experiences can significantly influence the eventual outcome in the ED. Using the same interviewing approaches as in other history taking, the spiritual history interview can and should be simple and mostly open-ended, with the objective of eliciting both baseline and in-depth information that reflects a patient's spiritual dimension. It is of utmost importance to get feedback from patients regarding their feelings about being asked spiritual history questions and about the kinds of questions they are being asked.

Personal Reflections

 In order to accomplish this initial phase of assessment, ED clinicians should first ask themselves certain questions for personal reflection and discussion, including the following:

- How comfortably do I feel about discussing spiritual and religious issues with patients?
- What roles are appropriate for me to take in this setting?
- What roles are inappropriate for me to take in this setting?

Taking the Spiritual History

One approach when taking a patient's spiritual history is the mnemonic **SPIRIT**, described in Table 24-1, which can be used as a guide for identifying important components of the spiritual history.

Examples of Religious and Spiritual Problems
Religious Problems
The loss of faith is mentioned in the DSM-IV-TR definition as a religious problem, but other religious problems can result from the loss of religious connection, including:

- Questioning of faith
- Change in denominational membership or conversion to a new religion
- Intensification of adherence to the beliefs and practices of one's faith
- Joining, participating in, or leaving a new religious movement or cult

Table 24–1

The Mnemonic SPIRIT

SPIRIT	**Inquiries**
S = Spiritual belief system	Do you have a formal religious affiliation? Can you describe this?
	Do you have a spiritual life that is important to you?
	What is your clearest sense of the meaning of your life at this time?
P = Personal spirituality	Describe the beliefs and practices of your religion that you personally accept. Describe those beliefs and practices that you do not accept or follow.
	In what ways is your spirituality/religion meaningful for you?
	How is your spirituality/religion important to you in daily life?
I = Integration with a spiritual community	Do you belong to any religious or spiritual groups or communities?
	How do you participate in this group/community? What is your role?
	What importance does this group have for you?
	In what ways is this group a source of support for you?
	What types of support and help does or could this group provide for you in dealing with health issues?
R = Ritualized practices and restrictions	What specific practices do you carry out as part of your religious and spiritual life (e.g., prayer, meditation, service, etc.)
	What lifestyle activities or practices does your religion encourage, discourage, or forbid?
	What meaning do these practices and restrictions have for you?
	To what extent have you followed these guidelines?

Continued

Table 24–1

The Mnemonic SPIRIT—cont'd

SPIRIT	Inquiries
I = Implications for medical care	Are there specific elements of medical care that your religion discourages or forbids? To what extent have you followed these guidelines?
	What aspects of your religion/spirituality would you like to keep in mind as I care for you?
	What knowledge or understanding would strengthen our relationship as physician and patient?
	Are there barriers to our relationship based upon religious or spiritual issues?
	Would you like to discuss religious or spiritual implications of health care?
T = Terminal events planning	Are there particular aspects of medical care that you wish to forgo or have withheld because of your religion/spirituality?
	Are there religious or spiritual practices or rituals that you would like to have available in the hospital or at home?
	Are there religious or spiritual practices that you wish to plan for at the time of death, or following death?
	From what sources do you draw strength in order to cope with this illness?
	For what in your life do you still feel gratitude even though ill?
	When you are afraid or in pain, how do you find comfort?
	As we plan for your medical care near the end of life, in what ways will your religion and spirituality influence your decisions?

Adapted with permission from Maugans TA: The SPIRITual History. Arch Fam Med 1997;5:11-16.

Generally people undergo such changes without any significant crisis or emergency; however, some individuals will experience significant distress and may seek emergency mental health assessment and treatment for these problems.

Spiritual Problems

Spiritual problems may be related to questioning of spiritual values, which can be triggered by an experience of loss of spiritual connection. That loss may occur in relation to traditional, comforting religious or spiritual tenets and community identification or to a more personal search for spiritual identity; it may be expressed as:
- Anger and resentment
- Emptiness and despair
- Sadness and isolation
- A certain degree of relief

Examples of Religious and Spiritual Emergencies
Illness Seen as Punishment

A willingness to elicit and address patients' spiritual concerns in an ED setting is essential in situations where the perception of an illness as a sin can affect treatment decisions. Patients may refuse to take their medications, including those prescribed for medical conditions, because of their beliefs about what the medications or illness itself signifies. Some patients may believe their symptoms can be cured through prayer, and others reject all treatment modalities because they firmly believe that their illness is a punishment from God and that they don't deserve to be relieved of their suffering. The spiritual issues that patients may bring up during these emergency situations are varied and may include hopelessness, anger at God, grief, and loss.

Through empathic and supportive listening, ED clinicians may play an essential role in helping patients to utilize their spiritual beliefs in coping with illness. Supportive interventions should focus on the restoration of hope, forgiveness, love, and other spiritual values that can enhance coping and healing.

Near-Death Experiences (NDEs)

NDE is a subjective event experienced by persons who either were close to death or were believed to be dead and then unexpectedly recovered. Others may have had an NDE during a potentially fatal event and then escaped uninjured. NDE usually is characterized by dissociation from the physical body, strong positive affect, and transcendental experiences. Several characteristic temporal sequences of stages have been described during an NED:

1. Peace and contentment
2. Detachment from physical body
3. Entering a transitional region of darkness
4. Seeing a brilliant light
5. Passing through the light into another realm of existence

Although positive personality transformations frequently follow NDEs, interpersonal difficulties may also arise. Many individuals report that they doubted their mental stability, and therefore did not discuss the NDE with friends or professionals for fear of being labeled as mentally ill. Even religious professionals are not always sensitive to the spiritual dimensions of such experiences.

ED clinicians need to be aware that because of advances in medical technology, an increasing number of persons survive nearly fatal outcomes and experience NDEs with at least some of the features described previously above. NDEs are now recognized as fairly common occurrences in intensive care units (ICUs), and they need to be differentiated from ICU psychoses—NDEs should not be "treated" with antipsychotics.

Breaking Away from a Spiritual Leader

Some spiritual leaders may be authoritarian and foster a culture of enmeshment and dependence in their followers. When individuals decide to leave such a spiritual leader to seek independent functioning, they may experience intense feelings of betrayal, anger, fear, worthlessness, and guilt. During this period of transition, these individuals may seek ED interventions. The emergency intervention may be directed toward meeting the challenge of restoring personal integrity.

ED clinicians need to know that many individuals who have left destructive spiritual teachers have reported that the experience ultimately contributed to their wisdom and maturity.

Meditation-Related Problems

Intensive meditation practices can lead to altered perceptions. The meditations can be delightful (false enlightenment) or frightening and accompanied by terrifying visions. These practices are usually associated with Eastern traditions but also have been transplanted to Western meditation practices. A specific mental disorder that Tibetans call *sokrlung* can result from practicing meditation related to the "life-bearing wind that supports the mind"; it occurs as a consequence of straining too tightly in an obsessive way to achieve "moment-to-moment awareness." Such changes are not necessarily pathologic and may reflect in part a heightened sensitivity; however, they may lead to anxiety, dissociation, depersonalization, agitation, and muscular tension.

ED clinicians need to distinguish between psychopathology and meditation-related experiences. The voluntarily induced experiences of depersonalization or derealization that are part of meditative and trance practices should not be confused with the psychiatric symptoms of depersonalization associated with dissociative disorders.

Mystical Experiences

Mystical experiences can be defined as transient, extraordinary episodes marked by intense feelings of unity, harmonious relationship to the divine and to all creation, as well as euphoria and sense of access to a hidden spiritual dimension. Loss of ego functioning, alterations in time and space perception, and the sense of lacking control may also characterize such events, which have been described as "upheaval of the total personality" and "spiritual force that seems to lift someone out of the self." Although mystical experiences are usually associated with well-being, in some cases mystical experiences are disruptive and distressing, leading to spiritual problems and a spiritual emergency.

 ED clinicians should be careful not to misdiagnose mystical experiences as mania, schizophrenia, or panic disorder and should attempt to integrate such experiences as a component of their own overall spiritual beliefs and practices.

Psychic Experiences

Psychic experiences are extrasensory occurrences, such as *clairvoyance*, in which people experience visions of past, future, or remote events, and *telepathy*, communication without apparent physical means. These experiences are associated with many spiritual paths and altered states of consciousness. Spiritual problems related to unpredictable psychic experiences can lead to a crisis requiring emergency intervention. Interventions by ED clinicians may be difficult due to the subjective nature of psychic experiences, and referral to reputable professionals trained in dealing with these issues is strongly advised.

Visionary Experiences

Visionary experiences involve the activation of the unconscious archetypal psyche, which then dominates consciousness. This activation is believed to be the part of the mind that produces dreams and also myths. Visionary experiences have played a pivotal role in the evolution of cultures, particularly when rapid cultural change is occurring due to outside interventions or indigenous changes. Cultural turmoil activates the psyches of many individuals, and sometimes creative cultural innovations emerge from this process.

When the psyche is activated to an intense degree during visionary experiences, the individual can appear psychotic. Beliefs that meet the DSM-IV-TR criteria for delusions, particularly grandiose ones, as well as hallucinations, are usually present, although for many patients, the experience became a turning point in their lives toward growth. During the acute phase, when psychotic symptoms usually are present, the individual may become seriously disabled and may experience crises that require emergency intervention.

ED clinicians may need to initiate treatment of the prominent psychotic symptoms until the acute phase of the visionary experiences subside.

Shamanic Crisis

Shamanism is one of humanity's oldest healing practices, dating back to the Paleolithic era. Originally, the word *shaman* referred specifically to a healer of the Tungus people of Siberia. In recent times, that name has been given to healers in many traditional cultures around the globe who use consciousness-altering techniques in their practice.

Historically, shamanism has been confused with schizophrenia because shamans often speak of altered-state experiences in the spirit world as if they were "real" experiences. The themes common to shamanic crises include descent to the realm of death, confrontations with demonic forces, dismemberment, trial by fire, communion with the world of spirits and mythical creatures, assimilation of elemental forces, ascension via the World Tree and/or Cosmic Bird, realization of a solar identity, and return to the Middle World (the world of human affairs).

Persons experiencing a shamanic crisis can decompensate and may seek emergency treatment. ED clinicians may apply principles of crisis interventions, as described in Chapter 1, when intervening in a shamanic crisis.

Alien Encounters

Alien encounters are usually described as abduction by aliens. These experiences are characterized by subjective memories of being taken secretly and/or against one's will by apparently nonhuman entities, usually to a location described as an alien spacecraft commonly referred to as a UFO (unidentified flying object). The content themes of UFO encounters are commonly described as capture, examination, communication with aliens, other-worldly journey, theophany (receipt of spiritual messages), and finally return to earth.

Although patients with schizophrenia and posttraumatic stress disorder (PTSD) have reported alien encounter experiences, many persons without psychiatric disorders have reported such experiences. Both positive and problematic aftereffects have been reported by persons claiming to have experienced alien encounters. These include injuries such as cuts, bruises, puncture wounds, eye problems, skin burns and irritation, gastrointestinal distress, equilibrium and balance problems, thirst, dehydration, and healing of a preexisting illness.

Other symptoms and potential problems in persons reporting encounters with UFOs include:

- Anxiety and irritability
- Intrusive thoughts about aliens and abduction
- Labile mood
- Disorientation, derealization, and depersonalization
- Psychic experiences presumed to be from an extraterrestrial source (e.g., telepathic messages)
- The belief that one's thoughts are being shared with extraterrestrial beings
- Change in spiritual or religious values, beliefs, and practices
- Fear, anticipation, and recurring nightmares
- Paranormal experiences and personality changes

Such extraordinary experiences, which to many seem sheer fantasy, are prevalent and cannot be ignored when individuals with symptoms attributed to UFO encounters present to the ED.

ED interventions should be supportive and based on enhancing coping strategies to deal with the aftereffects of the reported alien encounter rather than on attempting to discredit such occurrences.

Possession Experiences

In the DSM-IV-TR, *possession* and *possession trance* are listed under the diagnosis Dissociative Disorder Not Otherwise Specified. Possession trance is defined as a single or episodic alteration in the state of consciousness characterized by the replacement of the customary sense of personal identity by a new identity, which is attributed to the influence of a spirit, power, deity, or other person. The DSM-IV-TR also lists the related Dissociative Trance Disorder as a diagnosis requiring further study.

Possessed individuals enter an altered state of consciousness in which they feel that a spirit, power, deity, or other person has assumed control of their mind, body, and soul. Generally, there is no recall of these experiences in the waking state. Such experiences have a long human history, and many religions offer healing rituals to protect persons from unwanted possession.

The oldest theories about the etiology of mental disorders identifies spiritual possession as the cause. People with complaints of being possessed may present to the ED with associated clinical symptoms related to feelings of loss of control over bizarre behaviors such as choking, projectile vomiting, frantic motor behavior, wild spasms, and contortions along with grotesque vocalizations that are frightening for both the possessed person and those witnessing the symptoms.

 ED interventions should be supportive and based on symptomatic relief of distress and motivation and on the enhancement of coping strategies rather than on attempts to reverse the precipitating events that led to the possession episode. Medical workup with an electroencephalogram (EEG) and brain imaging may be obtained to diagnose frontal lobe dysfunction, which could present with a clinical picture that resembles possession experiences.

Spiritual Emergence

Spiritual emergence is a type of "born-again experience" in which some aspects of a person's life that were not yet encompassed by the fullness of life are integrated or challenged to be integrated into a fuller and deeper life. Although spiritual emergence is usually less disruptive than the other previously described spiritual emergencies, it can also lead persons to seek interventions to help integrate the newly found spiritual experiences. ED clinicians should promptly refer persons with spiritual emergence to qualified professionals, including clergy who belong to the same religious affiliation as the patient experiencing the spiritual emergence.

Differential Diagnosis of Religious and Spiritual Emergencies

Religious and spiritual emergencies can be associated with unusual experiences and behaviors, including visual, auditory, olfactory, and kinesthetic perceptions. These may appear to be psychiatric symptoms of delusions, loosening of associations, thought disorder, or disorganized behavior. Therefore, in many instances, making the distinction between religious and spiritual emergencies and certain psychiatric emergencies can be difficult (Table 24-2).

Table 24–2

Differences between Psychiatric Symptoms and Religious and Spiritual Emergencies

Psychiatric Symptoms	Religious and Spiritual Emergencies
Illusions and/or hallucinations prominent	Perceptual alterations coinciding with and overlapping with religious and spiritual experiences
Affect may be flat, restricted, neutral or incongruent with the underlying prevailing mood; mood frequently fluctuates	Mood described as "ecstatic"; experienced as "beyond words"; affect usually mood-congruent; prevailing mood persisting for several weeks
Delusions fixed and persistent	Sense of newly-gained knowledge
Conceptual disorganization in the form of incoherence and thought blocking	No conceptual disorganization; ideas lucidly expressed
Ongoing deterioration in functioning; presence of paranoia, grandiose delusions; social isolation	Positive outcome likely; life-changing experiences (e.g., enlightened, altruism)
High risk for homicide and/or suicide	Low risk for homicide and/or suicide

In religious and spiritual emergencies, social, psychological, and physical factors can be involved, and these also play a role in psychiatric disorders. The relationship between these concepts is therefore complex. Differential diagnostic skills may have a part to play in offering help to those whose problems may have a spiritual or a medical/psychiatric origin. Spiritual discernment by the ED clinicians is of at least equal, if not greater, importance when intervening in such matters.

Spiritual Issues and Comorbid Psychiatric Disorders

Traditionally, the clinical literature tended to regard religiosity in persons with mental disorders as a component of the pathology. There was even implied assertion that the less religious patients were, the more emotionally healthy they tended to be. Only in the past decade has psychiatry begun to address a bias against spirituality and religion that dates back to some of the writings of Sigmund Freud.

 The American Psychiatric Association (APA) has issued guidelines advising psychiatrists to be sensitive to patients' religious and spiritual beliefs. The guidelines state that "psychiatrists should not impose their own religious, antireligious, or ideological systems of beliefs on their patients, nor should they substitute such beliefs or rituals for accepted diagnostic concepts or therapeutic practices." Explicit and nonjudgmental attention to religious concerns can add significantly to the quality and effectiveness of clinical work. Indeed, struggles of faith are embedded in the life course of many patients in acute and emergency therapy, and in such cases, spiritual problems can be associated with the full range of mental disorders. In the DSM-IV-TR, the diagnosis Religious or Spiritual Problems is an Axis I condition and can be assigned along with coexisting other Axis I disorders. Following are some examples of comorbid Axis I disorders.

Substance Dependence

The founders of Alcoholics Anonymous (AA), Bill Wilson and Bob Smith, did not ponder whether religious and spiritual factors were important in recovery, but rather whether it was possible for alcohol-dependent persons to recover without the help of a higher power. They believed that when a spiritual awakening occurred in a recovering alcoholic, the craving for alcohol was the equivalent of the spiritual thirst of human beings for wholeness. Given the magnitude of the spiritual dimension in the case of substance dependence, some clinicians have approached all drug addictions as essentially spiritual crises rather than psychiatric disorders.

Because substance dependence may coexist with other religious and spiritual problems, the diagnosis Religious or Spiritual Problem should be coded as an Axis I disorder along with Substance Dependence.

It is significant that patients in alcohol and drug treatment programs who become involved with a religious community after treatment have lower relapse rates than those who do not.

Obsessive-Compulsive Disorder

Some individuals with obsessive-compulsive disorder present with what they consider scrupulous devoutness, but upon further assessment, their religiosity may be a metaphor for the expression of compulsiveness. Superficially, religious rituals and obsessive-compulsive behaviors share some common features, such as the prominent role of cleanliness and purity; the need for rituals to be carried out in specific ways and for a certain number of times; and the fear of performing the rituals incorrectly. The following criteria may be used for differentiating obsessive-compulsive behaviors from religious practices:

1. Compulsive behavior usually exceeds and goes beyond the letter of the religious practices.
2. Compulsive behavior is focused on one specific area and does not reflect an overall concern for all religious rituals and practices.
3. The choice of focus of obsessive-compulsive behavior is typical of the disorder—e.g., cleanliness for fear of contamination, checking for safety concerns, and obsessively fearful thoughts about blasphemy toward God or about illness.
4. In obsessive-compulsive disorder, almost all the important dimensions of religious practices are neglected, and the patient's life is totally consumed by these behaviors.

Psychotic Disorders

Coexistence of religious and spiritual problems and psychotic disorders may frequently occur, especially during manic episodes of bipolar disorder and in paranoid schizophrenia. In such cases, the diagnosis Religious or Spiritual Problem should be coded along with the concomitant Axis I disorder. It is important to treat the psychosis because during a psychotic episode patients are unable to differentiate their delusions and hallucinations from their spiritual and religious beliefs. When the psychotic symptoms subside, patients are often able to gain insight into their experiences and separate their beliefs from their psychosis.

By being nonjudgmental and discerning, ED clinicians can avoid the presumption of considering certain kinds of religious experience or behavior as being simply a manifestation of psychosis. Many mentally ill patients' experiences of the divine and the spiritual can be quite healthy—genuine, believable, and life-giving. Patients recovering from psychosis who have strong spiritual and religious beliefs may have renewed opportunities for spiritual growth, along with challenges to its expression and development. They will find much-needed support for the task when they are guided clinically by ED clinicians to explore their spiritual lives.

Interventions

The religious convictions of patients can be used effectively during psychiatric emergencies. Religion can be a usable support system for the patient even when ED clinicians believe that patients' spiritual and religious beliefs have no objective value. The mnemonic FAITH, described in Table 24-3, can help structure questions when ED clinicians are planning interventions.

Spiritual and religious beliefs have an important role in specific psychiatric interventions, such as depression, substance abuse, and coping with illness.

Depression

Religious commitment has been associated with a decreased prevalence of depression. Research has also demonstrated that, in addition to protecting against depression, higher levels of religious commitment may afford protection against suicide, the most severe outcome of depression. By tapping into the

Table 24–3

The Mnemonic FAITH

FAITH	Questions to Guide Interventions
F = Faith and Belief	Do you consider yourself spiritual or religious? or Do you have spiritual beliefs that help you cope with stress? If the response is "No," this question may be asked, What gives your life meaning? (Patients may respond with answers such as family, career, or nature.)
A = Affiliation	Are you part of a spiritual or religious community? Is this a support to you and how? Is there a group of people you really love or who are important to you?
I = Importance	What importance does your faith or belief have in your life? Have your beliefs influenced how you take care of yourself in this emergency? What role do your beliefs play in regaining your ability to cope with this emergency?
T = Treatment	How would you like this emergency to be addressed by the ED staff?
H = Help	At this point in the intervention, referral to churches, temples, mosques, or a group of like-minded friends can serve as systems of immediate and ongoing support for patients facing the emergency.

Adapted from Puchalski CM, Romer AL: Taking a spiritual history allows clinicians to understand patients more fully. J Pall Med 2000;3:129-137.

religious beliefs of patients with depression and suicidal ideation, the ED clinician may utilize these beliefs in implementing a plan of intervention that is congruent with the patient's spiritual and religious values.

Substance Abuse

Abuse of alcohol and other drugs has been linked to a lack of purpose in life, which often is associated with low levels of religious commitment. Individuals with a high degree of religious commitment are less likely to use alcohol and other drugs and, even if they do so, are less likely to engage in heavy use and suffer its multiple clinical and social complications. There are several possible reasons for this:

1. Attendance at religious services may influence individuals' adherence to the norms of religious groups that discourage alcohol and other drug use.
2. Religious attendance may influence individuals to develop friendships with peers who do not themselves abuse alcohol or other drugs.
3. Religious attendance may promote mental health and well-being, which militates against the initiation of substance abuse.

Coping with Illness

Religious commitment seems to become especially important once an illness, particularly a life-threatening illness, is diagnosed. Patients who become ill may rely heavily on their religious beliefs as a coping strategy. Those who use religious means of coping seem to cope more effectively with illness than those who do not. The relationship between an individual's religious commitment and coping seems to be most substantial among people with high levels of disability. Religious commitment also can moderate the relationship between disability and depression: as religious commitment increases, the relationship between disability and depression becomes weaker. The ED clinician needs to be aware of this correlation and apply it when intervening in an emergency related to coping with illness.

Recovery from Illness

Religious commitment may play a role in hastening recovery from illness. This observation has been documented in patients recovering from a life-threatening illness or undergoing extensive surgeries. Religious beliefs were also essential in preventing depression following recovery from physical illness. The ED clinician needs to utilize this relationship to enhance coping with emergencies during the recovery phase of an illness.

Specific Emergency Intervention Modalities

Because many religious practices are potentially meaningful and congruent with patients' own value systems, these practices may be valuable resources in the ED for enhanced prevention, coping, and recovery. The following techniques can help ED clinicians apply relevant aspects of patients' religious commitment to the intervention.

First, ask appropriate questions—that is, questions that can gain access to potentially valuable information on how to integrate religious factors into the care plans of patients suffering from chronic or severe medical illness that led to the psychiatric emergency.

Second, encourage patients to make use of potentially health-promoting religious resources from their own religious traditions. When appropriate, encourage patients to meditate; to increase their prayers, either individually or with others; to continue their usual religious and spiritual practices, including attending their church, synagogue, or mosque; and to engage in religiously based mourning rituals, seek and ask forgiveness from significant others, or to read holy scriptures. Refer patients to clergy or chaplains as an adjunct to standard emergency care. The involvement of clergy might be an especially important source of support for patients who, by virtue of their disability or suffering, need extra community support.

Also, when appropriate, encourage patients to meditate using the relaxation response technique. The effects of relaxation response and meditation in an emergency can be initiated with patients who hold firm religious or spiritual beliefs. The relaxation response is elicited by a simple two-step procedure: (1) repeating a word, phrase or muscular activity; and (2) passively disregarding any obtrusive thoughts that come to mind and returning to the repetition. When practiced regularly, this technique results in a reproducible set of physiologic effects and is effective therapy for many medical conditions. Box 24-1 summarizes some of these conditions.

It is notable that in one study, 80% of patients, when given the choice between a religious or secular phrase, voluntarily

Box 24–1. The Relaxation Response Technique

Technique

1. Repeat a word, sound, phrase, or prayer that has meaning for you (e.g., "one," "peace," "Om," "Sh'ma Yisroel," "The Lord is my shepherd," "Insha'allah," "Hail Mary, full of grace") or a physical activity that is calming for you (e.g., jogging, breathing techniques, knitting).
2. Passively disregard intrusive thoughts that come to mind and return to the repetitive focus.

Physiologic Effects

Decreased rate of breathing
Decreased blood pressure
Decreased muscle tension
Decreased heart rate

Conditions Responding to Relaxation Response Technique

Hypertension
Cardiac arrhythmias
Chronic pain
Anxiety
Insomnia
Mild to moderate depression
Infertility
Postoperative anxiety
Premenstrual syndrome
Migraine and cluster headaches
Low self-esteem
Symptoms of cancer and acquired immunodeficiency syndrome (AIDS)

Adapted from Anandarajah G, Hight E: Spirituality and medical practice: Using the HOPE questions as a practical tool for spiritual assessment. Am Fam Physician 2001;63:81-89; Benson H: Timeless Healing: The Power and Biology of Belief. New York, Scribner, 1996.

chose a religious phrase to elicit the relaxation response. One fourth of these patients described a feeling of increased spirituality as a result of practicing the technique. These same patients were more likely to have better measurable medical outcomes than those who did not experience increased spirituality. Other studies regarding the effects of spirituality on a patient's prognosis showed that prayers were more beneficial than the placebo effect.

Discussions about Spiritual Resources

Discussions about spiritual resources can flow naturally following discussion of other support systems. Appropriate timing for more in-depth discussion requires skillful interpretation of verbal and nonverbal cues from patients and families and the willingness to explore further with gentle, open-ended interview techniques. The topic of spirituality may be introduced during discussion of advance directives, diagnosis of severe illness, terminal care planning, addiction, chronic pain, chronic illness, domestic violence, or grieving.

The ED Clinician and Spiritual and Religious Practices

The adoption by ED clinicians of any spiritual and religious practices is likely to lead to enhanced coping during times of crises and emergency.

Spiritual Self-Understanding and Self-Care

Spiritual self-understanding and self-care can help ED clinicians cope with personal stress; equally important, it can increase the success of clinicians' interventions in spiritual and religious issues with patients.

ED clinicians need to understand their own spiritual beliefs, values, and biases in order to remain patient-centered and non-judgmental when dealing with the spiritual concerns of patients. This is especially true when the beliefs of the patient differ from those of the clinician. One way to promote self-understanding is to perform a spiritual self-assessment test using the tool HOPE, described in Table 24-4.

Spiritual self-care is integral to serving the multiple needs and demands of patients in the ED. Self-care can take the form of reconnecting with family and friends, spending time alone, community service, or religious practices.

Self-care and self-understanding can help clinicians respond sensitively and intelligently when patients make requests for prayer or spiritual guidance or ask difficult questions related to end-of-life issues or questions such as "Why is this happening to my child?"

Table 24–4

The Tool HOPE

HOPE	Concepts for Discussion
H	The sources of **h**ope, strength, peace, love, and feelings of connection
O	The role of **o**rganized religion, spiritual organizations (e.g., Alcoholics Anonymous)
P	**P**ersonal spirituality and **p**ractices
E	**E**ffects on medical care and end-of-life decisions

Adapted with permission from Anandarajah G, Hight E: Spirituality and medical practice: Using the HOPE questions as a practical tool for spiritual assessment. Am Fam Physician 2001;63:81-89.

Further Reading

American Psychiatric Association. Guidelines regarding the possible conflicts between psychiatrists' religious commitments and psychiatric practice. Am J Psychiatry 1995; 152 (suppl II): 64-80.

American Psychiatric Association. Diagnostic and Statistical Manual of Mental Disorders, 4th ed, Text Revision. Washington, DC, American Psychiatric Association, 2000, pp 731-742.

Anandarajah G, Hight E: Spirituality and medical practice: Using the HOPE questions as a practical tool for spiritual assessment. Am Fam Physician 2001;63:81-89.

Block SD: Assessing and managing depression in the terminally ill patient. ACP-ASIM End-of-Life Care Consensus Panel. American College of Physicians— American Society of Internal Medicine. Ann Intern Med 2000;132:209-218.

Brawer PA., Handal PJ, Fabricatore AN, et al: Training and education in religion/spirituality within APA-accredited clinical psychology programs. Prof Psychol 2002;33:203-206.

Bregman L: Psychology Sliding into Spirituality: An Examination of the Death Awareness Movement. Speech to be delivered to the American Academy of Religion, Person, Culture and Religion Group, 11/21/04. Retrieved 10/29/04 at http://pcr-ar.home.att.net/2004/bregman.htm

Ebaugh HR: Return of the sacred: Reintegrating religion in the social sciences. J Soc Scien Study Rel 2002;41:385-395.

Flanagan OJ Jr, Jackson K: Justice, care and gender: The Kohlberg-Gilligan debate revisited. Ethics 1987;97:622-637.

Frank A: The Wounded Storyteller—Body, Illness, and Ethics. University of Chicago Press, Chicago, 1995, pp 75-114.

Hathaway WL, Scott SY, Garvey SA: Assessing religious/spiritual functioning: A neglected domain in clinical practice. Prof Psychol 2004;25: 97-104.

Hill PC, Pargament KI: Advances in the conceptualization and measurement of religion and spirituality: Implications for physical and mental health research. Am Psychol 2003;5:64-74.

Koenig HG, Bearon LB, Hover M, Travis JL: Religious perspectives of doctors, nurses, patients and families. J Pastoral Care 1991;45:254-267.

Koenig HG, McCullough ME, Larson DB: Handbook of Religion and Health. New York, Oxford University Press, 2001.

Maugans TA: The SPIRITual History. Arch Fam Med 1997;5:11-16.

Miller WR, Thoresen CE: Spirituality, religion and health: An emerging research field. Am Psychol 2003;58:24-35.

Pargament KI, Koenig HG, Perez LM: The many methods of religious coping: Development and initial validation of the RCOPE. J Clin Psychol 2000;56:519-543.

Periyakoil VS, Hallenbeck J: Identifying and managing preparatory grief and depression at the end of life. Am Fam Physician 2002;65:883-890.

Puchalski CM, Romer AL: Taking a spiritual history allows clinicians to understand patients more fully. J Pall Med 2000;3:129-137

Rose S: Is the term "spirituality" a word that everyone uses, but nobody knows what anyone means by it? J Contemp Religion 2001;16:193-207.

Sloan R, Bagiella E, VandeCreek L, et al: Should physicians prescribe religious activities? N Engl J Med 2000;342:1913-1916.

Steinhauser KE, Christakis NA, Clip EC, et al: Factors considered important at the end of life by patients, family, physicians, and other care providers. JAMA 2000; 284:2476-2482.

POSTSCRIPT

Trust in the Lord with all your heart and lean not on
your own understanding. In all your ways acknowledge
Him, and He will make your paths straight.

Proverbs 3:5, 6

CHAPTER 25

Psychiatric Emergencies Not Otherwise Classified

Tirath S. Gill, MD

KEY POINTS

- The emergency department (ED) clinician must act in a calm and rational manner when patients present with unusual symptoms.
- Certain high-risk situations such as neuroleptic malignant syndrome, catatonia, and serotonin syndrome should be recognized early and treatment initiated with close monitoring on a medical unit or ICU.
- Medical causes of unusual psychiatric symptoms should always be sought before ascribing the symptoms to purely psychiatric phenomenology. Further diagnostic data may support a medical etiology.
- Every emergency presentation is a crisis for the patient and should be given serious attention and concern even when the symptoms are believed to be conversion symptoms or psychogenic.

Overview

Patients with unusual psychiatric and physiologic symptoms may present to the ED. Due to their relative rarity, these symptoms often arouse anxiety in patients, significant others, and sometimes the ED staff. The knowledgeable ED clinician recognizes this possibility and takes steps to reduce the level of anxiety felt by patients, family members, and other staff in the ED.

Because pharmacological treatment of psychiatric symptoms in the ED can be especially valuable in the emergencies discussed in this chapter, commonly used anxiolytic/hypnotic, antipsychotic, and antidepressant agents are briefly reviewed in Tables 25-1, 25-2, and 25-3, respectively.

The disorders discussed in this chapter are listed alphabetically. Some were mentioned briefly in another context elsewhere in this book; most are listed here for the first time because they are unusual presentations rarely seen in the ED.

Acute Intermittent Porphyria

Patients with acute intermittent porphyria may present with agitation, anxiety, and psychosis. Accompanying physical symptoms may include abdominal pain, peripheral neuropathy, seizures, and extrapyramidal syndrome (EPS). Laboratory studies may reveal elevated porphobilinogen levels in the urine and hyponatremia. The latter may be related to loss due to diarrhea or SIADH (syndrome of inappropriate antidiuretic hormone) and may lead to further complications. The peripheral neuropathy may be mild or profound.

Precipitating factors include the use of medications such as sulfonamides, barbiturates, carbamazepine, divalproic acid, dapsone, phenytoin, tolbutamide, and hydralazine. Acute intermittent porphyria may also be precipitated by fasting.

Management consists of a high-carbohydrate diet, removal of the offending agent, and treatment with intravenous (IV) glucose and hematin. Electrolytes should be gradually corrected. Too rapid a correction of the hyponatremia may also be associated with neurologic complications. Obtaining a complete history and noting the absence of other signs of acute abdomen such as leukocytosis or fever can avoid unnecessary surgery.

Analgesics may be provided for the acute pain. Opioid analgesics, antianxiety agents, and low doses of antipsychotic agents are considered relatively safe.

Agitated Relative of a Patient

This is one of those situations that most psychiatrists and mental health workers do not expect but will probably encounter at some point in their careers. Many factors make this occurrence a possibility; including a genetic diathesis for a psychiatric disorder and inability to contact the family physician due to the many layers of bureaucracy. Some staff may inadvertently antagonize the patient's relative by honoring confidentiality requirements of the patient. There also tends to be a general

Table 25–1

Commonly Used Anxiolytic and Hypnotic Agents

Drug	Approximate Equivalent Dose	Usual Dose	Comments
Diazepam	5 mg	10-20 mg	Lipophilic; some risk for addiction
Clonazepam	1 mg	1-4 mg	Anticonvulsant properties; useful in bipolar disorder
Lorazepam	1 mg	1-4 mg	Reliably absorbed after intramuscular injection; preferred in liver disease
Estazolam	0.5 mg	1-2 mg	Used as hypnotic
Temazepam	15 mg	15-45 mg	Preferred in liver disease
Phenobarbital	15 mg	15-60 mg	Long-acting agent; useful in alcohol detoxification; high risk for respiratory depression
Chloral hydrate	250 mg	250-1000 mg	May cause gastric irritation
Zolpidem	5 mg	5-20 mg	Take immediately before bedtime; not a benzodiazepine
Zaleplon	5 mg	5-10 mg	Similar action to zolpidem
Eszopicelone	1 mg	1-3 mg	Similar action to zolpidem
Ramelteon	8 mg	8 mg	Melatonin receptor agonist; do not give with fluvoxamine or other CYP1A2 inhibitors.

Table 25–2

Commonly Used Antipsychotic Agents

Drug	Usual Dose	Comments
Haloperidol	5-20 mg	High risk for dystonic reactions in young adults; give with benztropine
Fluphenazine	5-20 mg	Somewhat more sedating than haloperidol; similar risks for EPS side effects; similar precautions as advised when using anticholinergic medications in young adults
Risperidone	4-6 mg	Effective antipsychotic with low risk for weight gain
Olanzapine	10-20 mg	Effective for bipolar disorder and schizoaffective disorder with bipolar subtype
Quetiapine	600-800 mg	Low risk for EPS side effects
Ziprasidone	80-120 mg	Caution advised if using with agents that cause prolongation of QTc interval
Molindone	30-225 mg	Low risk for weight gain
Thiothixene	10-40 mg	Effective antipsychotic in the compliant patient; moderate side effect profile
Aripiprazole	10-30 mg	May exacerbate symptoms in some patients; low risk for weight gain

EPS, extrapyramidal syndrome.

distrust of the mental health system by many patients and their families. At times this lack of confidence may be well founded, as mental health budgets dwindle and the quality of mental health services declines.

The ED staff should make a concerted effort to empathize with agitated family members and contact them proactively after interviewing the patient. They may be a vital link in the cycle of recovery. They generally are appreciative of the help and information provided. Often, talking to family members about the concept of high expressed emotion is very helpful (family members who are hypercritical and overinvolved in the life of a psychiatric patient may be defined as having *high*

Table 25–3

Commonly Used Antidepressant Agents

Drug	Usual Daily Dose	Comments
Fluoxetine	20-60 mg	Long half-life; low risk for withdrawal symptoms
Paroxetine	10-40 mg	May raise levels of other medications; more sedating
Sertraline	50-150 mg	Possible GI side effects; useful in PTSD
Citalopram	20-60 mg	Low risk for GI side effects
Escitalopram	10-20 mg	Low risk for GI side effects
Amitriptyline	150-250 mg	Sedating, with anticholinergic side effects; risk for orthostasis
Desipramine	150-250 mg	Useful in ADHD; few anticholinergic side effects
Imipramine	150-250 mg	Anticholinergic; orthostatic side effects less than with amitriptyline; useful in panic disorder
Doxepin	150-250 mg	Strong antihistaminic effects that may be helpful in peptic ulcer disease and allergic conditions
Nortriptyline	100-150 mg	Relatively benign side effect profile
Phenelzine	45-60 mg	MAOI-related precautions needed
Tranylcypromine	20-30 mg	MAOI-related precautions needed
Mirtazapine	15-60 mg	Sedating; stimulates appetite
Bupropion	200-400 mg	Do not use more than 150 mg of immediate-release form or 200 mg of slow-release form at any one time; doses should be 8 hours apart
Trazodone	100-300 mg	Useful as an augmenting agent in treatment for insomnia; caution patient about risk for priapism, sedation, and orthostasis

ADHD, attention deficit hyperactivity disorder; GI, gastrointestinal; MAOI, monoamine oxidase inhibitor; PTSD, posttraumatic stress disorder.

expressed emotion (EE)). For example, family members may avoid loud, divisive arguments among themselves and with the patient when they realize that this behavior increases the chances for relapse.

Education of the family regarding concrete thinking (a common symptom of schizophrenia) is also helpful; they can be taught to communicate with a schizophrenic patient in simple straightforward sentences that don't involve abstraction.

If the agitated relative seems manic or psychotic, security may be called; however, this should be considered a solution of last resort. If such is the case, it may be prudent to consider alternative placement of the patient. The risk of relapse is high when the patient must return to live with a relative who has a personality disorder or major mental illness. Such a relationship may be emotionally toxic, and severance of the relationship may be the key to lasting change.

Agranulocytosis

See "Leukopenia and Agranulocytosis."

Anorgasmia

Anorgasmia can occur with the use of SSRIs such as citalopram, paroxetine, sertraline, and fluoxetine at higher doses. Certain antipsychotics such as risperidone, and some first-generation antipsychotics such as mesoridazine have also been associated with orgasmic problems in men and women.

Cyproheptadine, a serotonin antagonist, 8 to 12 mg, taken an hour before sexual activity may be helpful. Some clinicians report successful treatment using dopaminergic agents such as bupropion, 100 to 200 mg/day in divided doses. Bupropion should not be used in a dose greater than 150 mg at any one time because of the risk of seizures.

Aspiration Pneumonia

Aspiration pneumonia is an untoward side effect that may be due to impaired motility of the esophageal tract or impaired gag reflex caused by sedation from medications. The patient may present with gagging and choking; later, fever, dyspnea, and altered mental status may be seen. IV antibiotics may be required to treat the mixed flora that is present in such infections.

Bromide Poisoning

Potassium bromide is no longer used as a sedative. Bromide poisoning may occur in farm workers who are exposed to pesticides containing methyl bromide. Symptoms include a burning sensation in the throat and eyes and nausea and vomiting. Chronic exposure may lead to dermatitis and psychiatric symptoms such as impaired sensorium, irritability, dysphoria, mania, and psychosis. Laboratory studies may indicate abnormal chloride levels. Treatment usually consists of increased sodium chloride (table salt) intake, diuretics, and removal of the offending agent.

Catalepsy

Catalepsy is an immobile position that is maintained for long periods of time. It is a feature of catatonia due to schizophrenia and other causes. Lorazepam, 1 to 2 mg by the intramuscular (IM) route or by slow IV push, usually helps to resolve this. There are also case reports of successful interruption of the catatonic behavior with morphine sulfate, 3 to 5 mg, given by slow IV push. Monitoring of respiratory function is essential when morphine is combined with the lorazepam.

Cataplexy

Cataplexy is a temporary loss of muscle tone associated with extreme emotional stimuli such as distressing news or due to extremes of romantic love or to excessive laughter. It is often a feature of narcolepsy, and the person with narcolepsy may be prone to drop attacks of cataplexy. Cataplexy is believed to be associated with a deficiency in the neuropeptide hypocretin. Various drugs have been reported to be useful in its treatment, including tricyclic antidepressants, venlafaxine, SSRIs, modafinil, and sodium oxybate.

Charles Bonnet Syndrome

This is a syndrome of complex visual hallucinations comprising people, animals, and landscapes that occurs in individuals with failing eyesight or blindness. The hallucinations are vivid, elaborate, and well formed, and the person often retains insight that he or she is experiencing visions that are not real. This syndrome can be distinguished from other illnesses with the symptoms of hallucination by the absence of other criteria for delirium, dementia, and psychotic disorders. The patient usually is oriented, has no fluctuation of attention, has relatively intact cognitive function, and manifests no delusional thought content.

Charles Bonnet syndrome is reported to exist in up to 3.5% of elderly psychiatric patients and up to 15% of the visually impaired. With increasing life expectancy and risk of impaired eyesight in the elderly, ED clinicians may come across this more often. Visual disorders associated with this syndrome include cataracts, glaucoma, and macular degeneration.

The visual hallucinations may last for a few seconds to several hours. Patients often may not report the symptom for fear of having their illness misdiagnosed—this is not an unfounded fear. Delirium, dementia, or psychosis may be diagnosed in these patients, unnecessary tests and medications may be ordered, and they may be referred for psychiatric hospitalization.

If the patient is frightened by the hallucinations, verbal reassurance and use of a mild antianxiety agent is advisable. Antipsychotic medications should be avoided in view of their unproven efficacy and relatively high burden of side effects.

Decreased Libido

Decreased libido is a common problem in patients taking antipsychotics with strong dopamine-blocking properties or serotoninergic agents used for depression. This can be ameliorated by reducing the dose and/or switching agents (e.g., a dopaminergic agent such as bupropion). Medical causes of decreased libido should also be investigated, such as diabetes, chronic medical illness, hypogonadism, and undiagnosed and untreated depression.

Delusional Parasitosis

A patient may present to the ED with a delusional belief of being infested with a parasite. This can be a frustrating and difficult condition for the patient, who feels totally misunderstood and suffers in lonely anguish. It can also challenge the diagnostic acumen and treatment skills of the ED clinician because the literature discussing treatment of this rather rare condition can best be described as sparse. The patient harboring the delusion may in other ways be able to carry on a relatively normal life. Patience is golden when interviewing the patient; unresolved issues causing the delusion may be revealed by a careful and objective assessment.

It is also possible that the patient may actually have an infestation by mites that can cause dermatitis but are almost invisible to the naked eye. Skin scrapings and laboratory testing to rule out these possibilities are indicated. In addition a diagnostic workup should include a metabolic profile, urine drug screen, thyroid profile, and assay of erythrocyte sedimentation rate (ESR) and vitamin B_{12} and folate levels. A nutritional deficiency, hidden endocrinopathy, occult disease such as cancer, or undetected cerebrovascular or neurologic disease may coexist. If no physical cause is found, one must nevertheless be open to the possibility of a physical illness while searching for other causes in the psychiatric domain.

Delusional parasitosis may exist as an independent disorder or be associated with certain psychotic states, depression, and anxiety disorders. The psychosocial profile of an individual often will reveal a middle-aged individual of average intelligence who feels rejected by his or her social group and has feelings of loneliness and low self-esteem. Other social factors include belonging to a low socioeconomic group and being a single parent with children. There tends to be higher incidence of the disease in women. In younger patients, stimulant drugs of abuse may induce a tactile hallucination of insects crawling on the skin (formication) and related delusions of parasitosis.

Often, treatment of the primary physical or mental illness may resolve the parasitosis. In other cases, the use of a low-dose atypical antipsychotic or the drug pimozide along with an SSRI in modest doses may resolve the symptoms. Medications with antihistaminic properties may be helpful in decreasing some symptoms related to pruritus. More drastic measures may have to be taken if the patient is more floridly psychotic and shows a tendency for mutilation of skin or body to remove the nonexistent parasites.

Drugs and Weapons in the ED

A patient with antisocial personality may secretly collect weapons to be used for escape or violence against others.

Increased vigilance with these patients is recommended. Family members or friends may be coerced into delivering contraband to potentially violent patients, such as illicit drugs or weapons, and visitors should be carefully scrutinized by security before visitation. All outside food should be checked for contraband as well, and gifts of food should be limited to those in dire need such as anorexic, debilitated, or depressed patients who have a strong distaste for hospital food.

Dry Mouth

Dry mouth is a side effect due to many psychiatric medications, including low-potency antipsychotic agents, tricyclic antidepressants, and muscle relaxants. Management techniques include lowering the dose of the offending agent, instructing the patient to take frequent sips of water, chew sugar-free gum, or suck on candy. Pilocarpine, 5 mg qid, or cevimeline, 30 mg tid, may be useful in refractory cases.

ECT Patients

ECT (electroconvulsive therapy) is a life-saving intervention in cases of vegetative depressed state, of acute sustained manic agitation, catatonia, neuroleptic malignant syndrome, some cases of delirium, and acute suicidal depression. Patients presenting to the ED who are scheduled for ECT should be educated about its risks, side effects, and potential benefits. Patients and their families often are confused about the merits of this procedure and may have some anxiety about its psychological and physiologic effects.

Once their anxieties are quelled through education and support, patients should preferably be admitted overnight in the hospital. The typical workup prior to the ECT procedure is described in Box 25-1.

Group Hysteria

Group hysteria may be seen in the ED when people present with somatic symptoms after feared exposure to a toxic or infectious agent. The individuals may exhibit extremes of grief or other disruptive behaviors. The group should be dispersed, and each member of the group should be interviewed separately. Reassurance that there are no adverse effects usually is sufficient to

---

> ### Box 25–1. Workup of ECT patients
>
> 1. Complete physical examination
> 2. List of allergies
> 3. Complete history, including any history of adverse events under anesthesia in patient or family members
> 4. Complete blood count
> 5. Comprehensive chemistry panel with electrolytes
> 6. Chest x-ray
> 7. Spinal x-ray if indicated
> 8. Urinalysis
> 9. Electrocardiogram
> 10. CT scan of head if indicated by presence of atypical psychiatric symptoms or neurologic symptoms and deficits.

relieve anxiety. However, benzodiazepines and crisis-oriented therapy may be necessary in these situations.

Homicidal Threats by a Patient

Under the Tarasoff decision made in California in 1974, if a therapist (e.g., clinician) is aware of threats made against an individual by a patient, the individual must be informed of the threats. The patient may later recant threats made when his or her paranoia or delusions or anger due to other causes resolve. Nevertheless, it is prudent to let the threatened person know when the patient is to be discharged from the hospital.

The patient should be informed that making threats against another constitutes a charge of terroristic threats, an offence that is punishable by law, and that the presence of mental illness may not necessarily exempt the patient from legal charges and punishment.

Laryngeal Dystonia

 Laryngeal dystonia is a rare but deadly side effect of antipsychotic agents with dopamine-blocking properties; it constitutes a medical emergency because it may compromise the airway. Treatment consists of IV or IM diphenhydramine, 50 mg, or IV or IM Cogentin, 2 mg, stat. Benzodiazepines may be of some help in alleviating associated anxiety.

Leukopenia and Agranulocytosis

 A sore throat or a fever may be a subtle indication of this rare but dangerous side effect. Fever can be a direct side effect of medications such as Clozaril but usually indicates an opportunistic infection secondary to medication-induced leukopenia and agranulocytosis. Although a number of psychotropic agents are capable of inducing bone marrow suppression, the prime suspects in a drug regimen should be clozapine, Tegretol, valproic acid, various immunosuppressive drugs, and anticancer agents.

A white blood cell (WBC) count less than 3000 and a neutrophil count less than 1500 indicates a vulnerability for opportunistic infection. The suspected medication should be withheld and the WBC count should be monitored carefully. If fever and infection are present, transfer to an isolation room in the intensive care unit (ICU) is warranted. The usual infections are related to stomatitis, cellulitis, pneumonia, and septicemia.

Treatment consists of broad-spectrum antibiotics and isolation in a relatively germ-free atmosphere. Recent literature reports that clozapine may be reintroduced gradually at lower doses without inducing another case of leukopenia. Avoidance of other myelosuppressive agents is recommended. Some reports indicate that the use of beta blockers such as propranolol may be associated with an increased risk of precipitating leukopenia in patients maintained on clozapine.

Munchausen Syndrome

In this psychiatric condition, also known as *hospital addiction*, a person intentionally produces physical signs and symptoms to gain medical attention. Video monitoring and surveillance may reveal surreptitious manipulation of medical specimens or self-injurious behaviors that prolong the person's status as a patient. The person may have experienced the loss or absence in early childhood of a nurturing figure. The person may have some background and training in the medical field, or a family member may have a medical background.

Munchausen Syndrome by Proxy

Munchausen syndrome by proxy is a more sinister phenomenon in which a child is presented to the ED by a concerned, seemingly model parent (or in some cases an elderly person is presented by a caregiver). The child's symptoms may include seizures, vomiting, apnea, diarrhea, fevers, lethargy, dehydration or hematemesis, ataxia, hematuria, and unconsciousness, as well as symptoms related to intentional poisoning.

Clinical features that suggest this disorder include the following:
- The child will seem to get better in the absence of the parent
- The parent is not distressed by the possibility of painful and invasive testing of the child and even welcomes it.
- The physical symptoms do not follow any consistent pattern.

The parent may have had some medical training, and there may be other children in the family that have suffered or died from strange illnesses. There is a significant morbidity and mortality rate for these children, and if Munchausen syndrome by proxy is suspected, it is vital that the child be placed on protective watch.

The parent, most often the mother, should be referred for counseling and therapy. Often there is a childhood history of strife and abandonment and feelings of low self-esteem and depression beneath the "model parent" exterior. Some parents seem to show genuine remorse but remain at risk for repeating the behaviors. Alternative placement for the child and any other children should be strongly considered. Treatment consists of separation from the parent and ongoing follow-up for any depressive symptoms in the child caused by the separation and ambivalent feelings for the parent.

Obstipation

Obstipation is a state of severe constipation that can be caused by medications such as opiate analgesics, medications with anticholinergic effects, and calcium channel blockers. Medical conditions such as hypothyroidism, parkinsonism, and electrolyte disorders may be predisposing factors. It is best managed by reducing the dosage of the offending medication, if possible. A high-fiber diet, increased liquid intake, and increase in physical activity is recommended. Laxatives and enemas may be tried and repeated if necessary. Treatment of the underlying medical condition and correction of electrolyte imbalance are also recommended.

Obstructive Sleep Apnea

Patients with obstructive sleep apnea generally are middle-aged, obese males and present with personality changes, depression, and symptoms of fatigue. Many psychiatric medications may cause obesity, and this should be noted as an iatrogenic phenomenon with potentially serious consequences when making the ED assessment.

Treatment includes withdrawal of the medication causing obesity from the regimen and taking other measures to reduce body weight by 15% to 20%. The use of continuous positive airway pressure devices is helpful, but patients tend to become noncompliant over a period of time. Surgical procedures and orthodontic devices have been tried with varying degrees of success. Antidepressants may be used to treat depressive symptoms, and they may limit the apneic episodes by suppressing REM sleep.

PANDAS

PANDAS is an acronym for pediatric autoimmune neuropsychiatric disorders associated with streptococcal infections. It tends to present in a subset of children with features of obsessive-compulsive disorder (OCD), such as counting, excessive hand washing, and obsessive ruminations, and/or tic disorders, similar to Tourette's syndrome. The onset of symptoms is preceded by a sore throat caused by group A beta-hemolytic streptococci. These bacteria are better known as causes of rheumatic fever, rheumatic heart disease, and chorea.

The mechanism appears to be autoimmune in nature. The course tends to be episodic, and there is a risk of exacerbation, with subsequent cases of pharyngitis caused by this organism. A plausible explanation of PANDAS is an infectious etiology in combination with a genetic vulnerability that influences neurodevelopment through immunologic or direct tropic effects on parts of the developing nervous system.

Treatment is directed toward prevention of future infections. OCD symptoms can be treated with SSRIs, and motoric movements may respond to low doses of dopamine blockers. Plasmapheresis has shown benefit in decreasing OCD behaviors in some patients.

Postpartum Blues and Postpartum Depression

Postpartum blues ("baby blues"), with its accompanying dysphoria, is almost universal due to the shift of a large amount of fluids and fluctuations in hormone status following pregnancy and childbirth. It is a common temporary psychological state occurring soon after childbirth that responds to social support and encouragement.

Postpartum depression, on the other hand, is a much more serious condition that may grow to psychotic proportions and endanger the life of the patient and her child. Postpartum psychosis is a distinct illness with a high incidence of bipolar disorder or schizoaffective disorder in family members and patients. Some experts believe that postpartum depression and postpartum psychosis are manifestations of an underlying diathesis or disposition for mood disorder and schizoaffective disorder, respectively, and that the physiologic stress of pregnancy and childbirth brings about the expression of the latent illness.

If a woman has had postpartum depression or psychosis, there is a strong chance that it will recur in future pregnancies. There are several reports of mother and daughter both having postpartum depression or psychosis. A family history of postpartum psychiatric illness in a patient's mother or other female relatives or during prior pregnancies should be noted in the patient's history during antenatal visits. If such a history is present, close monitoring, support, and institution of medications that have been effective in the past are warranted. See Table 25-4 for differentiating features of postpartum disorders.

The Pregnant Patient

Presentation of pregnant patients to the ED is not rare, of course. It is listed here because it is an opportunity for ED clinicians to educate pregnant patients about the risk to the fetus of certain agents (teratogens). In fact, this is an issue that should be discussed with all female patients of childbearing age. Table 25-5 lists some common teratogens that pose a risk to the fetus.

Text continues on page 610.

Table 25–4

Differential Diagnosis of Postpartum Blues, Postpartum Depression, and Postpartum Psychosis

Finding	Postpartum Blues (Baby Blues)	Postpartum Depression	Postpartum Psychosis
Incidence	50% of women giving birth	10% of women giving birth	1 to 2 per thousand women giving birth
Time of onset	3 to 5 days after delivery	3 to 6 months after delivery	Within 6 weeks of delivery
Duration	Days to weeks	Months to years if untreated	Months to years if untreated
Associated stressors	None	Lack of support	Lack of support worsens outcome
Associated cultural influence	Present in all cultures and socioeconomic classes	Psychosocial stressors worsen outcome	May not be as influential but difficult circumstances worsen outcome
History of mood disorder	None	Strong association with previous depressive episodes	Increased incidence of bipolar disorder or schizoaffective disorder in patients
Family history of mental disorder	None	Some association with depressive symptoms in other family members at time of pregnancy	History of psychotic illness or bipolar disorder

Finding	Postpartum Blues (Baby Blues)	Postpartum Depression	Postpartum Psychosis
Tearfulness	Yes	Yes	Yes; hallucinations, delusions also present
Mood lability	Yes	Often present, but sometimes the mood is uniformly depressed	Often present; mood may be elevated or mixed
Anhedonia	No	Often	Anxiety and distress more prominent
Sleep disturbance	Sometimes	Nearly always	Always
Suicidal thoughts	No	May be present	May be present
Thoughts of harming the baby	Rarely	Often	May be a significant risk
Feelings of guilt, inadequacy	Absent or mild	Often present and excessive	May or may not be present

Table 25-5

Teratogens Associated with Birth Defects

Medication/Agent/ Substance	Birth Defect	Use during Lactation	Comments
Lithium	Epstein's anomaly (associated with a defect of the tricuspid valve)	Contraindicated	Ultrasound may detect defect in first trimester if exposure occurs
Valproic acid	Neural tube defects	Contraindicated	High risk for neonatal hepatotoxicity; folic acid supplementation may lower risk
Carbamazepine	Neural tube defects	Contraindicated	Folic acid supplementation helpful
Phenytoin	Cleft palate	Contraindicated	Folic acid supplementation helpful
Paroxetine	Associated with atrial septal and ventricular septal defects	May breast-feed with caution	FDA issued advisory that there may be a 1.5-2 times higher risk for defects compared with other antidepressants
Accutane	Associated with heart and central nervous system defects	Contraindicated	Female teenagers and young women must be informed of risk and educated about birth control; suicide and depression are significant side effects
Clozapine	May cause suppression of infant bone marrow	Contraindicated	Pregnancy should be avoided; substitute another antipsychotic

Medication/Agent/ Substance	Birth Defect	Use during Lactation	Comments
Methyl mercury from contaminated fish or from grains laced with methyl mercury used as fungicide	Encephalopathy resembling cerebral palsy	Contraindicated	Avoid eating fish from contaminated waters; limit fish intake if safety is unknown
Alcohol	Fetal alcohol syndrome	Contraindicated	Midfacial hypoplasia, wide philtrum, mental retardation
German measles	Heart disease, congenital cataracts	Not applicable	All females should be vaccinated prior to reaching age of menarche

Priapism

Priapism is persistent, usually painful erection of the penis that is not related to sexual arousal. It is an uncommon side effect of trazodone and other drugs that cause vasodilation by various mechanisms including blockade of peripheral alpha receptors located in the blood vessels. Certain medical conditions such as sickle cell trait may increase the risk for priapism.

Priapism is a urologic emergency if it lasts for more than 4 hours. The patient should be told that if priapism occurs, the medication causing it should be stopped. The patient should go immediately to the ED, where procedures to drain the corpus cavernosum can be undertaken.

Atenolol (up to 75 mg/day), Cogentin (up to 6 mg/day), and diphenhydramine (in doses of 50 to 100 mg) have been reported to be helpful in dealing with this condition before emergency interventions can be instituted.

Psychodermatologic Conditions

The bond between skin and the brain originates in the earliest period of human development when they share the common ectodermal plate. This close relationship, continued in adulthood, may be manifested in psychodermatologic conditions such as psoriasis, eczema, acne, alopecia areata, trichotillomania, atopic dermatitis, urticaria, dermatitis artefacta, and self-induced skin lesions. Self-induced skin lesions have a bizarre appearance and irregular margins and may be secondarily infected. The underlying cause often is conscious or unconscious emotional distress.

Treatment efforts are oriented toward resolving the underlying psychiatric issues as well as the skin condition. Therapeutic agents include topical and systemic anti-inflammatory agents such as antihistamines and corticosteroids. Strongly antihistaminic antidepressants such as Sinequan or doxepin are favored because of their efficacy in alleviating the pruritic itch that causes scratching and disfigurement. Psychotherapy and exploration of unstated conflicts and repressed emotions may have lasting benefits for some patients. In some cases, a low-dose antipsychotic agent such as risperidone may prove useful, possibly by decreasing the psychic anxiety and distress.

Renal Failure

Psychiatric patients tend to have higher rates of diabetes mellitus, hypertension, and with increasing age, decreasing renal function that can result in toxic accumulation of certain medications and their metabolites. ED clinicians should be aware of this when assessing patients with renal impairment. Medications to avoid when treating such patients include lithium, gabapentin, levetiracetam, chloral hydrate, and tricyclics with secondary metabolites such as imipramine and amitriptyline. Low-risk medications include loxapine, molindone, ziprasidone, phenytoin, tiagabine, citalopram, sertraline, escitalopram, and zaleplon.

Seasonal Affective Disorder

This is thought to be an accentuation of the winter blues and the proverbial spring fever. It is more common in the higher latitudes of both the northern and southern hemispheres, and individual susceptibilities may differ, with a somewhat higher incidence in women. The depression tends to recur every winter and may be marked by atypical symptoms of increased sleeping and eating. Other symptoms such as anergia, decreased concentration, and anhedonia may also occur. As with any depression, the risk of suicide should always be explored. The depression tends to clear with the return of the spring season.

A number of treatment options can be considered, including treatment with an SSRI antidepressant and individual and group psychotherapy. A subset of the population with cyclic mood swings may benefit from the addition of lithium or another mood stabilizer. Light therapy in the range of 10,000 lux for about 30 minutes per day has been found to be useful, but compliance tends to be poor. Direct glaring into the lamplight should be avoided and ultraviolet light should be filtered out to avoid damage to the retina. Most of the commercial lamps available for phototherapy are free of ultraviolet radiation. Accommodation of work schedules and vacations to sunnier climes may also help with management of this unique clinical state. Exposure to morning light for an hour a day or obtaining an office with a window that lets in daylight are other practical measures that can be undertaken. Careful exploration of other factors such as anniversaries of sad events or separation from significant others are subjects worthy of exploration in psychotherapy. The resolution of any unresolved grief surrounding the events may bring about lasting change. Seasonal affective disorder may indicate a vulnerability of some individuals to major depression or bipolar disorder, and the individuals should be provided education regarding the symptoms so that early intervention can be provided should these major illnesses emerge at a later point.

Treatment-Emergent Seizure

Treatment-emergent seizure may be related to a missed dose of an anticonvulsant agent or may be the result of unrecognized alcohol or sedative/hypnotic withdrawal. High doses of drugs such as clozapine, bupropion, mianserin, and dilantin may result in seizures as well.

Treatment usually consists of withholding the epileptogenic agent and adjusting the levels of anticonvulsant that the patient is taking. In the immediate situation, IM or IV lorazepam, 2 mg, may be given. Alternatively, diazepam, which is not reliably absorbed by the IM route, may be given, 5 to 10 mg, by slow IV push.

New onset of seizures should prompt a more thorough search for intracranial pathology. This may require a detailed neurologic examination and appropriate imaging studies such as magnetic resonance imaging and computed tomography.

Trichotillomania

Trichotillomania is a noncosmetic urge to pull hair and often is accompanied by swallowing of the hair. Patients with this relatively rare psychiatric condition may present to the ED in acute pain due to obstruction of the gastrointestinal tract by a bezoar (hairball) formed by the swallowed hair.

Trichotillomania is classified in the fourth edition of the *Diagnostic and Statistical Manual of Mental Disorders, Text Revision* (DSM-IV-TR) as an impulse control disorder associated with obsessive-compulsive spectrum disorders. Trichotillomania usually first appears in the prepubertal age group, and the incidence tends to increase in adolescence. There may be bald spots; the individual with trichotillomania often has a surprising lack of insight regarding this phenomenon and does not see it as a problem. The disorder may be associated with organic conditions such as parietal lesions.

There are many anecdotal case reports in the literature regarding the efficacy of various treatments, including SSRIs and other antidepressants, topical agents, behavioral therapy, and supportive therapy. One case of trichotillomania was reported to respond to the atypical anticonvulsant quetiapine.

The Unresponsive Psychiatric Patient

The ED clinician should treat the unresponsive psychiatric patient the same as any patient who may have a medically emergent basis for the lack of response. Determine whether the patient is OK by a loud verbal request first, and then by gentle shaking of the shoulder or extremity. If there is no response, check breathing and pulse. If either is absent, alert other staff members and initiate cardiopulmonary resuscitation. If the patient has a pulse and is breathing, check the pupils. If the pupils are constricted, consider the possibility of opiate intoxication. IV naloxone, along with thiamine and dextrose, will reverse opiate-induced or hypoglycemia-induced coma and give clues to the underlying problem. If a medical bracelet is present, it should be carefully inspected for any medical data to help with further care and disposition of the patient.

Further Reading

Fernandez Ibieta M, Ramos Amador JT, Aunon Martinc I, et al: Neuropsychiatric disorders associated with streptococci: A case report. An Pediatr (Barc) 2005; 62:475-478.

King RA: PANDAS: To treat or not to treat. Adv Neurol 2006;99:179-183.

Magalhaes PV, Pinheiro RT: Pharmacological treatment of postpartum depression. Acta Psychiatr Scand 2006;113:75-76.

Robertson E, Jones I, Haque S, et al: Risk of puerperal and non-puerperal recurrence of illness following bipolar affective puerperal (post-partum) psychosis. Br J Psychiatry 2005;186:258-259.

Singer HS, Hong JJ, Yoon DY, Williams PN: Neuropsychiatric movement disorders following streptococcal infection. Dev Med Child Neurol 2005;47:771-775.

Snider LA, Lougee L, Slattery M, et al: Antibiotic prophylaxis with azithromycin or penicillin for childhood-onset neuropsychiatric disorders. Biol Psychiatry 2005;57:788-792.

Steinetz BG, Brown JL, Roth TL, Czekala N: Association between streptococcal infection and obsessive-compulsive disorder, Tourette's syndrome, and tic disorder. Pediatrics 2005;116:56-60.

Swedo SE, Grant PJ: Antibiotic prophylaxis with azithromycin or penicillin for childhood-onset neuropsychiatric disorders. Biol Psychiatry 2005;57:788-792.

Thorpy MJ: Cataplexy associated with narcolepsy: Epidemiology, pathophysiology and management. CNS Drugs 2006;20:43-50.

von Somm S: Postpartum depression is not merely "Baby Blues." Pflege Aktuell 2005;59:140-144. [in German]

Zonana J, Gorman JM: The neurobiology of postpartum depression. CNS Spectr 2005;10:792-799, 805.

INDEX

Note: Page numbers followed by b indicate box(es); f, figure(s); t, table(s).